THE VETERAN'S GUIDE TO
PSYCHIATRY

DEBORAH Y. LIGGAN, MD

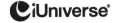

THE VETERAN'S GUIDE TO PSYCHIATRY

iUniverse books may be ordered through booksellers or by contacting:

iUniverse
1663 Liberty Drive
Bloomington, IN 47403
www.iuniverse.com
1-800-Authors (1-800-288-4677)

Because of the dynamic nature of the Internet, any web addresses or links contained in this book may have changed since publication and may no longer be valid. The views expressed in this work are solely those of the author and do not necessarily reflect the views of the publisher, and the publisher hereby disclaims any responsibility for them.

Any people depicted in stock imagery provided by Thinkstock are models, and such images are being used for illustrative purposes only. Certain stock imagery © Thinkstock.

ISBN: 978-1-4917-7504-2 (sc)
ISBN: 978-1-4917-8221-7 (e)

Library of Congress Control Number: 2015920456

Print information available on the last page.

iUniverse rev. date: 12/15/2015

Contents

Section Two: Mood Disorders

Section Three: Anxiety Disorders

Section Five: Disorders of Cognition

Section Six: Recovery from Mental Illness

Section 7: Emergency Psychiatry

Preface

The Veterans Administration (VA) has long played a central role in the provision of mental he alth services to those in need. Increasing knowledge about the spectrum of mental health illnesses will help better understand each disorder and its impact on the veteran's life.

This book is intended to be a practical guide for psychiatrists, psychologists, psychiatric social workers, and members of the other behavioral sciences, or those preparing to enter these fields, who are interested in achieving significant result in the diagnosis and treatment of severe forms of emotional illness. Nearly every diagnostic category and condition covered in this text is illustrated with a case example. And in conclusion of each chapter are ten questions of self-examination for review.

Section 1: Psychiatric Interviewing

Interviewing is an art, science, and a therapeutic tool all wrapped up in one complex package. The psychiatrist encourages a free-flowing exchange with the patient and then arrives at a diagnostic formulation few the patients' problems at the conclusion of the interview. The more accurate the diagnostic assessment, the more appropriate is the treatment planning. This section is the culmination of many years of working with medical students and residents to help them learn to interview psychiatric patients.

In the 1st Chapter, discuss the doctor -patient relationship. Then the specifics of meeting the patient and starting the interview takes place. How the student introduces him or herself and addresses the patient may seem to be small things, but they set the tone of the relationship. In this chapter important verbal and nonverbal information is obtained, as well as present a more formal discussion of psychiatric history and mental status examination.

In Chapter 2, the biopsychosocial model views the whole person, including the disease processes and how the illness may relate to the patient's personality and the society in which he or she lives. These three major areas of investigation- biological, psychological, and social- contribute to our understanding of the mental illness. How can the clinician utilize the biopsychosocial model in understanding the patient? The biological part emphasizes the anatomical, structural, and molecular substrates of disease. The psychological part examines the effects of psycho-dynamic factors, motivation, and personality on the experience of illness. And finality, the social part explains how the cultural, environmental, and familial conditions or experiences influence the expression and the experience of illness.

In Chapter 3, people have different ways of responding to stress and illness. The response is determined by a complex interaction of biologic propensities (which we often call temperament), past interpersonal interactions (the importance of childhood history), and the present situation. Individual's reactions are almost as varied as people, but reactions do fall into some general types. Therefore, the interview technique helps the patient cope with sometimes overpowering feelings.

Some patient's anxiety in the interview is great enough to be incapacitating. These patients need special help to feel more comfortable and enter into the interaction of the interview.

Interviews with depressed patients can be laboriously slow and unproductive. An interview with a patient who has attempted suicide or is believed to be suicidal is apt to be strained and unproductive if the suicidal attempts or thoughts are not acknowledged early in the interview. By far the best described somatic treatment is the Amytal interview. The structure of this interview begins when sustained rapid lateral nystagmus is present.

Section Two: Mood Disorder

Mood is a sustained emotional tone perceived along a normal continuum of sad to happy. In the section on mood disorders, DSM-5 requires at least 1 week of manic symptoms or bipolar I disorder. Bipolar II disorder is characterized by a clinical course of recurring mood episodes consisting of one or more major depressive episodes and at least one hypomanic episode. The dominant features common to these disorders are disturbances of the patient's mood and affect.

This section describes the clinical, diagnostic, epidemiologic, etiological, and treatment aspects of mood disorders. The criteria can be grouped into 5 general categories: (1) disturbances in mood: feelings of being sad, blue, depressed, hopeless, down in the dumps; (2) disturbances in cognition: loss of interest, difficulty concentrating, low self-esteem, negative thoughts, indecisiveness, guilt, suicidal ideation, delusions, hallucinations;(3) behavioral disturbances: social withdrawal, psychomotor retardation; (4) somatic disturbances: fatigue, sleep disturbance, changes in appetite, weight loss, or changes in weight gain; (5) if psychotic symptoms are present, delusions are often grandiose or paranoid and may also be mood-incongruent.

Chapter 4, Bipolar I Disorder, will give you a broad research-based, including its symptoms, course, diagnosis, treatment, and management. The most marked symptoms of bipolar disorder are significant shifts in mood from a high feeling, sometimes associated with irritability (mania), to sometimes severe feelings of sadness and hopelessness (depression). The patient reports a tremendous surge of energy- he feels like he could make love five times a day and write two or three symphonies at night. He became more talkative, experienced racing thoughts, and took on an excessive number of tasks at once. He doesn't need more than two or three hours of sleep, and he runs around the house like he's on speed.

In Chapter 5, Bipolar II Disorder, a mild or moderate level mania is called hypomania. In this state, the person feels good, may be more productive and function better than usual, and will tend to deny that anything is wrong, even when others around him or her learn to recognize the symptoms and confront the person with them. Episodes of hypomania often only last two to three days but can continue for a longer period. However, if left untreated, hypomania can develop into severe mania or switch to depression. Someone in a hypomanic state may stop taking medications because of the good feelings associated with this type of episode.

Chapter 6, Cyclothymic Disorder, discussed the notion of a bipolar spectrum and suggested that cyclothymic disorder may represent the lower end of this spectrum- that is, it produces mood swings of a lesser magnitude than those seen in either classical (type 1) bipolar disorder or in type II bipolar illness. The concept required that during a 2-year period of the disturbance the patient was never without hypomanic or depressive symptoms for more than 2 months at a time. Most classifications viewed cyclothymic as a personality disorder. It is often difficult to distinguish the cyclothymic patient from, for example, the labile borderline or histrionic patient.

In Chapter 7: Major Depressive Disorder is discussed. Depression is one other oldest recognized psychiatric illnesses that is still prevalent today. In chapter 7, symptomatology of depression can be viewed on a continuum according to severity of the illness. Mild depressive episodes occur when the grief process is triggered in response to the loss of a valued object. Moderate depression occurs when grief is prolonged or exaggerated. The individual becomes fixed in the anger stage of the grief response, and the anger is turned inward on the self. Severe depression is an intensification of the symptoms associated with the moderate level. The individual who is severely depressed may also demonstrate a loss of contact with reality. Finally, symptoms at the level of the continuum are established in transient depression as alteration in four spheres of human functioning: (1) affective, (2) behavioral, (3) cognitive, and (4) psychological.

In Chapter 8, previously known as depressive neurosis. Dysthymic disorder is to a major depression as cyclothymic is to bipolar disorder- it is, in effect, an attenuated form of major depression. Remember that dysthymic disorder may coexist with any of the Axis II personality disorders. The principal clues in distinguishing dysthymia from the Cluster B personality disorders – including histrionic, narcissistic, and borderline personality disorders—have to do with the onset, pervasiveness, and intermorbid dysfunction of the condition. This shows a persistent disturbance in appetite, energy, sleep, and concentration.

In Chapter 9, Seasonal Affective Disorder, the specifier "with seasonal pattern" may be appended to either unipolar or bipolar mood disorders, as a "course specifier." Depression that comes with shortened daylight in winter and fall and disappears during spring and summer; also known as seasonal affective disorder (SAD). It afflicts predominately younger women, displays many features of atypical depression (hypersomnia, weight gain, hyperphagia), and is often treated successfully with bright, artificial light (2-6 hours/day—response in 2-3 days, occasionally hypomania occurs).

Section Three: Anxiety Disorders

In Section III, anxiety is abnormal fear that is out of proportion to any external stimulus. Anxiety disorders are the most common of all psychiatric illnesses and result in considerable functional impairment and distress. It refers to a feeling of uneasiness or dread concerning some impending or anticipated ill. Often a distinction is made between state and trait anxiety. State anxiety whereas trait anxiety refers to a stable characteristic condition persisting across situations and over time. Anxiety may be regarded as pathologic when it interferes with effectiveness in living, achievement of desired goals or satisfaction, or reasonable emotional comfort, a number of elements, including psychosocial factors, biological influences and learning experiences most likely contribute to the development of these disorders.

In Chapter 10, this disorder is characterized by recurrent panic attacks, the onset of which is unpredictable, and manifested by intense apprehension, fear, or terror, often associated with feelings of impending doom and accompanied by intense physical discomfort. The attacks usually last minutes, or more rarely, hours. And the individual often experiences varying degrees of nervousness and apprehension between attacks. Panic disorder may or may not be accompanied by agoraphobia. Symptoms characterized by this disorder cause this disorder to experience a fear of being in places or situations from which escape might be difficult or in which help might not be available in the event that a panic attack should occur.

In Chapter 11, phobia refers to a specific kind of fear and is defined as an exaggerated and often disabling fear. Social phobia is an excessive fear of situations in which a person might do something embarrassing or be evaluated negatively by others. The individual has extreme concerns about being exposed to possible scrutiny by others and fears social or performance situations in which embarrassment may occur. In some instances, the fear may be quite defined, such as the fear of speaking or eating in a public place, fear of using a public restroom, or fear of writing in the presence of others. Exposure to the phobic situation usually results in feelings of panic anxiety, with sweating, tachycardia, and dyspnea. Specific phobia was formerly called simple phobia. The essential feature of this disorder is a marked, persistent, and excessive or unreasonable fear when in the presence of, or when anticipating an encounter with, a specific object or situation. Exposure to the phobic stimulus produces overwhelming symptoms of panic, including palpitations, sweating, dizziness, and difficulty breathing. In fact, these symptoms may occur in response to the individual's merely thinking about the phobic stimulus.

In Chapter 12, generalized anxiety disorder is characterized by chronic, unrealistic, and excessive anxiety and worry. Symptoms such as autonomic responses (palpitations, diarrhea, cold clammy extremities, sweating, and urinary frequency), insomnia, poor concentration, fatigue, sighing, trembling, hyper-vigilance, and marked apprehension occur. The symptoms have existed for 6 months or longer and cannot be attributed to specific organic factors, such as caffeine intoxication or hyperthyroidism. This text concentrates on the differences between anxiety and depression. There is a significant overlap between anxiety and depression in that patients with generalized anxiety disorder often are depressed and depressed patients often are anxious.

Chapter 13 addresses obsessive compulsive disorder. Recurrent intrusive ideas, impulses, thoughts (obsessions) or patterns of behavior (compulsions) that are ego-alien and produce anxiety if resisted. Obsessions are recurring ideas, thoughts, images, or impulses that seem senseless but continue to intrude into the patient's mind. Examples include images of violence, thoughts of doing violence to someone else, or fears of leaving on lights or the stove or leaving the door unlocked. Compulsions are behavior or rituals that are performed to dispel the anxiety brought up by obsessions. For example, the patient may wash his or her hands numerous times to dispel a fear of being contaminated, check the stove again and again to see if it is turned off, or look continually in the rear mirror while driving to assuage anxiety about having hit somebody.

In Chapter 14, the patient can acknowledge the traumatic event and the impact it has had on his or her life. PTSD can be caused by any traumatic event such as war, a car accident, abuse, or a natural disaster. People who have these kinds of experiences sometimes begin to suffer flashbacks, bad memories, or dreams, extreme irritability, trouble sleeping, along with other difficulties. We hope that everyone who treats the victims of PTSD –the war-wounded, military veterans, patients who have been assaulted or injured, and those who have lived through a natural or personal disaster—will read this chapter and put it to use in their lives.

Section Four: Psychotic Disorder

A psychotic disorder is a mental illness that causes abnormal and irrational thinking and perceptions. Psychotic illnesses alter a person's ability to think clearly, make good judgments, respond emotionally, communicate effectively, understand reality, and behave appropriately. People with psychotic disorders have difficulty staying in touch with reality and often are unable to meet the ordinary demands of ordinary daily life.

Chapter 15 addresses schizophrenia as the most common psychotic disorder. It generally has a prodromal phase, and active phase with delusions, hallucinations, or both. And most schizophrenics are psychotic for only a small part of their lives. Typically they spend many years in a residual phase during which time they display more minor features of their illness. Studies have been conducted to determine whether psychotic episodes may be precipitated by stressful life events. There is no scientific evidence to indicate that stress causes schizophrenia. However, it is very probable that stress may contribute to the severity and course of the illness. Finally, potential for suicide is a major concern among patients with schizophrenia. They estimate that approximately ten percent of patients with schizophrenia die by suicide.

In Chapter 16, this is a vague and poorly defined disorder meant for patients who have evidence of both schizophrenia and major affective disorder with depressed mood. The disorder can affect all aspects of daily living, including work, social relationships, and self-care skills (such as grooming and hygiene). People with schizoid-affective disorder can have a wide variety of symptoms, including problems with their contact with reality (hallucinations and delusions), mood (such as marked depression), low motivation, inability to experience pleasure, and poor attention. It can be hard for the person with the disorder to distinguish between reality and fantasy.

In Chapter 17, schizophreniform disorder is described as an illness which resembles schizophrenia in every respect except course.

Schizophrenia is a chronic, life long illness, but schizophreniform disorder is said to undergo a full, complete and spontaneous remission within six months. Psychotic symptoms are essentially identical to those seen in schizophrenia and include hallucinations, delusions, loosening of associations, bizarre behavior or catatonia. In some cases, these psychotic symptoms may be accompanied by considerable confusion or perplexity, or by flattening or blunting of affect. Prior to the onset, the patient's premorbid functioning may or may not have been normal.

In Chapter 18, brief psychotic disorder is a diagnosis for patients who experience psychotic symptoms lasting at least one day but no more than one month with gradual recovery. The psychotic symptoms may include disorganization, incoherence, loosening of associations, hallucinations, delusions, and catatonic behavior. Affective symptoms may be more common than the classic schizophrenic symptoms. Onset is acute but according to DSM-5, this syndrome is more likely to occur in patients who have severe personality disorders at baseline. While the patient's mental status may be indistinguishable from that of a patient with schizophrenia or a psychotic mood disorder, the diagnosis hinges on the history of brief duration and an identifiable stressor.

In Chapter 19, addresses shared psychotic disorder with the essential feature, common also called Folie-a-deux. The delusional symptoms develop in a second person as a result of a close relationship with another person who already has psychotic disorder with prominent delusions. The person with the primary delusional disorder is usually the dominant person in the relationship, and the delusional thinking is gradually imposed on the more passive partner. This occurs within the context of a long-term close relationship, particularly when the couple has been socially isolated from other people.

In Chapter 20, demonstrates delusional disorder as hallucinations that may or may not occur in paranoia. If hallucinations do occur, they are at most a minor part of the clinical picture and in general are consistent with the patient's delusions. Voices may be heard; the persecuted patient may hear execution day announced.

Visions, though less common than voices, may also occur. Tactile and olfactory hallucination may also occur, especially with patients with bodily concern. The patient convinced of an infestation may feel bugs on the skin, and the patient convinced of several halitosis may smell several foul odors. For the most part, delusional disorders appear to pursue a chronic, waxy and waning course. Whether spontaneous remissions ever truly occur is unclear; however in some instances partial remissions lasting months or years do occur, and symptoms may be quite minimal during these times.

Section Five: Disorders of Cognition

In this section, delirium, dementia, and amnestic disorder are the three major cognitive disorders. Each disturbance involves impaired memory, abstract thinking, or judgment that produces a clinically significant decline from a previous level of functioning. In delirium, attention is impaired and all of the cognitive processes are therefore also impaired. In dementia, attention is intact but the cognitive processes, particularly memory are impaired. When memory alone is lost and other cognitive powers remain largely intact, the delirium mental state is described as amnesia.

Chapter 21, presents a mental state characterized by a disturbance of cognition, which is manifested by confusion, excitement, disorientation, and a clouding of consciousness. Autonomic manifestations, such as tachycardia, sweating, flushed face, dilated pupils, and elevated blood pressure are common. Traditionally, two subtypes of delirium have been identified-one associated with agitation and the other with hypo activity. Change in arousal and level of vigilance may range from lethargy to agitation. In this phenomenon, called sundowning, reduced sensory input and fatigue combine to unmask organicity in night-time hours.

In Chapter 22, dementia is classified as impairment that is evident in abstract thinking, judgment, and impulse control. In the early stages of dementia, the individual loses the ability to perform some activities of daily living (ADLs). Independently, such as hygiene, dressing, and grooming and require some assistance to manage these ongoing basis. As the disease progresses urinary and fecal incontinence are common. Psychomotor symptoms include wandering, obsessiveness, agitation, and aggression. Symptoms seem to worsen in the late afternoon and evening – a phenomenon termed sundowning.

In Chapter 23, amnestic disorder is characterized by problems with memory function. Among the most common medically based amnestic disorder is so-called Wernicke-Korsakoff syndrome. Other causes of amnesia include: head trauma, hippocampal infarction, herpes simplex encephalitis, neoplasms, and anoxic injury. Another amnestic syndrome sometimes seen by psychiatrists is that of transient global amnesia. This syndrome presents as an acute period of memory loss consisting of two components. An ongoing anterograde amnesia that persists for several hours, and a retrograde amnesia that lasts a few weeks. The syndrome differs from dementia in that there is no impairment in abstract thinking or judgment, no other disturbances of higher cortical function, and no personality change.

Section Six: Recovery from Mental Illness

Mental health recovery is a journey of healing and transformation enabling a person with a mental health problem to live a meaningful life in a community of his or her choice while striving to achieve his or her full potential. When people begin to take responsibility for developing coping skills and learning ways to manage their illness, they have taken a significant step forward. It is when focusing on what they can do to improve their quality of life that things often begin to get better. In each chapter, caregivers are most helpful when they collaborate with people in meeting goals consumers set for themselves. Caregivers can also assist by offering education about mental illness, recovery, when services are available, medications, other forms of treatment, and the pros and cons of each.

We begin Chapter 24 with an overview of general principles relevant to the safe and effective use of psychotropic medications. Although each psychotropic medication affects neurotransmission, the specific drugs within each class have varying neuronal effects. For example, researchers hypothesize that most antidepressants work by blocking the reuptake of neurotransmitters, specifically serotonin and norepinephrine. And antipsychotic medications block dopamine receptors, while some affect muscarinic cholinergic, histaminergic, and alpha-adrenergic receptors. The atypical anti-psychotics block a specific serotonin receptor.

Chapter 25 addresses pain management when patients come to the clinic with their pain that they present with a marvelous opportunity. Their presence is the chance to understand symptoms, to understand symptoms, to understand how their pain is affecting their lives, the challenge of discovering what is causing their pain, and finally the opportunity to prescribe medications and lifestyle changes to help them gain relief from their pain. The studies tend to differentiate acute from chronic pain. Acute pain is associated with inflammation and activation of spinal pathways that send instructive pain messages to encourage future injury avoidance and cause protective muscle spasm. There is no question that the presence of pain greatly compromises the quality of life. Someone who is having pain is asked to match the perceived intensity of pain to a scale. And patients with chronic pain often report a variety of complaints, including pain, sleep abnormalities, mood disturbance, and interference with personal, social, and work relationships.

The main focus of Chapter 26, is primarily the method and the clinical principles of psychotherapy. It draws together these principles and gives them a theoretical foundation. It describes and contrasts the three predominant psychotherapeutic approaches psycho-dynamic, cognitive, and interpersonal techniques. The primary aim of psychotherapy is to alter pathological behavior, with treatment goals ranging from relieving specific symptoms, such as bed-wetting, to making fundamental changes in character structure and behavior patterns that affect important aspects of life, such as work, love, sex, and interpersonal relationships. The use of medication helped reduce aggression and enhanced communication, making psychotherapy a potentially more effective treatment for those patients. To some extent, managing aggression and enhancing communication remain among the most significant reasons to use medication in combination with psychotherapy, whatever the diagnosis. We described individual counseling or psychotherapy as a dyadic (two-way) interaction between a client who is distressed, and perhaps confused and frightened, and a professional helper whose helping skills are recognized and accepted by the client. In addition, group psychotherapy requires additional skills that are not learned through training and experience in individual psychotherapy.

In Chapter 27, the goal of nutrition counseling is to help a person make and maintain dietary changes. Mental Health can be influenced by several nutritional factors, including: overall energy intake, intake of the energy -containing nutrients (proteins, carbohydrates, fats) and intake of vitamins and minerals. Often deficiencies of multiple nutrients rather than a single nutrient are responsible for changes in brain functioning. Foods rich in high-quality protein include meats, milk and other dairy products, and eggs. Carbohydrates include starches, naturally occurring and refined sugars, and dietary fiber. Dietary intake of fats may also play a role in regulating mood and brain function. Some studies suggest that reducing fat and cholesterol in the diet may deplete brain serotonin levels, causing mood changes, anger, and aggressive behavior.

Relaxation therapy in Chapter 28 is an effective means of reducing the stress response in some individuals. Various methods of relaxation are described as follows: Deep relaxation can counteract the physiological and behavioral manifestations of stress. That is why deep breathing exercises involve inhaling slowly and deeply through the nose, holding the breath for a few seconds, then exhaling slowly through the mouth. In progressive relaxation, each muscle group is tensed for 5 to 7 seconds and then relaxed for

20 to 30 seconds during which time the individual concentrates on the difference in sensations between the two conditions. Mental Imagery uses the imagination in an effort to reduce the body's response to stress. The frame of reference is very personal, based on what each individual considers to be a relaxing environment. And finally, biofeedback is the use of instrumentation to become aware of processes in the body that usually go unnoticed and to help bring them under voluntary control. Biological conditions, such as muscle tension, skin surface temperature, blood pressure, and heart rate, are monitored by the biofeedback equipment.

Chapter 29, promotes electroconvulsive therapy (ECT), which remains one of the most effective treatments for depressive illness, especially for patients with medication-resistant depression, with psychotic symptoms or catatonia, at immediate and significant risk of harm to self or others, or with serious comorbid medical conditions, particularly in the elderly. In ECT, a bidirectional square wave lasting about 2 msec is applied through right (nondominant) unilateral or bilateral electrodes to produce a generalized electrical seizure in the brain lasting 20-150 seconds. A number of researchers have demonstrated that electric stimulation results in significant increases in the circulating levels of several neurotransmitters. These include serotonin, norepinephrine, and dopamine, the same biogenic amines that are affected by antidepressant drugs. Electroconvulsive therapy (ECT) is the oldest and most reliable of the modern somatic therapies for mood disorders. ECT has undergone fundamental changes since its introduction 75 years ago. It is no longer the bone-breaking, memory-stealing, fearsome treatment pictured in films. Anesthesia, controlled oxygenation, and muscle relaxation make the procedure so safe that the risks are less than those accompanying the use of several psychotropic drugs.

Section 7: Psychiatric Emergencies

People with a primary psychiatric complaint, such as depression and suicidal ideation or psychotic thought processes, are easily recognized by most emergencies personnel. According to the American Psychiatric Association, a psychiatric emergency is defined as," a situation that includes an acute disturbance of thought behavior, mood, or social relationship which require immediate intervention as defined by the client, family, or social unit." In setting priorities, the following life threatening emergencies should be identified and managed: agitated, menacing, self-destructive, and out-of- control behavior; serious and chronic self-neglect, and serious medical problems either co-existing with or causing psychiatric symptoms.

Suicide is intentional self-inflicted death. In Chapter 30, suicidal ideation and attempted suicide are among the most common of emergency presentations. That is why common themes in suicide includes a crisis that causes intense suffering and feelings of hopelessness and helplessness, conflict between survival and unbearable stress, a narrowing of the patient's perceived options, and the wish to escape. The assessment of suicide risk is one of the most important and difficult task in emergency psychiatry. Certain psychiatric or general medical illnesses also increase the risk of completed suicide. Important among the psychiatric illnesses are depression, (either of major depression or bipolar disorder), a mixed- manic episode, alcoholism, schizophrenia, and borderline personality disorder. The best hope for suicide prevention lies in the early detection and treatment of these contributory psychiatric disorders.

In Chapter 31, acute psychosis is a medical emergency. It is the psychiatric term for psychosis which is triggered by extreme stress. By definition, signs and symptoms of acute psychosis have developed rapidly, over a period of days or weeks. The patient usually has severe impairments of thought and judgment. Combined with agitation or hyper-activity, this impairment may result in violence, inadvertent self-injury, or suicide. The focus of this chapter is first, the method of evaluating acutely psychotic patient so that the differential diagnosis can be approached systematically and seconds the early steps in psychological and psycho-pharmacological management. The condition usually spontaneously resolves itself within 2 weeks, and the main goal of treatment is to prevent the patient from harming either themselves or others.

In Chapter 32, violence can be due to a wide range of psychiatric disorders, but it may also occur in aged appropriate people who cannot cope with life stresses in less severe ways. Why does age make a difference? There are probably many reasons, including biological and psychological ones, but a curious reason that is often ignored, for males, in particular, is an evolutionary one: by the age of twenty-five there is less reason for a man to be violent. Biological theories register areas of the brain that may be involved including the temporal lobe, the limbic system, and the amygdaloid nucleus. Specifically, studies show that various nuero-transmitters in particular norepinephrine, dopamine, and serotonin may play a role in the facilitation and inhibition of aggressive impulses. The next objective is to make a diagnosis that will lead to a treatment plan including measures to minimize the likelihood of subsequent violence.

Chapter 33 discusses the physical and behavioral manifestations and personal and social consequences related to the abuse of or dependency on alcohol, other central nervous system (CNS) depressants, CNS stimulants, opioids, hallucinogens, and cannibals. Many of the treatment samples that have been studied were drawn from substance abuse treatment programs in VA hospitals. There are at least two components to achieving a substance-free lifestyle. The first involves enhancing motivation for abstinence, and the second relates to teaching our patients how to rebuild their lives after redirecting the focus of their activities away from substance use.

Chapter 34 discusses the multitude of problems created by drinking. Alcohol abuse is the most serious drug abuse problem in the United States. A substantial proportion of patient presenting for emergency treatment have alcohol related problems, including alcohol intoxication and withdrawal, trauma, neurologic complaints, and alcohol-related illnesses (such as gastro-intestinal bleeding). These drinking habits usually result in depression and anxiety. This is important because it has been estimated that 25% of all suicides in the United States occur in alcoholics.

Acknowledgements

So much progress has been made in the mental health field at the VA just in the last decade. With our new knowledge of the brain, medications an treatment methods for mental illnesses have changed dramatically.

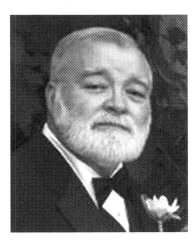

This book is dedicated in loving memory of Ismael Carlo, MD (1949-2015) for his wonderful contribution to psychiatry at the Michael Debakey Veterans of Affairs Medical Center in Houston, Texas. Without Dr. Carlo's clinical treatments and personal mentoring I would never have conceptualized this project.

Contributors

Contributors were selected not only because they are familiar with recent advances in their fields, but also because they are physicians who apply this information in daily patient care. This book would not have been possible without the help of many people who have taught me, guided me, and worked with me since I became involved in the mental health field. For all these things, I want to express my appreciation to each editor. Without the warm support, the careful reviewing, and the stimulating comments, this book would have been difficult to write.

Last but not least, I give thanks to my secretary Desiree F. Liggan, a gracious and patient contributors, who deciphered my handwriting and on her own free time typed my manuscript, much credit is due.

I wish to express my gratitude for permission to reproduce material that originally appeared in the following publications:

American Journal of Geriatric Psychiatry

American Journal of Psychiatry

American Journal of Public Health

American Journal of Emergency

American Journal of Clinical Nutrition

American Journal of Psychotherapy

American Emergency Medicine

Deborah Y. Liggan, MD

Archives of General Psychiatry

Archives of Internal Medicine

Archives of Neurology

Biological Psychiatry

British Psychiatry

British Journal of Psychiatry

British Journal of Medical Psychology

Comprehensive Psychiatry

Canadian Journal of Psychiatry

Canadian Journal of Neurological Sciences

Convulsive Therapy

Clinical Nutrition

Community Psychiatry

Current Psychiatry Reports

Clinical Psychology Review

General Hospital Psychiatry

International Journal of Neuro-Psychiatric Medicine

Journal of Affective Disorders

Journal of American Geriatric society

Journal of Consulting and Clinical Psychology

Journal of Nervous and Mental Disease

Journal of Neurophysiology

Journal of Neurology, Neurosurgery and Psychiatry

Journal of Psychiatric Research

Journal of Clinical Psychiatry

Journal of the American Medical Association (JAMA)

New England Journal of Medicine

Neuropsychology Review

Psychosomatic Medicine

Psychiatric Annals

Psychiatric Clinicals of North America

Section One

Psychiatric Interviewing

> *All the world's a stage, and all the men and women merely players; They have their exits and their entrances, And one man in his time plays many parts … That ends this strange eventful history. Is second childishness and mere oblivion, sans teeth, sans eyes, sans taste, sans everything.*
>
> *William Shakespeare (1564-1616)*

Patient interviewing is the core skill in medicine and psychiatry, and communication between doctor and patient is the basis of good; medical practice. In this section we outline the process of psychiatric interviewing and to give the reader some vicarious experience with interviewing patients by using selected examples.

Purpose of the interview is to (1)obtain historical perspective of patient's life, and (2) establish rapport and a therapeutic alliance, (3) develop mutual trust and confidence, (4) understand present functioning, (5) make a diagnosis, and (6) establish a treatment plan. The techniques deals with questions that come to mind as psychiatric patients that are interviewed and gives a "road map" to follow for the examination.

Chapter 1

The Psychiatric Interview

The purpose and conduct of a psychiatric evaluation depends on who requests the evaluation, why it is requested, and the expected feature role of the psychiatrist in the patient's care. A thorough evaluation of a psychiatric patient consists of a psychiatric history, mental status examination, complete physical examination, laboratory screening evaluation, and when indicated, specific psychological and biological tests.

The ability to conduct an effective interview is an important tool for a physician. A psychiatric interview has two important functions. One is to create an atmosphere for mutual exploration in which the patient feels free to say what is on his or her mind; the other is to obtain information necessary for diagnosis and treatment. An interview needs the skills to gather the data necessary to competently treat the patient and to obtain the patient's advice. Every interview has three main components, all of which demand specific techniques and skills: the beginning of the interview, the interview proper, and the closing of the interview.

Beginning the Interview

The mundane yet often neglected practice of shaking hands helps set the tone for the initial relationship between therapist and patient. Shaking hands firmly with a patient brings to the first moments of contact an element of personal warmth and respect. This simple gesture eases the tension preceding the initial interview and reassures the patient, who almost always approaches the doctor with a degree of apprehension.

Once the patient is seated, the therapist focuses his attention on facilitating in every way possible the patient's efforts to tell his story. Every aspect of the initial stages of the therapist-patient relationship can be measured against a single, simple standard" is the therapist, in his exchange of initial courtesies, as warm and respectful to the patient says he offers his hand; and takes pains to make the visitor welcome and comfortable.

From the first moment of contact, the doctor or therapist imitates a process that involves a multiplicity of factors within himself as well as within the patient and determines in large measure whether or not the patient recovers.

The Interview Proper

The psychiatric history includes information about the patient as a person, the chief complaint, the present illness, the premorbid adjustment, and the past history, the history of medical illnesses, a family history of psychiatric and medical disorders, and a development history of the patient. Through the interview the psychiatrist tries to learn how the patient experiences life events and to understand the patient's perceptions of how such events evolve. The major elements of this initial encounter are (1) the therapist's attitude toward the patient; (2) the therapist's emotional resources and standard of conduct; (3) the professional versus to social relationship; (4) the concept of resistance and therapeutic alliance and therapeutic alliance; (5) obstacles in the patient" manifestation of resistance' (6) feelings toward the therapist: reality and transference: (7) obstacles in the therapist: impediments to listening; (8) feelings toward the patient: reality and countertransference: (9) jargon and humor as obstacles: and (10) ethical considerations: sexual relations within therapy.

Harry Stack Sullivan said that the interview must always have in mind one question about the patient: "Who is this person and how did he come to be here? The generic answer is that a combination of his native endowments and personal experience has brought him to this pass." Reading about interviewing is only a first step toward becoming a competent interviewer. However, a critical problem in the assessment process is to determine whether any observed change in functioning is due to normal aging or whether it reflects some type of change within the central nervous system above and beyond what might be expected in the normal aging process.

The therapist's approach to the patient sets the tone for the initial interview. In the course of treating psychiatric patients, clinical observation and careful history taking are the most important tools possessed.

Interviewing Across Cultural Differences

Interviewing patients from different social, cultural, or language groups presents the interviewer with special challenges and opportunities. These include establishing rapport and adequate communication with someone different from oneself.

The cross-cultural doctor-patient relationship also provides the opportunity to learn about a person from a different group than one's own, to learn a modified set of interviewing skills and to learn about the culture itself. The three groups that will be discussed in this section are the poor (a social group), Blacks, and Spanish-speaking groups. This brings us to the first basic principle of interviewing across sociocultural differences: the physician must first acknowledge to himself or herself that differences exist and that certain emotions may be present but are acceptable. The emotion felt during this sort of encounter may vary: a sense of general discomfort and unease, irritability, frustration, perhaps even anger.

Mental Examination

It is critical that the clinician asses the mental status of the patient. This is accomplished by conducting a mental status examination, which is an objective report on the patient's current mental functioning as witnessed by the interviewer. Technically the mental status examination is conducted and reported on as a separate part of the clinical psychiatric interview. Patients frequently change with time, and the mental status examination establishes a baseline against which to measure this change. The mental status examination assists in understanding, diagnosing, and measuring the progress of or deterioration in patients and facilitates communication among professional. An overview of the major parts of the mental status examination follows. An outline of this material is presented in Box 1-1.

BOX 1-1 Outline of the Mental Status Examination

Presentation

- General Appearance
- Level of consciousness
- Attitude toward interview
- Motor Behavior
- Speech

Emotional State: mood and affect

- Range of emotional expression
- Appropriateness of emotions
- Biological indicators of affect

Perceptual disturbances

- Hallucinations and illusions
- Depersonalization and DE realization

Thought Processes

- Stream of thought
- Continuity of thought
- Content of thought

Cognitive State

- Orientation
- Attention and Concentration
- Memory
- Intelligence
- Reliability
- Insight and judgment

Mental Status Exam

The format proposed here is based on a consensus among professors of psychiatry from medical schools across the country on what they think essential in a mental status examination. The mental status examination varies with each patient.

1. General appearance. Specific characteristics of dress and grooming ought to be coted, as well as posture, gait, facial expression and gestures.
2. Attitude. What is the patient's attitude toward his illness, toward the interview, and toward the doctor?
3. Motor behavior. The posture and gait of the patient should be noted as well as tics, tremors, posturing, pacing, grimaces, and other abnormal movements.
4. Speech. Tone of voice, pitch, rate of speech (very fast and pressured as in a manic state or very slow as in a depressed state).
5. Affective states. What the patient is feeling at the moment, which may be flat or blunted with little emotion expressed. Anger, fear, euphoria, elation, ecstasy, depression, irritability, and other emotional states should be noted.
6. Thought Processes. From attending to the content of the patient's speech, to the structure and rate of associations, and in the flow of ideas.
7. Thought content. The patient's preoccupations, ambitions, repetitive dreams, and daydreams give ideas of this content.

8. Perception. The capacity to be aware of objects and to discriminate among them. Perceptions of reality include illusions and hallucinations as they constitute the more serious forms of perceptual distortion.

9. Intellectual functioning. A general impression of the patient's intellectual capacity will be gained from listening to his history. His general level of knowledge must be measured against the years of formal education he has completed sand his particular family and cultural background.

10. Orientation. Disorientation in terms of person, place, or time must be noted.

11. Memory. The patient's ability to recall past and recent events can be tested as the doctor elicits dates and other details of his life.

12. Judgment. The patient's ability to make and carry out plans, to take the initiative, to discriminate accurately, ad to behave appropriately in social and other situations reflects his judgment.

VIGNETTE

The AMSIT states whether the patient demonstrates increased psychomotor activity, distractibility, and flight of ideas, as well as loose associations, blocking, and concrete thinking. A description of how the patient relates to the examiner is included. For practical purposes, the emotion sustained for the duration of the interview may be considered the patient's mood. His affect changed repeatedly through the interview. Twice the patient asked the examiner to stop speaking so that he could hear what the voices were saying to him. Affect was described as blunted, which was moderately decreased range and intensity.

Thoughts were pressured and rapidly jumped form one thought to another, yet the associations ere clear. Blocking involves sudden stops in his train of thoughts, often in midsentence. At all points the patient's affect was appropriate to his thought content. His sensorium was correctly oriented for time and place. Recent memory was excellent as demonstrated by object recall, digit span, and his spontaneous description of recent events. His judgment was clearly impaired as evidenced by his behavior in the interview. His poor insight was indicated by his puzzlement over why anyone would think he needed to be hospitalized in a psychiatric unit.

Discussion. The mental status of AMSIT report is a systematic documentation of the patient's t thinking, feelings, and behavior at the time of the interview. Since the AMSIT organizes clinical findings into a systematic report written after the interview, it in no way suggests the sequence of topics in the interview.

BOX 1-2 Report on Patient's Current Mental Status: AMSIT

I.   General **A**ppearance, Behavior and Speech
II.   **M**ood and Affect
III. **S**ensorium
IV.   **I**ntellectual Function
V.   **T**hought

Discussion. Observation of abnormalities in any of these 12 general categories will guide the clinician toward ruling in or out a particular diagnosis or conclusion about the patient's mental status. Deterioration in grooming sometimes marks the onset of schizophrenia or depression. Overly fastidious dress and grooming may indicate obsessive-compulsive traits. Certain disturbances in attitude will alert the examiner to specific diagnostic possibilities. The suspiciousness, evasiveness, and arrogance characterize paranoid patients; the uncooperativeness or impatience of severely manic patients; the reserved, remote, and unfeeling attitude of the schizophrenic; the resistant, uncooperative attitude of the passive-aggressive patient; the apprehensive attitude of the patient suffering from acute anxiety neurosis; the apathetic, helpless attitude of the depressed patient; and the easily distracted, seemingly indifferent attitude of the patient suffering from an acute brain disorder.

A number of disorders may show themselves in motor abnormalities. Echopraxia is the pathological repetition, by imitation of the movements of another person; this motor disturbance is often seen in catatonic schizophrenics. In waxy flexibility a patient maintains his body position for long periods of time. Cataplexy is a temporary loss of muscle tone and weakness may be precipitated by laughter, anger, or surprise. Stereotypy, the persistent, mechanical repetition of speech or motor activity, is observed in some schizophrenics. Akathisia refers to the particular type of restlessness and uncontrolled motor activity associated with certain psychomotor activity drugs as the phenothiazines. A person with an obsessive-compulsive neurosis manifests obsessive ideas, pervasive doubts, and compulsive rituals, such as repeated hand washing or checking to see that the gas or lights have been turned off.

Abnormal speech. Like abnormalities in motor activity, abnormalities in speech are associated with particular disorders. Mutism is the refusal to speak for conscious or unconscious reasons and is often present in severely psychotic patients. Aphasia refers to a loss of previously possessed facility of language comprehension. Amnestic aphasia is the loss of the ability to name objects; in Broca's aphasia, the loss of the ability to produce spoken and written language, with comprehension retained; and Wernicke's aphasia, the loss of ability to comprehend language.

Closing the Interview

Toward the end of the interview, the doctor should say' "Our time is about up" or "We have about five minutes left." This gives patients a chance to regroup and to add other things that they may not have mentioned yet.

Don't feel bad about ending an interview. The doctor can always come back. If something seemingly important is brought up the end, you can say "We will have to stop, but perhaps the patient would like to talk about that next time." Sometimes the doctor gives the patient a short summary of what has taken place in the interview, but this is not always necessary. Whether or not to summarize at the end of each interview is something to be judged with each patient. In closing, the doctor ends it with a statement such as, "Well, we got a little more understanding of your past life today," which can give a patient a good feeling without promising too much. Many patients do not ask for anything at the end of an interview. They feel relieved by having someone listen to them and by being able to express some of their feeling. This probably is true with most patients and they need no closing statement about what might have happened in the interview.

Multiaxial System

The APA (2000) endorses case evaluation on a Multi-axial System, to facilitate comprehensive and systematic evaluation with attention to the various mental disorders and general medical conditions, psychosocial and environmental problems, and level of functioning that might be overlooked if the focus were on assessing a single presenting problem. Each individual is evaluated on five exes.

They're defined by the DSM-IV-TR in the following manner:

- **Axis I- Clinical Disorders and Other conditions that may be a focus on Clinical Attention.** This includes all mental disorders (except personality disorders and mental retardation).
- **Axis II-** Personality Disorders and Mental Retardation. These conditions persist in a stable form into adult life.
- **Axis III- General Medical Conditions.** These include any current general medical condition that is potentially relevant to the understanding or management of the individual's mental disorder.
- **Axis IV- Psychosocial and Enviromental Problems.** These are problems that may affect the diagnosis, treatment, and prognosis of mental disorders named on axes I and II.

- **Axis V- Global Assessment of Functioning.** This allows the clinician to rate the individual's overall functioning on the Global Assessment of Functioning (GAF) Scale.

Chapter 1: Psychiatric Interview Examination Review

1. Identify the emotional state of mood and affect outlines in the Mental Status Examination.

    A. Range of emotional expression
    B. Appropriateness of emotions
    C. Biological indicators of affect
    D. All of the above

2. What important functions is diagnosed in the psychiatric interview?

    A. Create an atmosphere for mutual exploration in which the patient feels free to say what is on his or her mind
    B. Argue with the patient concerning his diagnosis
    C. Gather information without asking questions during the interview
    D. Stop the conversation periodically to summarize key points

3. What disturbances in attitude will alert the examiner to specific diagnostic possibilities?

    A. The reserved, remote, and unfeeling attitude of the depressed person
    B. The resistant, uncooperative attitude of the schizophrenic
    C. The uncooperativeness or impatience of depressed patient
    D. The apprehensive attitude of the patient suffering from acute anxiety neurosis

4. Memory may be defined as the ability to recall to consciousness previously registered experiences and information. Which symptom involves past events and is not usually progressive?

    A. Hysterical amnesia
    B. Anterograde amnesia
    C. Retrograde amnesia
    D. Fugue amnesia

5. In bringing the initial session to a close, what advice is given for the examiner?

   A. Cut the patient off in the middle of an important part of his history so that he will have a thought to conclude next appointment
   B. Close by saying, "Let's continue here the next time."
   C. Notify the patient every 15 minutes that the hour is up
   D. Avoid seeing the patient again by summarizing the appointment every 15 minutes

6. In order to capture more of the complexity of real patients, DSM-5 allows then to be described in multiple axes, which basically correspond to domains of function.

   A. Axis I: Personality disorders
   B. Axis II: Clinical syndromes and V codes
   C. Axis III: Psychosocial and environmental problems
   D. Axis V: Global Assessment of Functioning

7. What is an insistent, repetitive, intrusive, and unwanted urge to perform an act that is contrary to the person's ordinary wishes or standards?

   A. Dipsomania
   B. Compulsion
   C. Necromania
   D. Catalepsy

8. What temporary loss of muscle tone and weakness, may be precipitated by laughter, anger, or surprise?

   A. Stereotypy
   B. Akathisia
   C. Cataplexy
   D. Hyperkinesia

9. Manic patients may be in constant motion with an apparent inexhaustible supply of energy. Which diagnosis describes the inability to walk or stand, both that are associated with hysterical conversion?

    A. Astasia-abasia
    B. Hysterical aphona
    C. Catatonic excitement
    D. Psychomotor retardation

10. Which abnormality in speech defines the refusal to speak for conscious or unconscious reasons and is often present in severely psychotic patients?

    A. Punning and rhyming
    B. Verbigeration
    C. Mutism
    D. Aphasia

Chapter 1: Psychiatric Interview Examination Answers

1. D
2. A
3. D
4. C
5. B
6. D
7. B
8. C
9. A
10. C

Chapter 2

Biopsychosocial Perspective

What is a **diagnostic formulation**? It is as close an approximation to understanding the whole person as a psychiatrist initially can achieve. It is a comprehensive attempt to utilize the biopsychosocial model (Engell 1977) in a practical clinical manner. Most important, perhaps the diagnostic formulation embodies all that is unique about psychiatry-for no other discipline strives so rigorously to uncover and integrate biological, psychological, and social components of mental illness.

Though significant in all medical specialties, the quality of the doctor-patient relationship becomes crucial in the practice pf psychiatry. Distinctive features of the psychiatric interview include examining feelings bout significant events in the individual's life, identifying significant persons and their relationship of the patient in the course of this or her life, and identifying and tracing the major influences in the biological, psychological, and social development of the individual (Weissman, 1933).

The diagnostic formulation must consider a host of factors related to the patient's psychiatric symptoms. In the biopsychosocial model the doctor patient relationship is one of the main tools for evaluation and therapy. The mental health field is far from a complete understanding of the biological, psychological, and sociocultural bases of development, but development clearly involves interplay among these influences.

How can the psychiatrist utilize the biopsychosocial model in understanding the patient? What are the bio-, psycho-, and social- parts of this model? What are the practical instances in which this model is useful? The cross-cultural interview has the potential of a more rewarding outcome because of altered expectations and heightened interest, concentration, and awareness. Lefley (1990) has summarized the many ways in which culture may affect chronic mental illness. The three groups that will be discussed in this section are the poor (a social group), Blacks, and Spanish-speaking groups. These three are the largest and some of the general comments about interviewing patient's form these groups may apply to others. Most physicians and medical students in the United States come from middle class backgrounds, speak English as their primary language, are white, and are obviously well-educated. However, the majority fo people that medical students will have as patient's during their years in training are form the lower class (medically indigent) and often are poorly educated. Blacks and other minority groups are overrepresented among the medically indigent. Thus, the interview across social class, cultural, and language differences is important. When the patient is form the same social class and ethnic group as the treating psychiatrist, therapy is often successful. (Foulks, 1980).

Do such socioeconomic or ethnic factors actually influence psychiatric diagnosis? Some research suggests that Blacks and other minorities are more often misdiagnosed than whites (Adebimpe 1981; Mukherjee et al 1982). The social part of our biopsychosocial approach also deals with the family unit, education and socioeconomic status, peer group relations, life stresses, and social role. The consequences of these factors showed an association between low socioeconomic status and the incidence of mental illness. In addition, Durkheim's (1897/ 1951) seminal investigation showed an inverse relationship between suicide and the individual's degree of integration into a network of enduring ties. More recently – and perhaps, more unexpectedly- Waitzkin (1984) has shown that doctor-patient communication is influenced by socioeconomic factors.

Specifically, the increased likelihood of hallucinations in Black and Hispanic patients with bipolar disorder may contribute to the misdiagnosis of schizophrenia in these groups (Lawson 1986).

Evan objective evidence may lead us into diagnostic error. For example, because the Minnesota Multiphasic Personality Inventory (MMPI) was not standardized on a Black population, Blacks tend to score higher on the paranoia and schizophrenia scales than do whites (Gyunther 1982).

Global Assessment of Functioning (GAF)

The patients highest level of social, occupational, and psychological functioning according to the GAF scale (Table 1-2). Examiners should use the 12 months prior to the current evaluation as a reference point and rate from 0 (inadequate information) to 1 (lowest) to 100 (highest).

Axis IV. Severity of Psychosocial Stressor. Rate the severity of stress in the patient's life. Use the twelve months prior to the current evaluation as a reference. Use **codes 1 (none) to 6 (catastrophic).**

Axis V. Global Assessment of Functioning. Rate the highest level of functioning of the patient according to Table 1-2.

Table 1-2. DSM-IV-TR Global Assessment of Functioning (GAF) Scale

100- 91	**Superior functioning in a wide range of activities, life's problems never seem to get out of hand, is sought out by others because of his or her many positive qualities. No symptoms.**
90-81	**Absent or minimal symptoms** (e.g. mild anxiety before an exam), **good functioning in all areas, interested and involved in a wide range of activities, socially effective, generally satisfied with life, no more than everyday problems or concerns (e.g. an occasional argument with family members).**

80-71	**If symptoms are present, they are transient and expectable reactions to psychosocial stressors** (e.g. difficulty concentrating after family argument); **no more than slight impairment in social, occupational, or school functioning** (e.g. temporarily falling behind in schoolwork).
70-61	**Some mild symptoms** (e.g. depressed mood and mild insomnia) **or some difficulty in social, occupational, or school functioning** (e.g. occasional truancy, or theft within the household), **but generally functioning pretty well, has some meaningful interpersonal relationships.**
60-51	**Moderate Symptoms** (e.g. flat affect and circumstantial speech, occasional panic attacks) **Or moderate difficulty in social, occupational, or school functioning** (e.g., few friends, conflicts with peers or coworkers).
50-41	**Serious Symptoms** (e.g. suicidal ideation, severe obsessional rituals, frequent shoplifting) **Or any serious impairment in social, occupational, or school functioning** (e.g., no friends, unable to keep a job).
40-31	**Some impairment in reality testing or communication** (e.g. speech is at times illogical, obscure, or irrelevant) **Or major impairment in several areas, such as work or school, family relation, judgment, thinking, or mood** (e.g. depressed man avoids friends, neglects family, and is unable to work; child frequently beats up younger children, is defiant at home, and is failing at school).
30-21	**Behavior is considerably influenced by delusions or hallucinations OR serious impairment, in communication or judgment** (e.g. sometimes incoherent, acts grossly inappropriately, suicidal preoccupation) **OR inability to function in almost all areas** (e.g. stays in bed all day, no job, home, or friends).
20-11	**Some danger of hurting self or others** (e.g. suicide attempts without clear expectation of death; frequently violent; manic excitement) **OR occasionally fails to maintain minimal personal hygiene** (e.g., smears feces) **OR gross impairment in communication** (e.g., largely incoherent or mute).

| 10-1 | **Persistent danger of severely hurting self or others** (e.g., recurrent violence) **OR persistent inability to maintain minimal personal hygiene OR serious suicidal act with clear expectation of death.** |

Let us now try to bring together a number of ethnic, social, and socioeconomic factors in a clinical vignette.

VIGNETTE

During the first few sessions of an evaluation, a 33 year old woman experienced great difficulty speaking to the doctor. She entered the office and immediately began to cry. She expressed confusion over her fear of the doctor and her inability to talk to him. When she apologized for her loss of control, the doctor waited patiently for her to regain her composure and encouraged her to express all her feelings. The patient's brother accompanied her and provided some information. She carried the diagnosis of borderline personality disorder based on her behavior was impulsive, labile, and often violent. She had several arrests for shoplifting and disorderly conduct. In addition, to charges she incurred while on active duty, she complained of frequent bouts of anxiety and depression. A school history revealed an inability to sit still in class, difficulty with attention, and rowdy behavior on the playground. Her parents related the patient's inability as a child to watch television, "for more than 5 minutes at a stretch." She participated in psychotherapy while in active duty, which revealed an inability to sit still in sessions, difficulty with attention, and rowdy behavior before and after sessions. A diagnosis of adult attention deficit disorder was made.

DISCUSSION. How do cultural factors impinge on a psychiatric diagnosis? The patient in this vignette was clearly depressed and in need of treatment, regardless of the cultural nuances in her belief system. There is good evidence that attention-deficit disorder has a strong biological component. Consequently, this patient has several sociocultural risk factors that predispose her to depressive illness. For example, her status as an immigrant, recent loss of job, and break up with her boyfriend. In addition, the family history revealed that the patient's father had died when the patient was 7 years old, and that afterward the patient seemingly became more withdrawn.

The Biopsychosocial Model

In 1960, George Engel, MD began to elaborate a unified concept of health and disease- a concept that evolved the biopsychosocial model. This model posits that whether a cell or a person, every system is influenced by the continuation of the systems of which each is a part (e.g., one's family, community, culture, and nation). It is not my intention to elaborate on Engel's concept, but to provide the specific clinical underpinnings of his model. What are the bio, psycho and social parts of this model? An important component of the "bio" part of this model is the intercurrent physical illness that may be affecting the patient's psyche. There is good evidence that attention deficit disorder has a strong biological component, as is also the care with Tourette's disorder. However, both conditions are affected by and in turn, affect the psychosocial milieu in which the child or adolescent develops. The biological part of the bio-psychosocial model is heavily influenced by a variety of neuroendocrine disorders (Box 2-1).

BOX 2-1. Neuroendocrine Disorders with Psychiatric Complications

- Hyper-, hypothyroidism
- Hyper-, hypoparathyroidism
- Adrenocortical insufficiency (Addison's Disease)
- Adrenocortical excess (Cushing's Syndrome)
- Pheochromocytoma
- Diabetes Mellitus
- Insulinoma

For example, a patient who becomes aware that he or she has a chronic unremitting illness may undergo a period of marked depression or regression. Let us summarize the biological component of our biopsychosocial model. The diagnostic formulation must consider a host of biomedical factors related to the patient's psychiatric symptoms. These include genetic endowment; pre-, post-, and neonatal traumata; neurological illness; neuroendocrine disorders; intercurrent medical illness; and substance abuse or withdrawal.

The ego psychosocial model emphasizes the defensive compromises mediated by the ego. For example, such compromises may occur in mediating among primitive wishes, superego constraints, and the demands of reality. This model is directly linked to Mac Kinnon's description of the ego functions. Thus the symptoms we develop are determined by the characteristic ego defenses at our disposal. The ego-psychological model explores these defenses in relation to the individual's unconscious wishes and fears. On some such days he would have angry outburst, shouting at his therapist, "You must be the most incompetent jerk in the whole damn field." The psychiatrist encourages a free-flowing exchange with the patient and then at the conclusion of the interview' arrives at a diagnostic formulation of the patient's problems. The more accurate the diagnostic assessment, the more appropriate the treatment planning (Halleck, 1991).

Ego Functions in Psychiatry.

A complete psychological understanding of the patient would include and appraisal of these functions, as well as the psychodynamic formulation- that is, the understanding of the core conflict. In which, the ego functions are outlined. The clinician can compress an assessment of these functions intoduce 16 basic questions, as follows:

Defense Formation

1. Do the patient's defense mechanisms successfully mediate between the id and superego demands?
2. Are the patient's defenses mainly primitive or mature?

Regulation and control of drives, affects and impulses

1. Can the patient tolerate delay, tension, and frustration?
2. Can the patient sublimate- that is, channel drives into acceptable substitute behaviors?

Relationship to others

1. Can the patient experience others as whole persons with both good and bad traits?
2. Can the patient form emotionally rich and enduring relationship?

Self- Representation/ Self-Esteem

1. Does the patient have a reasonable degree fo self-confidence and self-esteem?
2. Does the patient possess a balanced, holistic sense of self, incorporating both good and bad traits?

Synthetic-Intergrative Functioning

1. Can the patient reconcile inconsistent or contradictory aspects of self and others, and act appropriately in the face of such contradictions?
2. Can the patient integrate knowing gained form new experiences in a constructive way?

Stimulus Regulation

1. Can the patient screen out extraneous or excessive stimuli in order to pursue constructive goals (e.g, reading, job task, etc)?
2. Can the patient provide sufficient stimulation to maintain intra-psychic and interpersonal stability?

Adaptive regression in the service of the ego

1. Can the patient relax enough to enjoy sex, music, hobbles, and so forth?
2. Is the patient open to new experiences in these areas?

Reality testing and sense of reality

1. Can the patient maintain adequate boundaries between self and others?
2. Can the patient reason objectively to distinguish wish or imagination form external reality?

Chapter 2: Biopsychosocial Perspective
Examination Review

Match the following parts of their functions described in the right hand column.

1.	Frontal Lobe	A.	Associated with multiple feelings and behaviors
2.	Parietal Lobe	B.	The ability to judge spatial relationships such s distance and to see in three dimensions
3.	Temporal Lobe	C.	Voluntary body movement; expression of feeling
4.	Occipital Lobe	D.	Integrates all sensory input except smell
5.	Thalamus	E.	Concerned with visual reception
6.	Hypothalamus	F.	Hearing, short-term memory, and sense of smell
7.	Limbic System	G.	Regulates appetite and temperature

Select the answer that is most appropriate for each of the following questions:

8. At a synapse, the determination of further impulse transmission is accomplished by means of

   A. Potassium ions
   B. Interneurons
   C. Neurotransmitters
   D. The myelin sheath

9. A decrease in which of the following neurotransmitters has been implicated in depression?

   A. GABA, acetylcholine, and aspartate
   B. Norepinephrine, serotonin, and dopamine
   C. Somatostatin, substance P, and glycine
   D. Glutamate, histamine, and opioid peptides

10. The delusional belief that one is loved by another, usually a person higher social status who is, at most, a casual acquaintance of the person.

    A. Erotomania
    B. Socioeconomic factors
    C. Cultural sensitivity
    D. Depersonalization

Chapter 2: Biopsychosocial Perspective
Examination Answers

1. C
2. E
3. F
4. B
5. D
6. G
7. A
8. C
9. B
10. A

Chapter 3

Specific Interviewing Situations

Information about patient symptoms is necessary before a diagnosis is made, but it is not sufficient for effective treatment. A broader aim of the interview is to understand the patient more fully and to develop hypotheses about personality, life experiences, assets and liabilities, and reactions to illness. Starting an interview, with an open-ended question facilities the diagnostic process, because the answer that the patient chooses to give in response to the open-ended question has a special significance.

The Veteran Patient

The Veterans Administration (VA) of the United States has been forced to come to grips with the problem of an explosive increase in health care costs for veterans. Since the Veterans Administration serves veteran who have had wartime service. Its population of beneficiaries is not a smooth bell-shaped curve, but rather centers around certain wartime periods. These activities increased and in the 1930s the Veterans Administration was established. The Veterans Administration originated in the closing decades of the 19th century when, after a presidential edict issued by President Lincoln, six national homes for disabled volunteers soldiers were established to care for the veterans of the Civil and Indian wars who could no longer defray the cost of their medical care and whose injuries prevented them from earing a livelihood.

Following World War II the VA saw a great influx of new patients as it entered a period of rapid physical expansion. For example, the veterans of World War II, who number approximately 12 million, are in 1985, 65 years of age and older. The total number will eventually decline, but the umber and percentage of aging will continue t increase (Durham +Hopkins 1983; Mather+ Lawson 1984). In the decades following the close of World War II, the schools of medicine so this country and various VA hospitals became closely affiliated with medical schools. The VA's interest in continuous care for older veterans is relatively new. In 1964 Public Law 88-450 was passed, which mandated that the VA begin to address the problem of the aging veterans (Program + Analysis service, 1964).

The Anxious Patient

With patients who have high anxiety, one must continue to use a more directive interview. Sitting silently waiting for a frightened patient to respond only adds to the tension; therefore, the first interview with these patient may well be a series of direct questions may well be a series of direct questions with the patient replying with short answers. If a patient is fidgety, restless, or easily startled, seems nervous, or has a tremor in his or her voice, the patient may be anxious. Proceeding with the interview may be difficult until the anxiety is discussed. (see section three). In any instance of patient anxiety, the prescription is the same: the physician's responsibility is the elicit the source of the patient's concern, understand it, and take appropriate measures to diminish it. Patients get angry for numerous reasons, but they can be conveniently grouped into two categories. First, a patient may be angry because of something said or not done. The second possibility is that the patient is the source of the anger and would be angry whether or not the physician did something provocative.

Some patients' anxiety in the interview is great enough to be incapacitating. These patients need special help to feel more comfortable and enter into the interaction of the interview.

Patients are often frightened by their illnesses or by the proposed treatments and may use anger as a means of both discharging and denying such anxiety. Certain patients may never achieve this degree of comfort, but most can and there are ways of helping to reduce the anxiety. Since anxiety begets anxiety, the interview must be a t least minimally comfortable while interviewing. This doesn't mean free of anxiety. If students are aware of their anxiety, they can control it better and realize that it need not interfere too much with the relationship with the patient. Before discussing some ways of relieving a patient's anxiety, we should say something about anxiety itself.

Anxiety and fear have identical manifestations. Fear is defined as a response to a real danger. Anxiety, although having the same physiologic response, is defined as the fear of an imagined threat. Anxiety can diffuse or specific. With diffuse anxiety, we feel anxious but do not know why. There is a reason or reasons for the fear, but for the moment we are unaware of those reasons. Specific anxiety relates to something a person is afraid of, but knows there is no reason to be afraid.

An important anxiety symptom of the individual/ psychological domain is anger/fear. More specifically, the problem of identifying, feeling, and expressing these two powerful emotions occurs. Anger has the most face validity when discussing violence, particularly in the public's mind; that is, it seems logical to think of anger when one thinks of violence. But fear is a bit different. How could this emotion relate to violence? Well, think for a minute what happens when the patient is angry or scared. Both emotional states invoke deep feeling, and the feeling is also accompanied by a high state of autonomic arousal, especially if there is an imminent, life threatening event: pulse rate quickens, blood pressure increases, skin flushes, and muscles tense. The ideal way to handle an angry patient is to make a concerted effort to understand the nature of the anger. If a patient is covertly angry, the appropriate response of the physician is to use the technique of confrontation, just as a physician would do in the case of the patient's acknowledged anxiety or depression.

The Hostile Patient

In an occasional patient, hostility may get out of control. These patients are most often encountered in the emergency room or on a psychiatry inpatient service. They may have been brought in against their will or they may have come voluntarily because of their own fear of their violent impulses. We are most concerned here with hostility that threatens a constructive doctor-patient interaction, not the kind that results in physical violence. Possible diagnosis is frequently paranoid schizophrenia, bipolar mania, or an organic mental disorder.

IF the patient is unresponsive, several other avenues are open. He can sit silently with the patient for a few minutes, making a comment bow and then. But silence must be used carefully and only if the physician is comfortable and the patient appears not too anxious, because silence tends to increase, rather than decrease, anxiety. Nonverbal responses may become especially important. The examiner should watch facial expressions and body movement. These may show whether the patient is comprehending what is being said, and whether he or she is being attentive or even purposely inattentive.

Depression: The Dependent Patient

Depressed Mood is another common response to physical illness, one expressed in terms of hopelessness, guilt, low self-esteem, and fatigue. Interviews with depressed patients can be laboriously slow and unproductive. (See section 2) Commenting on the slow process of the interview gives the patient a chance to discuss his or her difficulty with the interview if he or she wishes. Acknowledging that the patient appears to be on the verge of crying effectively grants the patient permission to cry or not to cry and can open the door to important emotional material.

When they come to see the doctor, all patients will show some signs of what we could call dependent behavior. Looking for clues as to what to do and asking advice about their problems are signs of normal dependency. Some patients are overly dependent and either shows this directly or they react against their dependency by the opposite behavior: being overly independent.

We do not generally know the mechanisms by which such somatic factors act on the psyche. Thus, pancreatic carcinoma is associated with an unexpectedly high incidence of depression, long before the patient is aware of the diagnosis, and in excess of the depression associated with other abdominal factors.

The depressed patient may be propagandizing himself or herself with ideas such as "I must have everyone's love, or I am worthlessness," "I must do well at everything I attempt, or T am an incompetent jerk," and so on. By helping the patient alter these cognitions we can help him or her get better.

The Suicidal Patient

An interview with a patient who has attempted suicide or is believed to be suicidal is apt to be strained and unproductive if the suicidal attempts or thoughts are not acknowledged early in the interview. Some interviewers are fearful about bringing up the subject of suicide, as if mentioning suicide might increase its likelihood. On the contrary, most patients are willing to discuss their suicidal thoughts and may even be relieved to be asked about them. (see chapter 30).

For a patient who has not attempted suicide, but in whom suicidal thoughts are suspected, begin exploration by asking about depression: "Have you been feeling depressed lately?" The depression can be explored along with sleep patterns and other vegetative signs of depression, possible precipitating circumstances, and past episodes. It is simple, somewhere in the course of the exploration, to say, "Have you felt so depressed that you have considered ending it all?."

IF there have been actual plans for suicide, assess their let hality and the patient's knowledge of their lethality. A person who has brought a gun and bullets and picked a time for suicide is in great danger. If he or she has made a will and given away possessions, the danger is even greater.

It is important to interview the suicidal patient's family and significant others to learn about possible precipitating events, possible supportive individuals in their environment, and to assess recent changes in behavior.

If the physician is concerned about the magnitude of depressive affect, the patient's suicide potential should be assessed. Usually, it is best to begin indirectly, asking if the patient feels hopeless, derives any meaning from life, or has ever wished he or she were dead. If the patient senses that the physician is timid about asking of suicidal intent, he or she is more likely to give an evasive answer.

Eventually, if the answers convince the physician that the patient is contemplating suicide, direct inquiry must be made: "Have you thought about taking your life?" "Have you thought about how you would do it?" "Have you t thought about how other people would feel?." The more lethal the method contemplated, the easier the patient's access to the method, and the more vivid his or her fantasies about how others would be affected, the greater the risk.

Amytal Interview

The Amytal interview has been used in the diagnosis of "hysterical" symptoms and, in theory, could be useful in the diagnosis of somatization disorder. However, the available literature does not make mention of this.

The Amytal Interview may help the conversion disorder patient to re-experience the precipitation trauma, and permits the therapist to suggest that the conversion symptoms will soon go away (Kaplan and Sadock, 1988). By far the best described somatic treatment is the Amytal interview. Ford (1989) used a 5% solution of Amytal Sodium, infused intravenously at a rate of no faster than 1 cc per minute (50 mg per minute).

The interview begins when the patient's speech becomes slightly slurred or when sustained rapid lateral nystagmus is present.

The therapist begins with emotionally neutral topics and then progresses to areas of suspected trauma and repression. If the patient becomes severly agitated in the process of abreacting, it may be necessarily to terminate the interview. At the conclusion of the procedure, the therapist may suggest that "all will be remembered" or may administer enough additional Amytal to produced amnesia for the interview itself (Ford 1989). Contrainications to the Amytal interview include a history of porphyria, barbiturate allergy, concurrent intoxication, or severe hepatic, renal, or cardiac disease. Ford (1989) has review the complex medicolegal issues arising from material obtained during the Amytal interview; the clinicans is well advised to obtain legal counsel in cases involving criminal charges.

VIGNETTE

A thirty old male veteran was discharged with the diagnosis of antisocial personality disorder. Since early childhood, he lied, cheated at games, shoplifted, and stole money from his mother's purse. He even burglarized a church offering bowl. Despite an above-average IQ, his school performance was poor, and he was frequently in detention for breaking rules. Because of continued law-breaking, he was sent to a juvenile reformatory at age 16 for 2 years. During this time, he chain smoked and admitted to regular alcohol abuse. In addition, he had poorly cooperated with attempts at both individual and group therapy. There he admitted to having used marijuana, amphetamines, tranquilizers, cocaine, and heroin in the past.

He had never held a full-time job in his life; the longest job he had held lasted 60 days. He was currently doing bodywork on cars in his garage, but had not dome any work for several months. He reported that he was unable to provide support to his common-law-wife and four children. On active duty his behavior was still characterized by a pervasive pattern of violating social norms (e.g. criminal behavior), impulsivity, excessive emotionality, grandiosity, acting out (e.g. tantrums, self-abusive behavior, angry outbursts), or violating the rights of others.

Deborah Y. Liggan, MD

Discussion. Antisocial personality disorder was first recognized in the early nineteenth century. In DSM-1, the disorder was called sociopathic personality and was renamed antisocial personality disorder in DSM-III in 1980 (Reid and Burke, 1989). Personality disorders, according to DSM-IV-TR (American Psychiatric Association 2000), are patterns of inflexible and maladaptive personality traits that cause subjective distress, significant impairment in social or occupational functioning, or both.

There is no standard treatment for antisocial personality, and no medication targets the full syndrome. The ventral characteristic of antisocial personality disorder is a long-standing pattern of socially irresponsible behaviors that reflects a disregard for the rights of others. Many persons with this disorder engage in repetitive unlawful acts. The more prevailing personality characteristics include a lack of interest in or concern for the feelings of others, deceitfulness, and most notably, a lack of remorse over the harm they may cause others. These characteristics generally make these individuals fail in roles requiring fidelity (e.g. as a spouse or a parent), honesty (e.g. as an employee), or reliability in any social role. Individuals with antisocial personalities see themselves as victims, using projection as the primary ego defense mechanism. In their own minds, this perception justifies their malicious behavior, lest they be the recipient of unjust persecution and hostility form others. The clinician's task is to help patients understand how their maladaptive personality traits contribute to their ongoing troubles. They are restless and easily bored, often taking chances and seeking thrills, as if they were immune to danger.

Family Interview

Family assessment is relatively new compared with diagnosis of an individual. Family interview are designed to gain an understanding of family dynamics and the families; interaction with society as these relate tot the patient. Family interview and family therapy fit well with all psychiatric diagnosis and therapies. Usually, but not always, family members can help to evaluate a delusional system or to give additional information about the patient's behavior and symptoms at present, prior to, and at the time of onset of the illness.

In interviewing family members, one should always be aware that their perceptions are also colored by emotions and by their involvement with the patient. The basic principles of psychiatric interviewing already discussed also apply to interviewing a family member.

To maintain relationship with the patient, ask his or her permission to talk with a family member or interested other person and tell the patient that no confidential information will be given to that person. For example, one can say, "I would like to talk with your wife, who came with you today. How do you feel about that?." Then go on to say, "I want you to know that I won't tell her an of the things we talked about. They are confidential between us."

Help the person feel at ease and give the person an opportunity to say what s on his or her mind. After helping to reduce tension, one way to begin is to say, "I've seen your husband and he agreed that it would be good for me to talk with you."

Using mental status and psychiatric history for guidance, we can assess the family unit as a whole, make observations of individual members and their relationships, and learn something of important historical events in the family. This model can also be used to develop guidelines for recording the family interview. To paraphrase Harry Stack Sullivan, in gathering information about a family we want to know who is this family and how did they come to be here? (Sullivan, 1954).

Chapter 3: Specific Interview Examination Review

1. Open-ended questions involve:

    A. Are useful early in the interview and when new topics are introduced
    B. Limit the patient's response alternatives prematurely
    C. Involve the greatest level on interviewer control
    D. Are likely to confuse most patients

2. Which of the following statements regarding the interview techniques of facilitation is correct?

    A. The most powerful facilitating technique involves the use of silence
    B. Pointing our inconsistencies in the patient's story is an aspect of effective facilitation
    C. Facilitation is used mainly to elicit information and to guide the interview in the desired direction.
    D. In dealing with an angry patient, the physician should follow the natural tendency to defined himself or herself or retaliate in kind.

3. Which of the following statements regarding the handling of patient emotions is correct?

    A. The technique of confrontation is most useful at the beginning of the interview
    B. If a patient seems overly depressed about his or her illness, it becomes necessary to assess the patient's suicide potential
    C. When a patient is overcome with emotion, distraction or changing the subject is advised
    D. In dealing with an angry patient, the physician should follow the natural tendency to defend himself or herself or retaliate in kind.

4. Why on first contact with a physician, does a patient waits for clues which tell him or her how to respond?

    A. Verbally clues are given by facial expression and body position
    B. Don't start with "I'm just going to ask you some questions."
    C. The terms directive and nondirective refer to the interview's purpose.
    D. A directive approach allows patients to tell what is on their minds.

5. How is a broad sweep of what to look for in a psychiatric history?

    A. Throughout the entire history it is important to understand the patient's feelings
    B. Interviewing patients from different social, cultural, or language groups presents the interview with special challenges
    C. The emotion felt during this sort of encounter may vary: a sense of general discomfort and unease, irritability, frustration, perhaps even anger
    D. History tells all above

6. How is the mental status or AMSIT report when it is a systematic documentation of the patient's thinking, feelings, and behavior at the time of the interview?

    A. Clinical findings into a systematic report written after the interview
    B. No intellectual function
    C. No mood and / or affect
    D. Feel bad about the doctor does not come back.

7. When does a person have a feeling of being watched, discussed, or ridiculed by others?

    A. Delusions of reference
    B. Delusions of grandiosity
    C. Delusions of persecution
    D. Secondary delusion

8. Which of the following statements is correct?

    A. Flight of ideas is suggestive of acute dysphoria
    B. Clang associations are always pathological
    C. The confabulating patient has poverty of speech
    D. Echolalia is a condition in which the patient involuntarily responds to all questions in the same way

9. Which of the following statements is correct?

    A. Obsessions involve thoughts, whereas compulsions involve actions
    B. A clear sensorium suggests that the patient is not well oriented
    C. Remote memory is usually the first to fade with age
    D. Probably the best brief indicator of intelligence is a facility with math

10. What is important to determine whether the person's spirits are worse in the morning and improved during the day or vice versa?

    A. Inappropriate affect
    B. Diurnal variation
    C. Change in libido
    D. Change in appetite

Chapter 3: Specific Interview Examination   **Answers**

1. A
2. C
3. B
4. B
5. D
6. A
7. A
8. B
9. A
10. B

Reference Section-1

Adebimpe VR. Overview: White Norms and Psychiatric Diagnosis of Black Patients. American Journal of Psychiatry, 138; 279-285, 1981.

Akiskal HS, Webb WL. Psychiatric Diagnosis: Exploration of Biological Predictors. New York, Spectrum Publications, 1978.

Akiskal HS. Mental Status Examination: The Art and Science of the Clinical Interview. In Diagnostic Interviewing, ed. M. Hersen and S. Turner. 2nd Ed New York: Plenum Press, 1994.

Aldrich CK. The Medical Interview. New York. Subtitled, "A Manual for First or Second Year Medical Students, 1993.

American Psychiatric Association. Practice Guidelines for the Treatment of Psychiatric Disorders, Compendium. 2006.

Benson H. The Relaxation Response. William Morrow, 1975.

Blanchard EB and Young LD. Clinical Applications of Biofeedback Training. Archives General Psychiatry 30 (5): 573- 589, 1974.

Bloch S and Chondoff P. Psychiatric Ethics. New York: Oxford University Press, 1991.

Billings JA and Stoeckle JD. The Clinical Encounter: A Guide to the Medical Interview and Case Presentation, Chicago, 1989.

Birren JE and Sloane RB. Handbook of Mental Health and Aging. Englewood Cliffs, NJ: Prentice Hall, 1976.

Briggs GW. Some pitfalls of the Authoritarian Doctor- Patient Relationships in primary care medicine. Journal of Mississippi State Medical Associates, 1990.

Brown SL. Family Interviewing as a basis for clinical management. In: The Family: Evaluation and Treatment, Hofling CK, Lewis JM (Eds). New York: Brunner/ Mazel, 1980.

Butler RN. Geriatrics and Internal Medicine. Annals of Internal Medicine, 91: 903-908, 1979.

Butler RN and Lewis MI. Aging and Mental Health: Positive Psychosocial and Biomedical Approaches. St. Louis: Mosby, 1982.

Cooper AM and Ronnington E. Narcissistic Personality Disorder, in American Psychiatric Press review of Psychiatry, Vol 11. Washington DC, American Psychiatric Press, pp 80-97, 1992.

Cummings JL. Clinical Neuropsychiatry. Orlando, FL. Grune +Stratton, 1985.

Deutsch F and Murphy NF. The Clinical Interview. New York: International Universities Press, 1955.

Durham M and Hopkins D. toward a System of Comprehensive Care for the Aging Veteran. American Lake, WA: VA Medical Center, Geriatric Research Education and Clinical Center, 1983.

Elmore AM and Tursky B. The biofeedback hypothesis: An idea in search of a theory and method. Expanding dimensions of consciousness. New York: Springer, 1978.

Enelow AJ and Swisher SN. Interviewing and Patient Care, 3rd ed. New York, Oxford University, 1986.

Engel G. The Biopsychosocial Model. American Journal of Psychiatry. 137: 535-543, 1980.

Engel G. The need for a new medical model: a challenge for biomedicine. Science 196: 129-133, 1977.

Entralgo PL. Doctor and Patient. New York: Mc Graw-Hill, 1969.

Exon-Smith AN and Overstall PW. Geriatrics. Baltimore, MD: University Park Press, 1979.

Finesinger JE. Psychiatric Interviewing. American Journal of Psychiatry, 1948

Follette WC and Houts AC. Models of Scientific Progress and the role of theory and taxonomy development: a case study of the DSM. Journal Consulting Clinical of Psychology, 64. 1996.

Ford CV. Somatization, in Handbook of Psychiatric Diagnosis. PSG Publishing, 1987.

Foulks EF. The Concept of Culture in Psychiatric Residence Education. American Journal of Psychiatry. 137: 811-816, 1980.

Fuller GD. Biofeedback: Methods and Procedures in Clinical Practice. Biofeedback Press. 1977.

Gaarder KR and Montgomery S. Clinical biofeedback: A procedural manual for behavioral medicine. Baltimore: Williams and Wilkins. 1981.

Garrity T. Medical Compliance and the Doctor-Patient Relationship: A Review. Social Science Medicine, 1981.

Goodwin DW, Guze SB. Psychiatric Diagnosis. New York, Oxford University Press, 1984.

Gunderson JG. The borderline patient's intolerance of aloneness: Insecure attachment and therapist availability. American Journal of Psychiatry; 153.1996.

Gyunther MD. Is the MMPI an appropriate assessment device for Blacks? Journal of Black Psychology. 7: 67-75, 1981.

Halleck SL. Evaluation of the Psychiatric Patient: A Primer. New York, Plenum; 1991.

Herpertz S, Gretzer EM, Steinmeyer V, et al. Affective Instability and Impulsivity in Personality Disorder. Journal of Affective Disorder. 44: 31-37, 1997.

Hersen M and Turner SM. Diagnostic Interviewing 3rd Ed. Kluwer Academic Publishers, 2003.

Holland AL. Working with the aging aphasic patient: Some clinical implications. Lexington, MA: DC. Heath, 1980.

Hollingshead AB, Redlich FC. Social Class and Mental Illness. New York, Wiley, 1958.

Howells JG. Principles of Family Interviewing. New York: Brunner/ Mazel, 1975.

Jervis GA. Biomedical Types of Mental Deficiency, in American Handbook of Psychiatry, 2nd Ed. Vol. 4, New York, Basic Books. 1975.

Katz J. The Silent World of doctor and patient. New York: Free Press, 1984.

Kaplan HI and Sadock BJ. Synopsis of Psychiatry, 5th Ed. Baltimore MD, Williams & Wilkins, 1988.

Kaye AL and Shea MT. Personality Disorders, Personality Traits, and Defense Mechanism Measures. Handbook of Psychiatric Measures. pp 713-750.Washington, DC: American Psychiatric Press, 2000.

Kemperma I, Russ MJ, Shearin E. Self- injurious behavior and mood regulation in borderline patients. Journal of Personality Disorder 11: 146-157, 1997.

Kennie D.C. Good health care for the aged. Journal of the American Medical Association. 249: 770- 773, 1983.

Korsch BM, Negrete V. Doctor- patient communication. Scientific America. 227: 66-74, 1972.

Lamb H.R. Treating the Long-Term Mentally Ill. Jossey- Bass Publishers, 1982.

Lawson WB. Racial and Ethnic Factors in Psychiatric Research. Hospital Community Psychiatry. 37: 50-54, 1986.

Lefley HP. Culture and Chronic Mental Illness. Hospital Community Psychiatry 41, 1990.

Leon RL. Psychiatric Interviewing: A Primer. Elsevier/ North Holland, 1982.

Libow LS. Geriatric medicine and the Nursing Home: A Mechanism for Mutual Excellence. The Gerontolist, 22 (2); 134-141. 1981.

Luborsky L, Singer B, Luborsky L. Comparative Studies of Psychotherapies. Archive of General Psychiatry 32: 995-1008, 1975.

Mackinnon RA. Psychiatric History and Mental Status Examination, in Comprehensive Textbook of Psychiatric, 3rd Ed, pp 906-920, 1980.

Mather J. and Lawson MP. VA System: Health Care /Benefits. Conference on Complex Cube of Long- term care. Washington, DC: American Health Planning Association. 1984.

Meloy JR. Violence Risk and Threat Assessment: A Practical Guide for Mental Health and Criminal Justice Professionals. Specialized Training Services, 2000.

Meissner WW. The concept of therapeutic alliance. Journal American Psychoanalytic Association, 40. 1992.

Meyer A. The Common Sense Psychiatry. Life A (Ed). New York: McGraw-Hill, 1948.

Mukherjee S, Shukla S, Woodle J, et al. Misdiagnosis of Schizophrenia in bipolar patients: a multiethnic comparison. American Journal of Psychiatry 140. 1983.

Ouslander JG. Drug Therapy in the Elderly. Annals of Internal Medicine, 95: 711-722. 1981.

Othmer Ekkehard. The Clinical Interview using DSM IV. Vol 2. The Difficult Patient. Washington, DC: American Psychiatric Press, 1994.

Perry S, Cooper AM, Michels R. The psychodynamic formulation: Its purpose, structure, and clinical application. American Journal of Psychiatry. 144: 543-550. 1987.

Pies RW. Clinical Manual of Psychiatric Diagnosis and Treatment: A Biopsychosocial Approach. American Psychiatric Press, Inc. 1994.

Pinkofsky, H.B. Mnemonics for DSM-IV personality disorders. Psychiatric Services, 48, 1197-1198; 1997.

Pohl R, Lewis R, and Niccolini R. Teaching the Mental Status Examination: Comparison of Three Methods. Journal Medicine of Education. 57, 1982.

Program & Analysis Service. Caring for the older veteran—a shared visions for the future. Washington, DC: Veterans Administration, 1984.

Quill TE, Recognizing and Adjusting to Barriers in the Doctor-Patient Communication. Ann. Intern. Med, 1989.

Redlich F and Mollica RF. Ethical issues in contemporary psychiatry. American Journal of Psychiatry 133, 1976.

Rogers R. Handbook of Diagnostic and Structured Interviewing. The Guilford Press: New York, 2001.

Ross CA, Joshi S, Currie R. Dissociative experiences in the general population: a factor analysis. Hospital Community Psychiatry. 42: 297-301, 1991.

Shapiro D. Tursky B, Schwartz GE. Control of blood pressure in man by operant conditioning. Circulation Research, 26: 127-132.1970.

Smelson D.A. Evaluating the Diagnostic Interview: Obstacles and Future Directions. Journal Clinical of Psychology. 53. 1997.

Sullivan HS. The Psychiatric Interview. New York: Norton, 1954.

Stoyva JM and Budzynski TH. Biofeedback methods in the treatment on anxiety and stress disorders.

In Principles and Practice of Stress Management 2nd Ed. Pp 263-300. New York: Guilford, 1993.

Strub RI and Black FW. The Mental Status Examination in Neurology, 3rd Ed. Philadelphia: Davis, 1993.

Tyrer PJ and Alexander J. Classification of personality disorder. British Journal of Psychiatry, 135: 163-167. 1979.

Tyrer PJ, Fowler- Dixon R, Ferguson B, et al. A plea for the diagnosis of hypochondriacally personality disorder. Journal of Psychosomatic Research, 34: 637-642. 1990.

Tyrer PJ, Seivewright N, and Seivewright H. Long-term outcome of hypochodriacal personality disorder. Journal of Psychosomatic Research, 46: 177-185. 1999.

Waitzkin H. Doctor-Patient communication: Clinical Implications of Social Scientific Research. JAMA 252: 543-550,2441-2446, 1984.

Wallerstein RS. Defense, defense mechanisms, and the structure of the mind. Journal of American Psychoanalyst Association 31 (suppl): 207- 225. 1983.

Weissman MM. The epideology of Personality Disorders: a 1990 update. Journal of Personal Disorder. 7: 44-62. 1993.

Weitzel W, Morgan D, Guyden T, et al. Toward a More Efficient Mental Status Examination. Archives of General Psychiatry 128. 1973.

Weston A. A Rulebook for Arguments. 4th Ed. Hackett Publishing Company Inc., 2009.

Widiger TA. And Frances A. Interviews and Inventories for the Measurement of personality disorders. Clinical Psychology Review, 7: 49-75, 1987.

Williams TF. Rehabilitation in the Aging. New York: Raven Press, 1984.

Winokur G, Clayton PJ. The Medical Basis of Psychiatry. 2nd Ed. W.B. Saunders Company, 1994.

Wright RH, Cummings NA. Destructive Trends in Mental Health: The Well-Intentioned Path to Harm. Taylor & Francis Group, 2005.

Yudofsky SC, Silver JM, Jackson W, et al. The Overt Aggression Scale for the objective rating of verbal and physical aggression. American Journal of Psychiatry. 143: 35-39. 1986.

Zanarnini MC, Frankenburg FR, Chauncey DL, et al. The Diagnostic Interview for Personality Disorders: Interrater and test-retest reliability. Comprehensive Psychiatry, 28: 467-480. 1987.

Section Two

Mood Disorders

> *Smiles are associated with joy, relief, and amusement. But smiles are by no means limited to the expression of positive emotions: People of many different cultures, smile when they are frightened, embarrassed, angry, or miserable.*
>
> *Amy Cunningham*
> *Why Women Smile*

Mood is a pervasive and sustained emotion that may have a major influence on a person's perception of the world. In this text, affect is described as the emotional reaction associated with experiences manifested by mood disorders classified as either depressive or bipolar. Depression tolerates and alteration in mood that is expressed by feelings of sadness, despair, and pessimism. Dysthymic disorders describes mood as sad or "down in the dumps" which is viewed as a milder form of major depression. Then bipolar disorder is characterized by mood swings from profound depression to extreme euphoria (manic), with intervening periods of normalcy. The essential feature of cyclothymic disorder is a chronic mood disturbance of at least two year duration, involving numerous episodes of hypo-mania and depressed mood of insufficient severity or duration to meet the criteria for bipolar I or bipolar II disorder.

Chapter 4

Bipolar Disorder

Some of the greatest people in history were bipolar. I searched the internet for famous bipolar individuals and came up with an incredible list: Christopher Columbus, Virginia Woolf, Abraham Lincoln. Florence Nightingale, Andrew Carnegies, and of course Vincent Van Gogh just to name a few. (Wooton, 2005) Do bipolar patients have specific psychodynamic characteristics? What about their premorbid personality and ego defenses? Karl Abraham (1877-1939), Sigmund Freud (1856-1939), and Franz Alexander (1891-1964) all made important contributions to our psychodynamic concept of manic depressive illness.

Abraham- Comparing normal grief with melancholia- argued that in the latter, unconscious hostility toward a lost object becomes directed at the self.

Expanding on this, Freud suggested that in melancholia the ambivalently regard lost object is incorporated in to the ego Freud explained mania as a fusion of the ego and superego, freeing up the energy previously used in the conflict between these two parts of the psyche. (Arieti, 1974)

Alexander developed an interesting variant on the views of Abraham and Freud. He believed that in the depressed phase of manic depressive illness the individual punishes himself or herself for supposed transgressions. When this self-punishment begins to feel excessive, the individual again feels free to behave uninhibitedly and becomes manic.

Introduction. Let's begin by defining the syndrome of bipolar disorder. Its key characteristic is extreme mood swings, form manic highs to severe depressions. It is called a mood disorder because it profoundly affects a person's experiences of emotion and affects (the way he or she conveys emotions to others). It is called bipolar because the mood swings occur between two poles, high and low, as opposed to unipolar disorder, where mood swings occur along only one pole- the lows (Miklowitz, 2011). In the manic high state, people experience different combinations of the following: elated or euphoric mood (excessive happiness or expansiveness), irritable mood (excessive anger and touchiness), a decreased need for sleep, grandiosity (an inflated sense of themselves and their abilities), increased talkativeness, racing thoughts or jumping form one idea to another, an increase in activity and energy levels, changes in thinking, attention, and perception, and impulsive, reckless behavior. These episodes alternate with intervals in which a person becomes depressed, sad, blue, or down in the dumps, loses interest in things he or she ordinarily enjoys, loses weight and appetite, feels fatigued, has difficulty sleeping, feels guilty and bad about him- or herself, has trouble concentrating or making decisions, and often feels like committing suicide.

Diagnosis. The practices that work most significantly to dispel stigma fall into four specific categories: compassion, advocacy, recognition, and education, which form the acronym **C. A. R. E.** Compassion demonstrates and fosters connection with oneself and others, challenges isolation, and promotes healing. It involves a fully conscious choice and commitment to this way of being. Advocacy is a major activity in reducing stigma. Advocacy may involve the promotion of increased education, the funding of research, the support of legislation, or any a variety of activities that both directly and indirectly reduce stigma. Recognition of mood disorders is needed before we can put a face on mental illness. It is no surprise that movements to combat stigma associated with illnesses such as bipolar disorder were initiated by those who live with the conditions. Education combats stigma and promotes compassion by presenting facts that help to eliminate fear and ignorance.

Bipolar Episodes

Periods of manic or depressive symptoms are called episodes, and they typically last for several weeks but can sometimes only a couple days. According to the Diagnostic and Statistical Manual (DSM) definitions, depressive episodes have to last for at least two weeks, manic episodes last for at least one week, and hypomanic episodes last for at least four days. Some manic or depressive episodes last much longer, and some shorter episodes can be crippling as well. Depressive periods tend to be more common, and last longer, than manic hypomanic episodes. Historically, it was thought that people with bipolar disorder have manic or depressive episodes that come and go. Those episodes were believed to have beginnings, middle, and endings with essentially normal periods in between episodes. If the patient has manic episode but no depressions, there will still be diagnosed as bipolar I disorder.

Manic Episode. Manic patients typically have inflated self-esteem and grandiosity, which may reach delusional proportions. Manic patient may believe that they have special abilities or powers that clearly are outside the normal range for their educational background or intellectual achievement. The may develop plans to write books, record compact discs, lead religious movements, or undertake expansive business ventures. When the grandiosity reaches delusional proportions, patients may report that they are rock stars, famous athletes or politicians, or even religious figures such as the messiah. Manic often begins with a pleasurable sense of heightened energy, creativity, and social ease. People with mania lack insight, deny anything is wrong, and angrily blame others for pointing out a problem. In manic state, some or all of the following symptoms are present for a t least one week, and the person has trouble functioning in a normal way:

- Heightened mood and exaggerated optimism and self-confidence
- Decreased need for sleep, without fatigue
- Grandiose delusions, inflated sense of self-importance
- Excessive irritability, aggressive behavior
- Increased physical and mental activity
- Rapid, pressured speech, flight of ideas form one topic to another, distractability
- Poor judgment, impulsiveness
- Reckless behavior such as spending sprees, rash business decisions, erratic driving, sexual indiscretions

Manic Episodes; DIGFAST
Elevated mood with three of these seven, or irritable mood with four of these seven, for 1 week signify a manic episode:

- Distractability
- Indiscretion (DSM-IV-TR's excessive involvement in pleasurable activities)
- Grandiosity
- Flight of Ideas
- Activity Increase
- Sleep Deficit (decreased need for sleep)
- Talkativeness (pressured speech)

Table 4-1. DSM-5.
Diagnostic Criteria Bipolar I Disorder: Manic Episode

A. A distinct period of abnormally and persistently elevated, expansive, or irritable mood and abnormally and persistently increased goal-directed activity or energy, lasting at least 1 week and present most of the day, nearly every day (or any duration if hospitalization is necessary).

B. During the periods of mood disturbance and increased energy or activity, three (or more) of the following symptoms (four if the mood is only irritable) are present to a significant degrees and represent a noticeable change form usual behavior.

1. Inflated self-esteem or grandiosity
2. Decreased need for sleep for sleep (e.g. feels rested after only 3 hours of sleep)
3. More talkative than usual or pressure to keep talking
4. Flight of ideas or subjective experience that thoughts are racing
5. Distractability (i.e. attention too easily drawn to unimportant or irrelevant external stimuli)
6. Increase in goal-directed activity (either socially, at work or school, or sexually or psychomotor agitation
7. Excessive involvement in activities that have a high potential for painful consequences (e.g. engaging in unrestrained buying sprees, sexual indiscretions, or foolish business investment)

C. The mood disturbance is sufficiently severe to cause marked impairment in social or occupational functioning or to necessitate hospitalization to prevent others, or there are psychotic features.

D. The episode is not attributable to the physiological effects of a substance (e.g. a drug of abuse, a medication, other treatment) or to another medical condition.

Bipolar/ Depression. Common symptoms of the depressive phase of bipolar disorder include: prolonged feelings of sadness, anxiety, or hopelessness, sense of impending doom or disaster, reduced enjoyment and pleasure, loss of energy and motivation, low self-esteem, feelings of worthlessness or guilt, indecisiveness, reduced concentration, slow thinking, significant changes in appetite and /or sleep patterns, social withdrawal, recurrent thoughts of death or suicide.

Depression. Writer Kay Redfield Jamison, who has bipolar disorder and knows the horror of deep depression intimately, describes "the black dog" in *An Unquiet Mind:*

Depression is awful beyond words or sounds or images … It bleeds relationships through suspicion, lack of confidence and self-respect, the inability to enjoy life, to walk or talk or think normally, the exhaustion, the night terrors, the day terrors. Depression gives you the experience of how it must be to be old, to be old and sick, to be dying; to be slow of mind; t be lacking in grace, polish, and coordination; to be ugly; to have no belief in the possibilities of life, the pleasures of sex, the exquisiteness of music, or the ability to make yourself and others laugh.

Depression is flat, hollow and unendurable … tiresome people cannot abide being around you … You are tedious … irritable and paranoid and humorless and lifeless and critical and demanding and no reassurance is ever enough. You're frightened, and you're frightening.

Table 4-2. DSM-5. Diagnostic Criteria for Bipolar I Disorder: Depressive Episode

A. Five (or more) of the following symptoms have been present during the same 2 eel period and represent a change from previous functioning; at least one of the symptoms is either (1) depressed mood or (2) loss of interest or pleasure.

1. Depressed mood most of the day, nearly every day, as indicated by either subjective report (e.g. feels sad, empty or hopeless) or observation made by others (e.g. appears tearful)
2. Markedly diminished interest or pleasure in all, or almost all, activities most of the day, nearly every day
3. Significant weight loss when not dieting or weight gain (e.g. a change of more than 5% of body weight in a month), or decrease or increase in appetite nearly every day.
4. Insomnia or hyper-insomnia nearly every day.
5. Psychomotor agitation or retardation nearly everyday (observable by others; not merely subjective feelings of restlessness or being slowed down).
6. Fatigue or loss of energy nearly every day.

7. Feelings of worthlessness or excessive or inappropriate guilt (which may be delusional) nearly every day (not merely self-reproach or guilt about being sick).
8. Diminished ability to think of concentrate, or indecisiveness, nearly every (either by subjective account or as observed by others).
9. Recurrent thoughts of death (not just fear of dying), recurrent suicidal ideation without a specific plan, or a suicide attempt or specific plan for committing suicide

Personality Disorders. Psychiatric disorders often confuse bipolar disorder with personality disorders which are long-lasting patterns of disturbance I thinking, perceiving, emotional response, interpersonal functioning, and impulse control. The physician can diagnose both simultaneously with mood disorder on Axis I and personality disorder on Axis II. There are several parallels between borderline personality disorder and bipolar disorder, particularly the rapid cycling forms, but there are also discernible difference.

Borderline personality disorder can sometimes present with a manic-like picture. The patient may appear irritable, sometimes giving a history of excessive spending or sexual activity. However, the borderline patient's mood is more labile than that of the manic patient. Grandiose delusions are less common in borderline personality disorder, in which psychotic symptoms tend to be more paranoid in nature. Furthermore, the borderline patient tends to show more inter-morbid impairment than does the bipolar patient. Finally, one's counterference toward the borderline patient is generally more negative than that toward the manic patient. These mood states tend to last for only a few hours or, at most, a few days. **Histrionic** personality disorder can occasionally present with manic-like features. These histrionic patient may be, for example, inappropriately sexual or seductive, or excessively emotional, self-centered, and demanding, thus mimicking some of the features of the manic patient. The histrionic patient does not typically give a history of acutely decreased need for sleep, racing thoughts or self-defeating actions (such as wild spending sprees) that have compromised social or vocational function. Morever, the histrionic patient will not demonstrate the persistently elevated energy level or rapid, pressured speech of the genuinely manic patient. Instead, he or she (more commonly she) will exhibit rapidly shifting and shallow expressions of emotion. Patients with true bipolar I disorder give a history of one or more episodes of mania and usually one or more bouts of major depression. Let's consider the following vignette.

VIGNETTE

A 50 year old male veteran gave a history in the E.R. of mood swings going back to age 25. He described his high periods as times when he feels like a cross between King Kong and Einstein, with markedly pressured speech, flight of ideas, and inappropriate sexualizing with staff. He was irritable at the interview and demanded consideration be given for his special powers (for example, his ability to read people's minds). Three years after being diagnosed, he began a period of rapid cycling that seemed to be provoked by an on –again, relationship with his girlfriend. During the past 6 months his rapid cycling intensified. His psychiatrist gave him a combination of lithium and divalproex (Depakote), which helped even out his cycles, but he still experienced unpleasant ups and downs. During these periods, which typically lasted or 4 weeks, he reported a tremendous surge of energy. He felt he could make love five times a day and he could write two or three symphonies at night. He does not need more than two or three hours of sleep, and then he runs around the house like he was on speed. In fact, the patient ws talented composer who got most of his creative work done during the early, mellower phase of his highs. During this phase, the patient typically became more talkative, experienced racing thoughts, and took on an excessive number of tasks at once.

Discussion. For bipolar I disorder, the patient must have had at least one manic or mixed episode, with elated mood and there other associated symptoms of mania (grandiose thinking, decreased need for sleep, pressured speech, increased activity or energy level, racing thoughts, flight of ideas, distractibility, or impulsive behavior) that lasted a week or more and / or required that the patient receive emergency treatment. If his/her mood was irritable and not elated, four or more associated symptoms are required. DSM-IV-TR requires a t least 1 week of manic symptoms for bipolar I disorder, unless hospitalization or other emergency treatment was necessary, in which case there is no time requirement. There must also be evidence of deterioration in work or family life (for example, major family arguments, loss of job). In most cases, a person with bipolar I disorder will also have had, at some point in life, a minimum 2 week period with five or more symptoms of major depressive illness (depressed mood, loss of interests, weight loss or change in appetite, loss of energy or fatigue, motor agitation or retardation, loss of concentration, feelings of worthlessness, insomnia or hypersomnia, suicidal thoughts or actions) during which there was a deterioration in everyday functioning.

Approximately 50 % of patients with bipolar I disorder manifest a psychosis (the inability to distinguish reality form fantasy or belief). These patient's frequently manifest poor judgment, impulsive behavior, and total lack of insight into their illness. Consequently, they may refuse treatment.

Mood Altering Foods. If your patient eats junk, he or she will have a body that's short on the nutrients it needs to do its daily tasks. Due to diagnosing mental illness, the need is to eat foods that are high in nutrients and nourish his/her brain, maximize its functions, and improve mood episodes. To maintain ideal health, it helps to eat the right combinations of minerals, amino acids, fatty acids, vitamins, fiber, and protein. For patients living with bipolar disorder specific nutrients have been found to help manage moods, while other substance, such as alcohol and caffeine, disturb moods. Sugar, caffeine (found in chocolate, coffee, and some teas, such as green and black teas), alcohol and chocolate have been shown to influence mood. These substances influence brain chemistry in ways that may trigger a bipolar episode. They may also interact negatively with any medications that the patient may be taking.

Certain foods, such as oil rich fish, fruit, vegetables, and whole grains, may help keep moods stable. In addition, there is some evidence that the B vitamins, zinc, and vitamin C also help stabilize moods. (Kaplan et al, 2007). Omega-3 supplements are more effective with depressive symptoms than with mania, because they elevate mood. A healthy diet is particularly important for people with bipolar disorder because obesity is common in those who have this condition, with up to 50 percent being overweight or obese. This is probably partly due to depression, which leads some to have binge-eating problems. In addition, several of the medications used to treat bipolar disorder can cause weight gain.

Biological Implications. The symptoms of mood disorders, as well a biological research findings, support the hypothesis that mood disorders involve pathology of the limbic system, the basal ganglia, and the hypothalamus.

Treatment

We have known for a long time that medication is the first-line treatment for bipolar disorder. We know that people with bipolar disorder remain well longer if they take medication regularly. Mood stabilizers are usually given during the acute phase and continued during the maintenance phase of treatment. To be defined as a mood stabilizer, a medication has to be effective in treating acute manic, mixed, and /or depressive episodes of bipolar disorder without causing a switch to the opposite pole of the illness or rapid cycling. Increasingly, people are being treated with atypical (second-generation) antipsychotics instead of or in addition to mood stabilizers. Given the suffering and impairment caused by bipolar depressions, most clinicians believe they should be kept as an option, especially if the patient has not responded to mood stabilizers. There has been some alarmism about the use of antidepressants for individuals with bipolar depression. One concern is that they cause people to become suicidal. Another is that antidepressants can bring on hypomanic, manic, or mixed states and cause rapid cycling.

Box 4-1. The Objectives of Psychotherapy for Persons with Bipolar Disorder

- To help the patient make sense of current or past episodes of illness
- To discuss long-term planning, given vulnerability to future episodes
- To help acceptance and adaption to a long-term medication regimen
- To identify and develop strategies for coping with stress or mood cycles
- To improve functioning in school or the workplace
- To deal with the social stigma of the disorder
- To deal with comorbid disorders like alcohol abuse or other addictive behaviors
- To improve family or marital/ romantic relationships

Like medications, psychotherapy comes in different sizes, shapes, and dosages. Individual therapy is most often recommended once the patient has started to recover from an episode of bipolar disorder, so it's is considered a maintenance rather than an acute episode treatment. Cognitive-behavioral therapy (CBT), a treatment designed by Aaron Beck, is the most well-established psychotherapy for depression. Published studies of CBT, while also taking medications, are less depressed and have fewer days of depression than those who take medications only (Miklowitz and Scott, 2009). Sometimes bipolar disorder is best treated in a family or couple context. The advantage of therapy with the patient's close relatives is that they can be educated about their disorder and taught coping skills for managing bipolar disorder often have high levels of family or relationship conflict or tension.

Chapter 5: Bipolar I Examination Review

1. Which of the neurotransmitter systems are believed to be important in mood regulation?

    A. Serotonin
    B. Norepinephrine
    C. Dopamine
    D. All of the above

2. What center of the brain controls memory and determines emotional reactions such as elation, excitement, anxiety, agitation, rage and aggression?

    A. Hypothalamus
    B. Amygdala
    C. Cerebellum
    D. Cingulate Gyrus

3. What ability reflects on oneself and recognize one's feelings, having a vocabulary for labeling those feelings, and understanding the relationships between thoughts, feelings, and reactions?

    A. Self-Awareness
    B. Personal Decision making
    C. Insight
    D. Managing Feelings

4. In the spirit of self-help, what key factor aids in achieving the necessary strength and confidence?

    A. Empowerment
    B. A proactive role
    C. Euphoria
    D. Out-of-body sensations

5. Which one of the following individuals is most likely to have a first degree relative with a mood disorder?

    A. A woman with major depressive disorder
    B. A man with major depressive disorder
    C. A woman with bipolar I disorder
    D. A woman with cyclothymia

6. A patient believes that his evil thoughts caused the recent death of his mother. His belief about his mother would best be described as

    A. Thought broadcasting
    B. A mood-congruent delusion
    C. Thought insertion
    D. A melancholic symptoms

7. What is the clinical difference between bipolar I and II disorder?

    A. In bipolar I disorder the patient experiences at least one episode of hypomanic disorder
    B. In bipolar II disorder the patient experiences at least one episode of manic disorder
    C. In bipolar II disorder, a person alternates between major depressive episodes and hypomanias
    D. Bipolar disorder with rapid cycling is determined by two episodes of major depressive disorder in any one year.

8. In what way does completing management of bipolar disorder require working together of emotion and intellect in order to move forward?

    A. Optimism
    B. Hope
    C. Transcendence
    D. Knee-jerk response

9. What is the most important element in putting bipolar "in order" instead of "disorder." If life is a journey and plans are your map then this practice is how to know where you are on the map?

   A. Acceptance
   B. Introspection
   C. Brainstorming
   D. Reflection

10. What are the foods that affect the patient's mood?

    A. Sugar and starch in carbohydrate foods boost a powerful brain chemical called "serotin."
    B. Spicy food makes the patient agitated
    C. Starchy vegetables such as potatoes help with feeling relaxed and calm
    D. All of the above.

Chapter 5: Bipolar Examination Answers

1. D
2. B
3. A
4. A
5. C
6. B
7. C
8. C
9. B
10. D

Chapter 5

Bipolar II Disorder

Diagnostic Features. Bipolar II disorder is characterized by a clinical course of recurring mood episodes consisting of one or more major depressive episodes (criteria A-C under Major Depressive Episode) and at least one hypomanic episode (criteria A-F under Hypomanic Episode). The major depressive episode must last at least 2 weeks, and the hypomanic episode must last at least 4 days to meet the diagnostic criteria. A diagnosis conveys the cluster of symptoms that characterize a disorder. Some people in hypomanic states of bipolar II is characterized by the confidence and energy so that they may be very charismatic, interesting, and uplifting to be with. These individuals rarely perceive such states as pathological, but instead tend to value the increased levels of energy that flow during these episodes. There are many reasons why bipolar disorder can be hard to distinguish from other disorders. First, moods can vary for any number of reasons, which can include hormones, personal stress, sleep problems, diseases of the brain, or ingestion of drugs or alcohol. Second, people with the disorder often have trouble describing their mood states to others and giving accurate histories of their disorders, Third, mental health professional are not always adequately trained to recognize the more subtle forms of the disorder (for example, mixed states, rapid cycling, mild depressions, hypomania). Lastly, mood variability is a key feature of borderline personality disorder.

There is an association between bipolar disorder type II and eating disorders, with a higher rate of binge eating occurring in people with bipolar disorder that in the general community. People with binge-eating problems feel an uncontrollable urge to eat large amounts of food (beyond feeling full). Binge eaters often develop this habit as a way to deal with stress and depression, finding comfort in eating but often feeling sad about their loss of control and resulting weight gain. These feelings cause them to eat more, continuing the vicious cycle.

Bipolar II Disorder: Hypo-manias. In bipolar II disorder, a person alternates between major depressive episodes and hypo-manias. Hypo-manias are milder forms of mania that may not last as long as full manias (the minimum requirement for the diagnosis is 4 days), but the number of symptoms required is the same (that is, three if the mood is elated, four if the mood is irritable). People with hypomania experience the first of the three stages of mania, but they do not go beyond this: they have sleep problems, irritability, increased activity, and an inflated sense of themselves, but not to the dangerous levels of the fully manic person. Generally, hypomanic episodes do not cause bug problems in work, family, or social life, but the patient may still experience some interpersonal difficulties when in this state (for example, more arguments with your spouse or kids). Hypo-manias do not require hospitalization.

Hypo-manic episodes can be quite enjoyable to the person experiencing them. In general, others will be baffled and put off by your energetic, hypersexual, and driven quality when hypomanic. Your family members or friends may also be relieved by what they perceive to be the disappearance of the depressive states that often precede the energized one.

Chapter 5 Bipolar II Disorder (Hypomanic Periods)

Some people in hypomanic states- characterized by euphoria, optimism, and increased confidence and energy- may be very charismatic, interesting, and uplifting to be with. They sometimes exercise leadership, convince others, and make excellent salespeople of both things and ideas. These individuals rarely perceive such states as pathological, but instead tend to value the increased levels of energy, confidence, and creativity that flow during these episodes. Consequently, people in a hypomanic state may view hypomania as a normal pattern of behavior and refuse any treatment that might compromise their energy ad creativity.

A milder form of mania, hypomania has similar but less severe symptoms and impairment. It is characterized by increased energy, increased activity, decreased need for sleep, increased confidence, sexual drive, poor judgment, impulsive behavior, euphoria or irritability, and sometimes grandiosity, but without psychosis. Friends and relatives notice that the behavior is not usual for the individual. Psychosis (e.g. delusions of having special powers) is not present in hypomania, but is present in mania in about 50 percent of cases. In bipolar II disorder, a person alternates between major depressive episodes and hypomania's. In its most severe forms, depression not only involves constriction in thinking and emotions, but may also be reflected in the person's physical demeanor through muscular rigidity, slowness in movement, and diminished fluidity in facial expression.

Table 5-1. DSM-5. Diagnostic Criteria
Bipolar II Disorder: Hypomanic Episode

A. A distinct period of abnormally and persistently elevated, expansive, or irritable mood and abnormally and persistently increased activity or energy, lasting at least 4 consecutive days an present most of the day, nearly every day.

B. During the period of mood disturbance and increased energy and activity, three (or more) of the following symptoms (four if the mood is only irritable) have persisted, represent a noticeable change from usual behavior, and have been present to a significant degree:

   1. Inflated self-esteem or grandiosity
   2. Decreased need for sleep. (e.g. feels rested after only 3 hrs of sleep)

3. More talkative than usual or pressure to keep talking.
4. Flight of ideas or subjective experience that thoughts are racing.
5. Distractibility (i.e. attention too easily drawn to unimportant or irrelevant external stimuli)
6. Increase in goal-directed activity (either socially, at work or school, or sexually) or psychomotor agitation.
7. Excessive involvement in activities that have a high potential for painful consequences (e.g. engaging in unrestrained buying sprees, sexual indiscretions, or foolish business investments).

C. The episode is associated with an unequivocal change in functioning that is uncharacteristic of the individual when not symptomatic.

D. The disturbance in mood and the change in functioning are observable by others.

E. The episodes is not severe enough to cause marked impairment in social or occupational functioning or to necessitate hospitalization. If there are psychotic features, the episode is, by definition, manic.

F. The episodes is not attributable to the physiological effects of a substance (e.g. a drug of abuse, a medication, or other treatment).

Let's consider the following Vignette.

Vignette

A 30 year old married female gave history of mood swings going back to age 25. In the interview she talked and laughed a lot, usually very loudly and often inappropriately. Her thought process was disorganized, with both tangential responses and periods of blocking. She reported depressed mood most of the day or markedly diminished interest or pleasure in all or almost all activities for most of the day, lasting for at least two weeks. Symptoms that make it difficult to function include significant changes in appetite or sleep patterns, loss of energy, or persistent lethargy. The patient's chief complaint was that "I just don't enjoy life … I don't have any interest in doing things, and I have no energy even if I wanted to do them." These symptoms had been present for at least the past two years, but the patient added, "I really can't remember the last time I felt happy." Although she was functioning as a salesperson in an electronics store, the patient felt like she had to drag herself through the day. She had few friends at work and remained socially isolated even from her husband and two children. Friends and relatives notice that her behaviors is euphoria or irritability but without psychosis. At times, she would snap at them for absolutely nothing. She had difficulty making decisions at work and had lost the chance of a promotion recently. This prompted feelings of intense guilt on the patient's part and the belief that "I've never amounted to anything and I never will." Her symptoms were not sever enough to mandate hospitalization, even though there were some interference in her normal level of functioning. However, the patient denied suicidal ideation or intent. There was no history of any serious medical disorder, and the patient denied any alcohol or other substance abuse.

Discussion. The diagnosis of bipolar II disorder is frequently missed due to its subtleties. It is characterized by episodes of hypomania alternating with even longer periods of major depression that can be very severe and threatening. Although these people exhibit symptoms that re commonly recognized as abnormal by either the patients or their families, their symptoms are generally not severe enough to mandate hospitalization, even though there may be some interference in their normal level of functioning. However, these patients do not manifest psychosis and may not even recognize, or report, their symptoms of hypomania, choosing only to remember their depressive episodes.

Chapter 5 Bipolar II: Woman

If the patient is a woman, bipolar disorder presents unique challenges in addition to those covered in earlier chapters. In particular, various stages and events in a woman's reproductive life and affect and are affected by the disorder.

Box 5-1. The Course of Bipolar Disorder in Woman

- Women have longer, more frequent, and more treatment resistant depressions than men.
- Mixed episodes, rapid cycling, and bipolar II disorder are more common I women.
- Women have more manic or hypomanic episodes brought on by anti-depressants.
- Women are more likely to have physical disorders an pain condition than men.
- For women, mood medications are more likely to cause weight gain, insulin resistance, and elevations in blood lipids.
- The disorder itself- not just the treatments for it- can affect woman's functioning during pregnancy and the post-partum period, as well as the regularity of the menstrual cycle.
- Women are more likely to ruminate when depressed, where as men are more likely to become aggressive or irritable.

Typical menstrual abnormalities include absence of a period (amenorrhea), and cycles that are irregular form month to month. Most women report that their mood symptoms- notably their depression and anxiety- get worse prior to and during their periods. But women with bipolar disorder have more extreme menstrually related mood variations.

Treatment

Just as the cause of bipolar disorder is not fully understood, there is no known cure for the illness, but it can be managed with medication, education, and psychotherapy, which is the classic three-pronged method for treating the disease. Other strategies for managing the disease include stress reduction, exercise, good sleep habits, and a diet high in Omega-3 fatty acids.

Medications. Antidepressants are medications that treat depression. Major classes include the following: tricycle antidepressants; selective serotonin reuptake inhibitors; serotonin-norepinephrine reuptake inhibitors; and heterocyclic anti-depressants. The major anti-manic agents include the following: lithium; anti-convulsants, neuroleptics; and electroconvulsive therapy (ECT).

Psychotherapy. Cognitive and behavioral therapy tend to be combined to one degree or another. Cognitive therapy works on thought patterns that are disabling. Behavior therapy works on behavior patterns that cause problems in life. Family therapies include family- focused therapy with focus on educating the family, and others emphasize smoothing out relationship issues. Interpersonal and social rhythms therapy is based on the observation that some people with bipolar disorder often end up living isolated lives and that both their social and their physical routines get disorganized, making the depression or even manic symptoms worse.

Keep in mind what different diagnostic subtypes may mean for your patient's treatment. If the patient has bipolar II instead of bipolar I disorder, the illness may be less severe. But he/she still needs to be careful: hypo-manias, while fun and exciting, can herald the development of a severe depression, or even of rapid cycling, especially if he/she is not protected by mood-stabilizing medications. Ongoing depressions appear to be the major difficulty experienced by people with Bipolar II Disorder.

Chapter 5: Bipolar II Disorder Examination Review

1. Identify the basic types of Insomnia.

    A. Initial Insomnia- trouble falling asleep than is normal
    B. Middle insomnia-occurs with waking up during the night and having trouble getting back to sleep.
    C. Terminal insomnia-waking up an hour or more earlier in the morning than intended and cannot go back to sleep.
    D. All of the above are accurate

2. What symptoms determine the range of severity of mood swings?

    A. Bipolar II disorder is defined as having periods of major depression and periods of hypomania
    B. Dysthymia is an acute but severe depression
    C. Cyclothymia is a severe form of bipolar disorder
    D. All of the above are accurate

3. What vegetative signs characterize mania?

    A. Increased libido
    B. Weight loss and anorexia
    C. Insomnia (expressed as no need to sleep)
    D. All of the above

4. What symptoms present mania with highly distractable, difficulty concentrating; memory if not to distracted, generally intact; abstract thinking generally intact?

    A. Affect
    B. Sensorium
    C. Euphoric mood
    D. Erratic behavior

5. What electrolytes are reported to be abnormal in bipolar illness?

    A. Sodium
    B. Magnesium
    C. Calcium
    D. All of the above

6. Hypomania is characterized by

    A. Decreased energy
    B. Increased need for sleep
    C. Increased confidence
    D. Presence of psychosis

7. What is an association between bipolar disorder type II and eating disorders?

    A. People with binge –eating problems feel uncontrollable urge to eat
    B. Binge eaters often develop a habit as a way to deal with stress
    C. People find comfort in eating but often feel sad about their loss of control and resulting weight gain
    D. All of the above

8. In bipolar II disorder, how is hypo-manias a milder form of mania?

    A. The minimum requirement for the diagnosis is 4 days
    B. The number of symptoms required is three if the mood is elated
    C. The number of symptoms required is four if the mood is irritable
    D. All of the above

9. If the patient is a woman, what symptoms are unique to her bipolar disorder?

   A. Mood mediations are more likely to cause weight gain in men

   B. Women have shorter and less frequent symptoms than men

   C. Women are more likely to ruminate when depressed, whereas men re more likely to become aggressive or irritable

   D. Rapid cycling and bipolar II disorder are more common in men.

10. In the spirit of self-help, what key factor aids in achieving the necessary strength and confidence?

    A. Empowerment
    B. A proactive role
    C. Euphoria
    D. Out-of –body sensations

Chapter 5: Bipolar II Disorder Examination Answers

1. D
2. A
3. D
4. B
5. D
6. C
7. D
8. D
9. C
10. A

Chapter 6

Cyclothymic Disorder

To make symptoms even more complicated, the patient can have a fluctuating form of mood disorder marked by short periods of hypomania alternating with short, mild periods of depression. Does the patient have short periods of feeling active, irritable, and excited? Short periods of feeling mildly depressed? There is a tendency to alternate back and forth between the two? About one in every four people with cyclothymic progress to bipolar I or II disorder (that is, they develop full-blown manic episodes, longer hypomania, or major depressive episodes) over periods of 2 to 4 years (Birmaher et al, 2009; Kochman et al, 2005). When the veteran's diagnosis was changed to bipolar II disorder with cyclothymic disorder; One can be diagnosed with both!

To have cyclothymic disorder, the patient must have alternated between high and low periods for at least 2 consecutive years and never been without mood disorder symptoms for more than 2 months at a time. It is noteworthy that the condition appears to occur more often in women than men, in contrast to full-blown bipolar disorder, which affects both sexes equally. We discussed earlier the notion of a bipolar spectrum and suggested that cyclothymic disorder may represent the lower end of this spectrum- that is, it produces mood swings of a lesser magnitude than those seen in either classical (type I) bipolar disorder or in type II bipolar illness. How is this different from bipolar II disorder? The patient's depressions had been worse and /or required hospitalization, the diagnosis would have been changed to bipolar II disorder with cyclothymic disorder. The term cyclothymia was coined by Kahlbaum in the mid-19th century. Cyclothymia was then described as a chronic mood disturbance of tat least 2 years duration. The patient was never without hypomanic or depressive symptoms for more than 2 months at a time. DSM-IV-TR also gave exclusionary criteria, such as no evidence of a chronic psychotic disorder or organic factors. However, it ws Kraepelin who first recognized cyclothymia as a form of manic-depressive illness, contending that certain temperaments are rudiments of manic-depressive insanity (Kraepelin, 1921) Akiskal and colleagues (1979) apply to four temperamental disturbances.

Table 6-1. Akiskal's Four Temperamental Disturbances

- **Hyperthymic:** chronically cheerful, overly optimistic, exuberant, extraverted, stimulus seeking, overconfident, meddlesome.
- **Cyclothymic:** frequent mood shifts form unexplained tearful to giddiness, eith variable sleeping patterns and changing levels of self-esteem.
- **Dysthymic:** chronically sad, tearful, joyless, lacking in energy
- **Depressive mixed:** simultaneously anxious, speedy, irritable, restless, and sad, with fatigue and insomnia.

Research views cyclothymia as a disturbance of temperament that predisposes people to bipolar disorder (Akiskal et.al., 2006).

This characterized by depressive periods lasting weeks or months and then mild hypomanic periods during which the person experiences increased energy, mental alertness, confidence, and decreased need for sleep that may make considerable success attainable. Periods of depressed and elevated mood may be separated by periods of normal mood lasting as long as several months. Many people with a history of depression and hypomania do not seek treatment for several years. In fact, these individuals may be quite creative and successful in their careers.

Table 6-2. DSM-5: Diagnostic Criteria for Cyclothymic Disorder

A. For at least 2 years (at least 1 year in children and adolescents) there have been numerous periods with hypomanic symptoms that do not meet criteria for a hypomanic episode and numerous periods with depressive symptoms that do not meet criteria for a major depressive episode.

B. During the above 2 year period (1 year in children and adolescents), the hypomanic and depressive periods have been present for at least half the time and the individual has not been without the symptoms for more than 2 months at a time.

C. Criteria for a major depressive, manic, or hypomanic episode have never been met.

D. The symptoms in criterion A are not better explained by schizoaffective disorder, schizophrenia, schizophreniform disorder, delusional disorder, or other specified schizophrenia spectrum and other psychotic disorder.

E. The symptoms are not attributable to the physiological effects of a substance (e.g. a drug of abuse, a medication) or another medical condition (e.g. hyperthyroidism).

F. The symptoms cause clinically significant distress or impairment in social, occupational, or other important areas of functioning.

Cyclothymia often presents a problem in differential diagnosis. Symptoms such as hyperactivity and distractibility that are part of cyclothymic hypomanic periods are easily confused with Attention Deficit/ hyperactivity Disorder (ADHD). The key difference is that when these symptoms are part of cyclothymia, they are more episodic and more characterized by rapid swings in attention and activity level than when they are part of ADHD. Cyclothymic disorder was originally classified as a personality disorder with mood swings that were not clearly manic or depressed. The impulsive, reckless behaviors (e.g. shoplifting, substance abuse, hostility) seen in cyclothymic hypomanic periods can also be mistaken for Antisocial Personality Disorder. Borderline personality disorder is associated with marked shifts in mood that may suggest cyclothymic disorder. If the criteria are met for both disorder and cyclothymic disorder may be diagnosed. Her, we acknowledged that the association of these behaviors with elevated or irritable mood states as central to the differential diagnosis. Again, psychotic symptoms are not present with cyclothymic disorder.

The cyclothymic disorder diagnosis is not made if the pattern of mood swings is better explained by schizoaffective disorder, schizophrenia, schizophreniform disorder, delusional disorders, in which case the mood symptoms are considered associated features of the psychotic disorder.

Vignette

A 30 year old women who, since adolescence, had experienced a pattern of alternating between 3 day periods during the week I which she cried a lot and felt sad and less interested in things, followed by weekends in which she would feel irritable, energetic, and talkative. She gave a 3 year history of real bad mood swings, characterized by occasional wrist cutting or violence directed at others. As she put it, "when I feel down I cut. When I feel high, I punch." In addition, she reports going to bed in a cheerful mood and waking up "down in the dumps." She had never been hospitalized for wither her depressive or hypomanic symptoms, nor had she been suicidal or unable to concentrate. Her boyfriend sometimes complained about her moodiness and rage. Although it was more difficult for her to work when she was depressed, she had never lost a job because of it.

Discussion. We discussed earlier the notion of a bipolar spectrum and suggested that cyclothymic disorder may represent the lower end of this spectrum-that is, it produces mood swings of a lesser magnitude than those seen in either type I or in type II bipolar disorders. It is also of note that cyclothymic patients experience their irritable, angry episodes as ego-dystonic with a sociopathic personality.

The patient in this vignette received a diagnosis of cyclothymia rather than bipolar disorder. Had her depressions been worse and /or required hospitalization, her diagnosis would have been changed to bipolar II disorder with cyclothymic disorder. One can be diagnosed with both. The psychiatrist Hagop Akiskal viewed cyclothymia as a disturbance of temperament that predisposes people to bipolar disorder (Akiskal et al. 2006) In fact, cyclothymia has a lot in common with bipolar I and II disorders in terms of its pattern of inheritance and its presumed biology. Cyclothymia is listed in DSM-IV-TR as a mild form of bipolar disorder. About one in every four people with cyclothymia progress to bipolar I and II disorder (that is, they develop full blown manic episodes, longer hypo-manias, or major depressive episodes) over periods of 2 to 4 years.

Treatment

Many patients with cyclothymia never seek diagnosis or treatment. They may function well, with some interruption during periods of mild to moderate depression alternating with mild hypomania and increased activity. In many instances, the elevated mood swings of cyclothymic disorder do not require psychiatric intervention; indeed, because the patient often experiences these up periods as a relief, engagement in psychotherapy may be minimal. The depressed phases of cyclothymic disorder may benefit from supportive or cognitive behavior therapy. Even more important, long-term treatment with mood-stabilizing medications (notably lithium) decreases the chances that a person with mood disorder will commit suicide. It remains to be seen whether other mood-stabilizing agents, such as carbamazepine, clonidine, or calcium channel blockers, will find a role in treating cyclothymic disorder.

Chapter 6: Cyclothymic Disorder Examination Review

1. What is the precise biochemical relationship between the full-blown mood disorder and their milder alter-egos?

    A. Cyclothymic disorder is a sort of low-grade bipolar disorder

    B. Cyclothymic disorder is viewed as a milder form of major depression

    C. Dysthymic disorder is viewed as a low-grade bipolar disorder

    D. Dysthymic disorder is manifested by both bipolar disorder and major depression

2. The features of cyclothymia must be differentiated from the mood swings seen in what disorder?

    A. Seasonal affective disorder

    B. Dysthymic disorder

    C. Borderline personality Disorder

    D. Cyclothymic Disorder

3. The diagnosis of cyclothymic disorder requires which one of the following criteria?

    A. Repeated episodes of hypomania and depression

    B. A minimum duration of 6 months

    C. At least one prior major depressive episode

    D. At least one prior manic episode

4. The diagnosis of cyclothymic disorder requires which one of the following criteria?

    A. Repeated episodes of hypomania and depression

    B. A minimum duration of 6 months

    C. At least one prior manic episode

    D. Comorbid substance abuse

5. What symptoms do cyclothymic disorder require in accordance with DSM-IV- TR?

    A. Symptoms must be at least 2 years duration
    B. Periods of depressed and elevated mood may be separated by periods of normal mood lasting as long as several months
    C. Psychotic Symptoms are not present
    D. All of the above

6. Which of Akiskal's temperamental disturbances is characterized by frequent mood shifts form unexplained tearful to giddiness?

    A. Hyperthymic
    B. Cyclothymic
    C. Dysthymic
    D. Depressive mixed

7. What type of personality disorder is described by Emil Kraepelin in addition to cyclothymic disorder?

    A. Depressive (gloomy)
    B. Manic (Cheerful and uninhibited)
    C. Irritable (labile and explosive)
    D. All of the above

8. What symptoms result in one in every four people with cyclothymia causes progression to bipolar I or II disorder?

    A. The patient develops presents with longer hypomanias
    B. The patient presents with longer hypomanias
    C. Major depressive episodes over periods of 2 to 4 years
    D. All of the above

9. Which symptoms characterize Akiskal's Four Temperamental Disturbances?

   A. Depressive mixed: chronically cheerful, overly optimistic, over confident
   B. Cyclothymic: frequent mood shifts from unexplained tearfulness to giddiness with variable sleep patterns
   C. Dysthymic: chronically cheerful, extraverted, and stimulus seeking
   D. Hyperthymic: Irritable, restless, with fatigue and insomnia

10. What personality disorder is associated with marked shifts in mood that may suggest cyclothymic disorder?

    A. Antisocial Personality Disorder
    B. Dependent Personality
    C. Borderline Personality Disorder
    D. Narcissistic Personality Disorder

Chapter 6: Cyclothymic Examination Answers

1. A
2. C
3. A
4. A
5. D
6. B
7. D
8. D
9. B
10. C

Chapter 7

Major Depressive Episode

Depression is characterized by an alteration in mind that is expressed by feeling of sadness, despair, and pessimism. There is a loss of interest in usual activities, and somatic symptoms may be evident. Changes in appetite and sleep patterns are common.

There has been remarkable consistency in the descriptions of depression since ancient times. The condition that today we label depression has been described by a number of ancient writers under the classification of "melancholia." The first clinical description of melancholia was made by Hippocrates in the fourth century B.C. He also referred to swings similar to mania and depression.

The cardinal signs and symptoms used today in diagnosing depression are found in the ancient description: disturbed mood (sad, dismayed, futile); self-castigations (the accursed, hatred of the gods); self- debasing behavior (wrapped in sackcloth or dirty rags); wish to die; physical and vegetative symptoms (agitation, loss of appetite and weight, sleeplessness); and delusions of having committed unpardonable sins.

The psychodynamic understanding of depression defined by Sigmund Freud and expanded by Karl Abraham is known as the classical view of depression. That theory involves four key points:

1. Disturbances in the infant –mother relationship during the oral phase (the first 0 to 18 months of life) predispose to subsequent vulnerability to depression
2. Depression can be linked to real or imagined object loss
3. Introjection of the departed objects is a defense mechanism invoked to deal with the distress connected with the object's loss
4. Because the lost object is regarded with a mixture of love and hate, feelings of anger are directed in ward at the self.

Melanie Klein understood depression as involving the expression of aggression toward loved ones. And Aaron Beck postulated a cognitive triad of depression that consists of

1. Views about the self-a negative self-precept
2. About the environment- a tendency to experience the world as hostile and demanding
3. About the future- the expectation of suffering and failure

Depression Symptoms
Daily Warning Signs Chart

Warning Signs	Mon	Tues	Wed	Thur	Fri	Sat	Sun
Overeating							
Lack of Appetite							
Lethargy							
Difficulty Exercising							
Fatigue							
Unwillingness to ask for things							
Low Self- Esteem							
Low Self-Confidence							
Procrastination							
Avoiding Crowds							
Irritability							
Negative Attitude							

Insecurity						
Difficulty getting up						
Insomnia						
Poor Judgment						
Obsessive Thoughts						
Repeating Things						
Inability to Concentrate						
Destructive Risk Taking						
Suicide Thoughts						
Paranoia						
Inability to Feel Pleasure						

Hamilton and White(1959) performed a factor analysis on data obtained from severely depressed patients who had been evaluated with the use of Hamilton's rating scale (1960). The first of the four factors obtained included such clinical features as depressed mood, guilt, retardation, loss of insight, suicidal attempt, and loss of interest.

Symptoms of Depression

Symptomatology of depression can be viewed on a continuum according to severity of the illness. Mild depressive episodes occur when grief process is triggered in response to the loss of a valued object. This can occur with the loss of a loved one, pet, friend, home, or significant other. As one is able to work through the stages of grief the loss is accepted, symptoms subside, and activities of daily living are resumed, usually within a few weeks. If this does not occur, grief is prolonged or exaggerated, and symptoms intensify.

Major depressive disorder is an example of severe depression. Symptoms at the severe level of depression include:

- **Affective:** Feelings of total despair, hopelessness, and worthlessness; flat (unchanging) affect, appearing devoid of emotional tone; prevalent feelings of nothingness and emptiness; apathy; loneliness; sadness; inability to feel pleasure

- **Behavioral:** Psychomotor retardation so severe that physical movement may literally come to a stand still, or psychomotor behavior manifested by rapid, agitated, purposeless movements; slumped posture; siting in a curled-up position; walking slowly and rigidly; virtually nonexistent communication (when verbalizations do occur, they may reflect delusional thinking); no personal hygiene and grooming; social isolation is common, with virtually no inclination toward interaction with others.
- **Cognitive:** Prevalent delusional thinking, with delusions of persecution and somatic delusions being most common; confusion, indecisiveness, and an in ability to concentrate; hallucinations reflecting misinterpretation of the environment; excessive self-deprecation, self-blame, and thoughts of suicide.
- **Physiological:** A general slowdown of the entire body, reflected in sluggish digestion, constipation, and urinary retention; amenorrhea; impotence; diminished libido; anorexia; weight loss; difficulty falling asleep and awakening very early in the morning and somewhat better as the day progresses. This may reflect the diurnal variation in the level of neurotransmitters that affect mood and activity.

Major Depression: **S-I-G-E-C-A-P-S**

Four out these eight, with depressed mood or anhedonia, for a t least 2 weeks signify major depression:
S--Sleep Disorder (either increased or decreased sleep)
I--Interest deficit (anhedonia)
G--Guilt (worthlessness, hopelessness, regret, regret)
E--Energy Deficit
C--Concentration Deficit
A--Appetite disorder (either decreased or increased appetite)
P--Psychomotor retardation or agitation
S—Suicidality

This mnemonic, devised by Dr. Cary Gross of the Department of Psychiatry, refers to what might be written on a prescription sheet for a depressed, anergic patient. Negative symptoms of depression refer to symptoms that reflect a loss or diminished capacity in functions ordinarily present in individuals such as social with draw, difficulty experiencing pleasure (and anhedonia), low motivation, blunted affect, and problems with attention and concentration. Positive symptoms reflect the presence of perceptions, thoughts, or behaviors I the patient that are not usually present such as hallucinations (false perceptions, such as hearing voices), delusions (false beliefs, such as paranoid delusions), bizarre behavior, or speech that is odd or difficult to follow.

There are several reasons why the negative symptoms of depression are a greater problem for relatives than the positive symptoms. First, negative symptoms tend to be more stable over time than positive symptoms. And positive symptoms usually occur during symptoms exacerbation and then subside or go into remission following pharmacological intervention. In contrast, negative symptoms are more likely to be present during residual phases of the disorder and improve less form pharmacological treatments. Second, positive symptoms are more readily recognized as manifestations of depression, because of its conspicuous presence and hits are assumed by relatives not to be under the patience control. Negative symptoms on the other hand are frequently misinterpreted by relatives as laziness or a sign of character weakness rather than as symptoms of depression and are a common source of criticism from relatives. Third, by their very nature negative symptoms tend to reflect deficits in social functioning that are more likely to impinge on the social lives of relatives than positive symptoms which are more personal and experiential. This, the severity of the patience negative symptoms and the associated problems in social functioning ot the burden of depression on other family members.

The body language of depression includes sitting slumped over, arms folded, mouth turned down, and eyes closed or down cast.

In addition, vegetative symptoms include disturbances in three major areas: sleep, appetite, and sexual function.

Sleep Disturbance. Change in sleep pattern is extremely common in all forms of mood disturbance. The insomnia of depression tis typically described as early morning awakening (i.e. waking earlier than usual and being unable to fall back to sleep). Sleep disturbance is common in depression and this may not be simply the effect of the depression itself. The principal EEG abnormalities noted in major depression include shortened REM latency (i.e. Time between sleep onset and first REM period), reduced delta sleep, and increased total REM and percentage of REM sleep during the early REM periods of the night (Gillin et al. 1979). A phase advance of REM sleep could explain the decreased REM latency; in effect, depressed patients are getting their first REM period too soon. Such phase changes and de-synchronization of other important biorhythms (such as temperature and cortisol secretion) may actually be causal in depression and mania (Wehr et al. 1987). Interestingly, the decreased REM latency and higher REM density found in depressed patients are often reversed by tricyclic antidepressants.

<u>Loss of Libido.</u> Some loss of interest in sex, whether of an auto-erotic or heterosexual nature correlated most highly with loss of appetite, loss of interest in other people, and depressed mood.

<u>Loss of Appetite.</u> For many patients, loss of appetite is often the first sign of an incipient depression and return of appetite may be may be the first sign that it is beginning to lift.

Table 7-1. DSM-5: Criteria for Major Depressive Episode

A. Five (or more) of the following symptoms have been present during the same 2 week period and represent a change from previous change functioning; at least one of the symptoms is either (1) depressed mood or (2) loss of interest of pleasure. NOTE: Do not include symptoms that are clearly due to a general medical condition, or mood incongruent delusions or hallucinations.

(1) Depressed mood most of the day, nearly every day, as indicated by either subjective report (e.g. feels sad or empty) or observation made by others (e.g. appears tearful).

(2) Markedly diminished interest or pleasure in all, or almost all, activities most of the day, nearly every day.

(3) Significant weight loss when not dieting or weight gain (e.g. a change of more than 5% of body weight in a month), or decrease or increase in appetite nearly every day.

(4) Insomnia or hypersomnia nearly every day

(5) Psychomotor agitation or retardation nearly every day

(6) Fatigue or loss of energy nearly every day

(7) Feelings of worthlessness or excessive or inappropriate guilt (which may be delusional nearly every day (not merely self- reproach or guilt about being sick).

(8) Diminished ability to think or concentrate, or indecisiveness, nearly every day

(9) Recurrent thoughts of death (not just fear of dying), recurrent suicidal ideation without a specific plan, or a suicide attempt or a specific plan for committing suicide

B. The symptoms do not meet criteria for a mixed Episode

C. The symptoms cause clinically significant distress or impairment in social, occupational, or other important areas of functioning.

D. The symptoms are not due to the direct physiological effects of a substance (e.g. a drug of abuse, a medication) or a general medical condition (e.g. hyperthyroidism).

E. The symptoms are not better accounted for by bereavement, i.e. after the loss of a loved one, the symptoms persist for longer than 2 months or are characterized by marked functional impairment, morbid preoccupation with worthlessness, suicidal ideation, psychotic symptoms, or psychomotor retardation.

Table 7-2. Medical Conditions associated with depression

Drugs and toxins: reserprine, alpha-methylopa, propranolol, cimetidine
Infectious Disease: mononucleosis, influenza, viral pneumona
Neoplasm: pancreatic bronchogenic carcinoma, brain tumor, lymphoma
Cardiovascular: hypoxia, mitral valve prolapse
Nutritional: pellagra, thiamine deficiency, B12/ folate deficiency
Collagen- vascular: systemic lupus erythematosus rheumatoid arthritis, giant cell arteritis
CNS Disease: Parkinson's disease, Huntington's disease, chronic subdural hematoma, temporal lobe epilepsy, stroke
Miscellaneous: Wilson's disease, psoriasis, amyloidosis

Multiple meanings of depression

Depression is an interesting word that has multiple meanings. Let's take a look at some of the ways it's used in everyday language:

- Sadness: A state of unhappiness and hopelessness
- Psychiatric disorder: A disorder characterized by symptoms such as feelings of hopelessness and dejection, poor concentration, lack of energy =, disturbed sleep or appetite, self-critical thinking, and sometimes suicidal tendencies
- Economic slump: A period in which an economy is greatly affected by unemployment, low output, inflation, and widespread poverty
- Reduced activity: A lowering of activity, quality, vitality, or force
- Hollow: A geographical formation that's lower than the surface area surrounding it
- Low pressure area: An area of low barometric pressure that often brings rain

Biological Theories. How does stress trigger depression? Researchers have found that upsetting situations arouse a part of the brain called the amygdala, a small, almond shaped region that recognizes and regulates emotions, especially fear and anger, and another region at the very base of the brain called the hypothalamus. If these brain regions overreact to stress, perhaps because of a genetic vulnerability, they may produce a chemical chain reaction that leads to depression.

Researchers believe that decreased amounts of serotonin and other neurotransmitters are involved in depression, causing the sleep problems, irritability, anxiety, fatigue, and despondent mood that characterize the illness. In addition, decreased serotonin activity may be linked to suicidal behavior, according to autopsies of suicide victims. And according to the biochemical theory of depression, the catecholamine hypothesis is that in depression the supply of active norepinephrine is depleted.

Areas of the brain affected by depression and the symptoms that they mediate include the following:

- **Hippocampus:** Memory impairments, feelings of worthlessness, hopelessness, and guilt
- **Amygdala:** Anhedonia, anxiety, reduced motivation
- **Hypothalamus:** Increased or decreased sleep and appetite: decreased anergy and libido
- **Other limbic structures**: Emotional alterations
- **Frontal Cortex**: Depressed mood; problems concentrating
- **Cerebellum**: Psychomotor retardation/Agitation

Let's look at a clinical vignette that draws together some of the main psychosocial factors in depression.

Vignette

A thirty year old female nurse has struggled with depression since early adolescence. She was over- weight even as a child and was often teased by kids at school. She felt ashamed of the way she looked and pushed away boys who expressed an interest in her.

She felt that other students talked about her behind her back and made fun of her weight. In college, she tended to steer away form social settings and continued to gain weight.

Her efforts to create a sense of comfort and pleasure centered on cooking and eating, and she tipped the scales at over two hundred pounds by the time she was thirty years old. She met a man in a cooking class, and they dated for six months and eventually had intimate relations. She was sure he had been turned off by how she looked naked, and she vowed to never be hurt by a man again. She continued to gain weight, physical activity became increasingly uncomfortable for her. At age thirty, she was diagnosed with diabetes and her depression spiraled out of control. She over dosed on medication ne night, hoping to go to sleep forever, and woke up in the emergency room.

She was started on an anti-depressant medication and a psychotherapy weekly that helped her realize that what she really wanted most in life was a partnership with a special person who would accept her for who she was and who would be a good parent and companion. She made a commitment to start dating again and practiced letting go of her preoccupation with her physical appearance. She also decided to do thirty minutes of fast walking a day so she could improve her overall health, and she committed to eating healthy meals on a regular basis and to stop snacking when she felt nervous, stressed, or depressed. This was difficult because she'd been thinking and behaving in this way for so long that it was almost automatic. Her diabetes, which had been out of control due to inactivity and snacking on junk food, started t o moderate, and this made her more optimistic about her future.

Discussion. As demonstrated in this case, there are five main ways that most people experience the downward spiral of depression: feelings, sensations, thoughts, memories, and behaviors.

<u>Feelings.</u> Depression often involves chronic sadness, anger and irritability, but in a more blunted and free-floating fashion than we usually experience emotions. Sometimes feelings seem to

come out of the blue, particularly crying spells when there seems to be nothing to cry about. Depression also involves a sense of emotional numbness and constriction. When a depressed person experiences positive emotions, they are often muted. This is referred to as anhedonia, which literally means the inability to experience pleasure. When negative emotions are in play, they seem to arise quickly and with great force.

<u>Sensations.</u> Depression also produces a variety of unpleasant physical symptoms, such as abdominal pain, chest pain, headaches, or various other pains and bodily discomforts. Breathing pattern may be shallow, resulting in less oxygen in the blood, so concentration and focus may be a problem. Tension may increase, and this can cause more restlessness, particularly at night. Fatigue is common, resulting in less desire to engage in physical activities and more problems with muscle aches and pains. In addition, depression is associated with increased risk of illness and disease, suggesting that it impacts the immune system in various ways. Depressed people tend to view themselves as unhealthy in the physical sense of the world.

<u>Thoughts.</u> Depressed thinking is characterized by a black and white flavor, and perfectionist, self-critical thoughts are common, such as "I'm a loser," "I'm unlovable," or "I'm damaged goods." Thinking is often focused on past setbacks and disappoints; guilt and feelings of shame are common. In a depressed state, people spend an excessive amount of time reviewing past mistakes, blaming themselves for letting other down, and imagining negative outcomes in the future. Another thinking pattern in depression is to ruminate about being depressed in the first place, repeatedly experiencing thoughts like "What's wrong with me?" or "Why can't I be happy some of the time, like other people?."

<u>Memories.</u> Depressed people spend a lot of time remembering events, particularly those that trigger depressed feelings. Research on memory in depression suggests that it is skewed in a negative events more easily than they do positive events. Additionally, their memory for life events is more vague and general in nature.

This tendency toward imprecise memories can trigger a vicious cycle of distorted thinking.

Behaviors. Depression both affets daily behavior patterns and is affected by them, Depressed people may engage in excessive amounts of certain behaviors, such as eating, sleeping, or consuming alcohol, and neglect behaviors like exercise, leisure pursuits, or spending time with friends or family.

All patients suffering from a major depressive episode, regardless of diagnostic type, require careful psychologic management. The clinician should communicate with the patient in a clear, empathetic, and hopeful manner. During the interview the clinician should try to establish a trusting relationship that will facilitate the patient's cooperation in participating in the proposed treatment. Many patients will feel some relief when the clinician successfully communicates that he or she understands the patient's problem; and the patient realizes that help is forthcoming. Patients may express the feeling that they do not deserve help or that they are reluctant to accept help. This attitude is a frequent symptom of depression.

Since many patients suffering from depression experience significant stresses prior to the evaluation, it may help the patient to identify these stresses and provide reassurance that they are manageable. It often helps to remind patients who, in the midst of their depression, feel as if the depression will never end, in fact within a reasonable time they will feel better.

Whenever possible, family members or friends should be included bot h in the assessment of the patient and the t reatment. Families oft en present more detailed and accurate historical information than the depressed patient and accurate historical information than the depressed patient because the latter may be too forgetful, agitated, or psychotic t o give a good history. It is also critical to disposition planning for the clinician to obtain an impression of the family's ability to support, supervise, and encourage the patient if he or she returns home.

Biological Theories. How does stress trigger depression? Researchers have found that upsetting situations arouse a part of the brain called the amygdala, a small, almond shaped region at the very base of the brain called the hypo thalamus. If these brain regions overact to stress, perhaps because of a genetic vulnerability, they may produce a chemical chain reaction that leads to depression. Researchers believe that decreased amounts of serotonin and other neurotransmitters are involved in depression, causing the sleep problems, irritability, anxiety, fatigue, and despondent mood that characterize the illness. In addition, decreased serotonin activity may be linked to suicidal behavior, according to autopsies of suicide victims. And according to biochemical theory of depression, the catecholamine hypothesis is that in depression the supply of active norepinephrine is depleted.

Treatment of Depression:

- Psychotherapy (see chapter 26)-There are many types of therapy available today including cognitive-behavior therapy, interpersonal therapy and psychodynamic psychotherapy.
- Medication (see chapter 24)- There are a variety of antidepressant medications available today including selective serotonin reuptake inhibitors (SSRI's) serotonin and norepinephrine reuptake inhibitors (SNRI's), bupropion, Mirtazapine, trycyclic anti-depressants, and monoamine oxidase inhibitors (MAOI's).
- Electroconvulsive Therapy (ECT) (see chapter 29)- For very severe depression that does not respond to treatment, ECT can be very successful.

Senescence. Depression is the most common psychiatric disorder of the elderly, who make up 12.4 percent of the general population of the United States (Administration on Aging, 2005). This is not surprising considering the disproportionate value our society places on youth, vigor, and uninterrupted productivity. These societal attitudes continually nurture the feelings of low self-esteem, helplessness, and hopelessness that become more pervasive and intensive with advanced age.

Symptoms of depression in the elderly are not very different from those in younger adults. However, depressive syndromes are often confused by other illnesses associated with the aging process. Symptoms of depression are often misdiagnosed as senile dementia, when in fact the memory loss, confused thinking, or apathy symptomatic of senility actually may be the result of depression. The early awakening and reduced appetite typical of depression are common among many older people who are not depressed. Compounding this situation is the fact many medical conditions, such as endocrinological, neurological, nutritional, and metabolic disorders, often present with classic symptoms of depression. Many medications commonly used by the elderly, such as anti-hypertensive, corticosteroids, and analgesics, can also produce a depressant effect.

Depression accompanies many of the illness that afflict older people, such as Parkinson's disease, cancer, arthritis, and the early stages of Alzheimer's disease. Treating depression in these situations can reduce unnecessary suffering and help afflicted individuals cope with their medical problems.

The most effective treatment of depression in the elderly individual is thought to be a combination of psychosocial and biological approaches. Anti-depressant medications are administered with consideration for age-related physiological changes in absorption, distribution, elimination; and brain receptor sensitivity. (see chapter 24)

In summary, Electroconvulsive therapy (ECT) remains one of the safest and most effective treatments for major depression in the elderly (see chapter 29). It may be considered the treatment of choice for the elderly individual who is an acute suicidal risk or is unable to tolerate anti-depressant medications.

Race and Culture. Studies have shown no consistent relationship between race and affective disorder. One problem encountered in reviewing racial comparisons has to do with the socioeconomic class of the race being investigated. That is why sample population of non-white clients are many time predominantly lower class and are often compared with white populations form middle and upper social classes.

Other studies suggest a second problematic factor in the study of racial comparisons. Clinicians tend to underdiagnose schizophrenia in clients who have racial or cultural backgrounds different from their own (Sadock & Sadock, 2003).

The Merck Manual of Diagnosis and Therpay (2005), states that, cultural factors seem to modify the clinical manifestations of mood disorder. For example, physical complaints, worry, tension, and irritability are more common manifestations in lower socio-economic classes; guilty ruminations and self-reproach are more common characteristics of depression Anglo-Saxton cultures; and mania tends to manifest itself more floridly in some Mediterranean and African countries and among black Americans.

Chapter 7: Major Depressive Disorder
Examination Review

1. What term is often used for short-term feelings of depression?

    A. Present-moment awareness
    B. Dysphoria
    C. Emotional avoidance
    D. Suppression

2. What is an area of study in psychology in which giving a person hidden verbal cues designed to influence the person's behavior in some type of simulated situation?

    A. Priming
    B. Aggression
    C. Intuition
    D. Implicit association

3. A category of particularly toxic evaluations involves trying to determine who or what is responsible for an unwanted outcome. How does the assignment feel extremely important when negative life outcomes are present?

    A. Right and wrong'
    B. Good and bad
    C. Fair and unfair
    D. Responsibility and blame

4. What form of self-awareness regards a perfect stance for promoting willingness to experience both positive and negative aspects of mental life?

    A. Mindfulness
    B. Rumination
    C. Observer self
    D. Intuition

5. The antidote for situations that cause development of habits that allow ACT (accept, choose, and take action). Which mental processes can act as cues for the ACT habit?

    A. Visualization: using chosen phrases or quotes as simple reminders
    B. Recalling: mentally practicing ACT strategies for specific situations
    C. Pairing: using a daily event, such as lunch, to trigger specific ACT strategies
    D. Mental Rehearsal: remembering previous positive experiences using ACT strategies

6. What symptoms of depression are grouped according to negative self-concept, pessimism, and negative interpretations of experience?

    A. Affective Group
    B. Motivational Group
    C. Cognitive Group
    D. Physical and Vegetative symptoms

7. A 64 year-old make presents to his internist believing that his evil thoughts caused the recent death of his mother. The patient's belief about his mother would best be described as

    A. Thought insertion
    B. Thought broadcasting
    C. A mood-congruent delusion
    D. A melancholic symptom

8. Another name for the inability to experience pleasure is

    A. Grandiosity
    B. Anhedonia
    C. Melancholia
    D. Hypomania

9. What division of dichotomies attempts to establish the basic etiology of depression?

   A. Endogeneous Vs. Exogenous
   B. Autonomous vs. Reactive
   C. Agitated vs. retarded
   D. Psychotic vs. Neurotic

10. What types of generalized somatic disorders are likely to be complicated by depression?

   A. Infectious disease such as hepatitis, influenza, and pneumonia
   B. Psychosomatic disorders such as ulcerative colitis, asthma, and rheumatoid arthritis
   C. Anemias
   D. All of the above

Chapter 7: Major Depressive Disorder
Examination Answers

1. B
2. A
3. D
4. A
5. C
6. C
7. C
8. B
9. A
10. D

Chapter 8

Dysthymic Disorders

Major Depressive disorder represents the classic condition in this group of disorders. It is characterized by discrete episodes of at least 2 weeks duration (although most episodes last considerably longer) involving clear-cut changes in affect, cognition, and neuro-vegetative functions and inter-episode remissions. Careful consideration is given to the delineation of normal sadness and grief from a major depressive episode. Bereavement may induce great suffering, but it does not typically induce an episode of major depressive disorder.

In "mourning and melancholia" Sigmund Freud asserted that an interpersonal disappointment early in life can cause a vulnerability to depression that leads to ambivalent adult love relationships; real or threatened losses in adult life then trigger depression. Persons prone to depression are orally dependent and require constant narcissistic gratification. When deprived of love, affection, and care, they become clinically depressed; when they experience a real loss, they internalize or introject the lost object and turn their anger on it and thus, on themselves.

Individuals with dysthymic disorder describe their mood as sad or "down in the dumps." He said he felt enveloped by a sense of gloom that was nearly always with him. He said he felt empty, going through life without any sense of direction, ambition, or passion.

Dysthymic disorder is an example of moderate depression. It occurs when grief is prolonged or exaggerated. The individual becomes fixed in the anger stage of the grief response, and the anger is turned inward on the self. All of the feelings associated with normal grieving are exaggerated out of proportion, and the individual is unable to function without assistance. Symptoms associated with dysthymic disorder include (Akiskal, 1983):

- **Affective:** Feelings of sadness, dejection, helplessness, powerlessness, hopelessness; gloomy and pessimistic outlook; low self-esteem; difficulty experiencing pleasure in activities
- **Behavioral:** Slowed physical movements (i.e. psychomotor retardation); slumped posture; slowed speech; limited verbalization, possibly consisting of ruminations about failures or regrets in life; social isolation with a focus on the self; increased use of substances possible; self-destructive behavior possible; decreased interest in personal hygiene and grooming.
- **Cognitive:** Retarded thinking processes; difficulty concentrating and directing attention; obsessive and repetitive thoughts, generally portraying pessimism and negativism; verbalizations and behavior reflecting suicidal ideation.
- **Psychological**: Anorexia or overeating; insomnia or hypersomnia; sleep disturbances; amenorrhea; decreased libido; headaches; backaches; chest pain; abdominal pain; low energy level; fatigue and listlessness; feeling best early in the morning and continually worse as the day progresses. This may be related to the dlurnal variation in the level of neurotransmitters that affect mood and level of activity.

This chapter is less severe form of depression that is usually caused by identifiable event or loss (also caused by depressive neurosis). But neurosis is no longer a separate category of disorders in the DSM-IV-TR (APA,2000). And DSM-5 fifth edition Diagnostic and Statistical Manual of Mental Disorders (2013), dysthymia is known as Persistent Depressive Disorder. A chronic disturbance of mood, involving depressed mood, for at least two years. In addition to depression, two or more of the following symptoms are necessary: decreased appetite or over-eating, hypersomnia or insomnia, fatigue, poor self-esteem, impaired concentration or difficulty with decision making, and feelings of hopelessness. The dysthymic patient generally does not have the profound neuro-vegetative changes seen n major depression (McNeil, 1987). In studies, dysthymia was also more common in women under age 65, unmarried persons, and young persons with low income. It is also common for a dysthymic patient to say, "I've been depressed for a s long as I can remember."

Dysthymic disorder was introduced in DSM-III to indicate a non-episodic chronic depression that was thought to be less severe than major depression. Some investigators have asked whether dysthymic disorder properly belongs on Axis II. Remember that dysthymic disorder may coexist with any of the Axis II personality disorders.

The diagnosis of dysthymic disorder should not be made if the chronic course has been interrupted by a period of formal mood lasting more than a few months. Individuals usually describe mild to moderate impairment in social and occupational functioning due to the chronicity rather than the severity of the depressive symptoms. Frequently, individuals come to the physician or emergency department because of significant stress in their personal or work life that exacerbates the depressed feelings. Patients may give histories of chronic feelings of inadequacy, low self-esteem, emptiness, or boredom. However, they of not have psychomotor changes or psychotic symptoms unless there is a superimposed disordered or intoxication.

Dysthymic disorder was introduced in DSM-III to indicate a non-episodic chronic depression that was thought to be less severe than major depression. The cardinal feature of dysthymic disorder is a chronically depressed mood that is present most of the day, for more days than not, for at least 2 years.

According to the text revision of the fourth edition of Diagnostic and Statistical Manual of Mental Disorders (DSM-IV-TR), the most typical features of the disorder are feelings of inadequacy, guilt, irritability, and anger; withdrawal from society; loss of interest; and inactivity or lack of productivity.

What is the real difference between major depressive disorder and dysthymic disorder? As demonstrated in Table 8-1, dysthymic disorder is distinguished from major depressive disorder by the fact that patients complain that they have always been depressed.

Table 8-1. Dysthymic Disorder versus Major Depressive Disorder

DYSTHYMIC DISORDER	MAJOR DEPRESSIVE DISORDER
2 Year Duration	2 Weeks Duration
Depressed Mood (plus two additional symptoms)	Depressed Mood (plus four additional symptoms)
More Cognitive Symptoms And Mild onset may be followed After 2 years by a major depression	More Vegetative Symptoms And Onset may begin with more Severe symptoms

As defined by DSM-IV-TR, dysthymic disorder is a chronic condition that has been present for at least 2 years. Individuals describe persistent depressed mood or loss of interest or pleasure in almost any activity, although there may be short periods of normal mood lasting a few days to weeks. The diagnosis should be made if the chronic curse has been interrupted by a period of normal mood lasting more than a few months.

Table 8-2. Diagnostic Criteria of Dysthymia

This disorder represents a consolidation of DSM-IV-TR defined chronic major depressive disorder and dysthymic disorder.

A. Depressed mood for most of the day, for more days tha not, as indicated by either subjective account or observation by others, for at least 2 years.

B. Presence while depressed, of two (or more) of the following:

    1. Poor appetite or overeating
    2. Insomnia or hypersomnia
    3. Low energy or fatigue
    4. Low self-esteem
    5. Poor concentration or difficulty making decisions
    6. Feelings of hopelessness

C. During the 2 year period of the disturbance, the individual has never been without the symptoms in Criteria A and B for more than 2 months at a time.

D. Criteria for a major depressive disorder may be continuously present for 2 years

E. There has never been a manic episode, and criteria have never been met for cyclothymic disorder.

F. The disturbance is not better explained by a persistent schizoaffective disorder, schizophrenia, delusional disorder, or other specified or unspecified schizophrenia spectrum and other psychotic disorder.

G. The symptoms are not attributable to the physiological effects of a substance (e.g. a drug abuse, a medication) or another medical condition (e.g. hypothyroidism).

H. The symptoms cause clinically significant distress or impairment in social, occupational, or other important areas of functioning.

Neurosis is no longer a separate category of disorders in the DSM-IV-TR (APA, 2000).

The following are common characteristics of people with neurosis:

- They are aware that they are experiencing distress.
- They are aware that their behaviors are maladaptive.
- They are unaware of any possible psychological causes of the distress.
- They feel helpless to change their situation.
- They experience no loss on contact with reality.

Dysthymia: **ACHEWS**

Two out of these six with depressed mood, for 2 years signify dysthymia

Appetite disorder (either decreased or increased)
Concentration deficit
Hopelessness
Energy deficit
Worthlessness
Sleep disorder (either increased or decreased)

Next we will use the more general term "dysthymia" interchangeably with the official term dysthymic disorder.

VIGNETTE

A 35 year old veteran male presented to the outpatient clinic with the complaint of "feeling like ending it all." He described his mood as bleak, stating that he had felt this way most of his life. His chief complaint was that "I just don't enjoy life … I don't have any interest in doing things, and I have not energy even if I wanted to do them." These symptoms had been present for at least the past 5 years, but the patient added, "I really can't remember the last time I felt Happy." He described some difficulty falling asleep for many years and occasional midcycle awakening. His appetite had never been robust, but there was no recent history of weight loss. He gave a family history that appeared to be positive for major depressive illness. He had a few friends at work and remained socially isolated even from his wife and to children. He had difficulty making decisions at work and had lost the chance of a promotion recently. There was no history of mood swings, psychiatric hospitalization, or bouts of depression resulting in missed work, suicide attempt, or severe weight loss. On mental status examination, the patient appeared sad looking, but was well groomed. Despite his gloom, he maintained his sense of humor throughout much of the interview, although at times he seemed on the verge of tears. There was no significant psychomotor retardation or agitation, although the patient showed some inattentiveness to questions. A full physical and laboratory examination revealed no significant abnormality. Klerman (1980) has noted that divorce, unemployment, and business or professional failure may often be the consequence of dysthymic disorder. These same occurrences can worsen or precipitate depressive downswings n dysthymic individuals.

The vignette considers a familial pattern. Dysthymic Disorder is more common among first-degree biological relatives of people with Major Depressive Disorder that among the general population. The risk of acute onset or a major depressive disorder following a stroke (CVA) within 1 day to a week of the event, appears to be strongly correlated with lesion location, with greatest risk associated with left frontal strokes and least risk apparently associated with right frontal lesions in those individuals who present within days of the stroke.

Biological Factors. If dysthymia is an attenuated form of major depression, we might expect to find in the etiology and expression of these two disorders. It has been hypothesized tht depressive illness may be relatied to a dieficiency of the beurotransmitters norepinephrine, serotonin, and dopamine, at functionally important receptor sites in the brain. A number of brain regions (e.g. prefrontal cortex, anterior cingulate, amygdala, hippocampus) have been implicated in persistent depressive disorder. About 25% to 50% of adults with Dysthymic Disorder have some of the same polysomnographic features that are found in some individuals with Major Depressive Disorder. This includes reduced rapid eye movement (REM) Latency, increased REM density, reduced slow-wave sleep, and impaired sleep continuity.

Associated Features and Disorders: Dysthymic Disorder may be associated with Borderline, Histrionic, Narcissistic, Avoidant, and Dependent Personality Disorders. However, the assessment of features of a personality Disorder is difficult in such individuals because chronic mood symptoms may contribute to interpersonal problems or be associated with distorted self-perception. Some dysthymic patients, particularly those with a family history of affective illness short REM latency, and relatively stable personality will respond fairly well to tricyclic antidepressants (Yerevanian and Akiskal, 1979).

Treatment

Dysthymic Disorder is to major depression as cyclothymia is to a bipolar disorder it is, in effect, an attenuated form of major depression. In chapter 8, characteristics of this mood disturbance are similar to, if somewhat milder than, those ascribed to major depressive disorders. Because there is no evidence of psychotic symptoms, somatic complaints, such as headache, edema, backache, and breast tenderness, as well as changes in appetite and sleep patterns, are common. Patients may not fully recover from a chronic depressive episode without treatment, and remain generally lacking in energy with a negative outlook on life. Premenstrual Dysphoric Disorder (PMDD) is characterized by a constellation of affective and somatic symptoms that are manifest during the late luteal phase of the menstrual cycle and resolve shortly after the onset of menses. Unlike other mood disorders, the mood disturbances associated with PMDD are cyclical and tightly linked to the menstrual cycle; hence the occurrence of symptoms ceases during pregnancy and after menopause.

Chapter 8: Dysthymic Disorder Examination Review

1. When is dysthymic disorder an example of moderate depression?

    A. When grief is prolonged or exaggerated
    B. When the patient is highly functional with self-esteem
    C. When increasing pleasure occurs in all activities
    D. When increased interest in personal hygiene and grooming

2. What cognitive symptoms are associated with dysthymic disorder?

    A. Difficulty concentrating and directing attention
    B. Obsessive and repetitive thoughts
    C. Verbalizations and behavior reflecting suicidal ideation
    D. All of the above

3. When does a person with dysthymic disorder feel the best?

    A. Early in the morning and continually worse as the day progresses
    B. When mood is accompanied by slowed physical movements
    C. When activities demonstrate retarded thinking process
    D. At meal times when characterized by anorexia

4. What is the cardinal feature of dysthymic disorder?

    A. Acute depression that was more severe than major depression
    B. A chronically depressed mood that is present most of the day, for more days than not, for at least 2 years
    C. Depressed mood with vegetative symptoms for at least 2 weeks duration
    D. Acute depressed mood with severe symptoms for 2 months duration

5. How do individuals with dysthymic disorder describe their mood?

    A. Usually described severe impairment in social functioning
    B. As sad or down in the dumps
    C. As being characterized by voices or other psychotic symptoms
    D. As more severe than those ascribed to major depressive disorder

6. What examples demonstrate the profound neurovegetative changes seen in the dysthymic patient?

    A. Significant weight loss
    B. Early morning awakening
    C. Psychomotor retardation
    D. All of the above

7. In studies, when was dysthymia most common for most of the day for at least two years?

    A. In men under age 40
    B. In women under the age 65
    C. In married persons
    D. In elderly persons with higher income

8. In what manner is Premenstrual Dyshporic Disorder characterized by a constellation of affective and somatic symptoms?

    A. Symptoms increase during pregnancy
    B. Symptoms increase during the first ten years after menopause
    C. Symptoms that are manifest during the late luteal phase of the menstrual cycle
    D. Symptoms accompany with the onset of menses

9. What is referred to as anhedonia in a depressed person's experience of positive emotions?

    A. When thoughts arise quickly ad with great force
    B. Imprecise memories that trigger a vicious cycle of distorted thinking
    C. The inability to experience pleasure
    D. Fatigue is common, resulting in less desire to engage in physical activities

10. What symptoms of depression can be described as alterations in the spheres of human functioning by slowed physical movements in which psychomotor retardation and slumped posture occur?

    A. Affective
    B. Behavioral
    C. Cognitive
    D. Physiological

Chapter 8: Dysthymia Disorder Examination Answers

1. A
2. D
3. A
4. B
5. B
6. D
7. B
8. C
9. C
10. B

Chapter 9

Seasonal Affective Disorder

Seasonal Affective Disorder was initially described by Rosenthal et al. (1984) as a condition in which patients experience recurrent depressions in autumn and winter, alternating with non-depressed periods in spring and summer. Many people living in climates in which there are marked seasonal differences in the length of the day have seasonal changes in mood, sleep, and energy (Hellekson 1989; Kasper et al. 1989). Also, seasonal variations occur in most mood disorders. For example, unipolar depression is more likely to recur in the spring, whereas bipolar depression is more likely to recur during the summer (Barbini et al., 1995).

The original defining criteria for SAD were as follows (Rosenthal et al. 1984): (1) a history of at least one episode of major depression by Research Diagnostic Criteria; (2) recurrent fall-winter depressions, at least two of which occurred during successive years, separated by non-depressed periods in spring and summer; (3) no other DSM-III Axis I psychopathology; and (4) the absence of regularly occurring psychosocial variables that might account for the regular seasonal depression.

Biological. Scientists now believe that SAD is related to how much light is hitting the retina of the eye. The less light, the more of a natural sleep hormone is circulating in the body. In scientific experiments, when lab animals were injected with this hormone they overate, overslept, and became lethargic.

Depressed people also experience abnormalities in hormones that affect appetite and sex drive. In women, hormonal imbalances related to menstruation, pregnancy, childbirth, and menopause have been related to depression. These findings suggest that or hormones may also be regulated by the neurotransmitters that regulate moods. Individuals afflicted with seasonal affective disorder (SAD)- a form of depression – become gloomy as nights become longer. As if getting ready to hibernate for the winter, they crave carbohydrates and become lethargic. They oversleep, gain weight, and feel generally fatigued during fall and winter months. Dr. Norman E. Rosenthal of the National Institute of mental Health in Bethesda, one of the first to identify SAD as an illness, explains that light and latitude have much to do with this type of depression.

There is growing evidence that some individuals may receive significant benefit from medicines that are helpful in the more obvious mood disorders. For example, some find their predisposition to depression is triggered y the seasons, with reduced energy, downcast mood, excessive sleep and weight gain occurring during the dark winter months, to be followed by rapid improvement and euphoria in the spring, a condition that has been named seasonal affective disorder, or winter depression. A correlation may exist between abnormal secretion of melatonin from the pineal gland and mood disorder with seasonal pattern, in which individuals become depressed only during the fall and winter months when the secretion of melatonin increases in response to o decreased amounts of daylight. The limbic brain predicts the coming of the seasons and sets our behavior accordingly. Seasonal cycles of energy and reproductive behavior are adjusted by the signals form the brain clocks to the pineal, an endocrine gland about the size of a pea that nestles just outside just outside the brain. The pineal secretes the messenger hormone melatonin, an important chemical regulator of sleep and seasonal behavior which is carried through our the bloodstream to all the organs I the body, including across the blood-brain carrier to the brain itself. In many studies, melatonin has been called the Dracula hormone because it is produced mainly during darkness.

Each evening, the level of melatonin in the blood stream rises and then falls again in the early morning. Through the long days of winter the nighttime peak of melatonin is extended, shortening dramatically with the onset of spring. This rhythmic production of melatonin guides many seasonal activities.

Symptoms. When the seasons change from spring and summer to fall and winter, does a patient develop the following symptoms? Check off the symptoms that are familiar. (Rosenthal, 2006)

- Lower energy than usual
- Awakening feeling tired, even though he sleeps more
- Mood changes such as feeling more anxious, irritable, sad, or depressed
- Diminished productivity or creativity
- Feeling that you have little control over your appetite or weight
- More memory and concentration problems
- Lowered interest in socializing
- Lessened ability to cope with stress
- Less enthusiasm about the future or reduced enjoyment in your life

The symptomology of SAD, which reminds the clinician of a syndrome of a syndrome that is delineated in the following vignette.

VIGNETTE

The patient was a 30 year old married female who gave a 5 year history of bad depression everytime it starts getting cold outside. In fact, she began to experience here depression in mid –November. Each depressive bout was characterized by excessive eating (especially cakes and cookies), excessive sleeping, and what she calls "a bad habit of biting people's head off when they cross me."

The patient noted that many of these symptoms also occurred during the 4 or 5 days prior to her menstrual flow, although less consistently. She also noticed irritability just before her menstrual period that seemed to increase during the winter months.

Discussion/ PMS. As suggested in the vignette, many persons with SAD also have Premenstrual Syndrome (PMS); As many as 25% of women develop significant psychological discomfort during the 4 – 5 days prior to menses, ending shortly after flow begins. The severity of depression in the postpartum period varies from a feeling of the blues, to moderate depression, to psychotic depression or melancholia. Women who give birth, approximately 70% experience an emotional letdown following delivery. (APA,2005). Symptoms usually begin 3 to 4 days after delivery, generally do not impair functioning, and resolve spontaneously within a couple of weeks. Symptoms of moderate postpartum depression have been described as depressed mood varying from day to day, with more bad days that good, tending to be worse toward evening and associated with fatigue, irritability, loss of appetite, sleep disturbances, and loss of libido. Premenstrual syndrome differs form premenstrual dysphoric disorder in that a minimum of five symptoms is not required, and there is nor stipulation of affective symptoms for individuals who have premenstrual syndrome. Postpartum psychosis is considered to be a mental health emergency an therefore requires immediate medical attention.

Light Therapy. In contemplating the use of light therapy, several factors mist be considered. How depressed is the patient? What is the time of year? What are the patient's daily habits: the time of sleep onset and waking; the amount of time in the morning before the patient has to leave home; the patient's work setup? What is the patient's financial status (light fixtures can e quite costly)? When is the patient likely to be able to use the light box? All of these questions will prove relevant to the clinical recommendations.

For instance, if a patient presents in the autumn with mild symptoms of SAD, it may be appropriate to start with a short duration of light therapy (about 10-15 minutes in the morning) and gradually increase the duration as the season deepens. On the other hand, if a patient presents with severe symptoms in mid-winter, it may be best to start with much more light therapy (about 45 minutes in the morning and 20 minutes in the evening), monitoring symptoms closely, and adjust treatment accordingly.

Seasonal Effective Disorder was initially described by Rosenthal (1984) as a condition in which patients experience recurrent depressions in autumn and winter, alternating with non-depressed periods in spring and summer. SAD most commonly begins in the 20's, and the peak time for presentation to research programs usually has been the late 30's and early 40's, by which age many cycles of winter depression have occurred.

Although isolated cases of what in retrospect appears to have been SAD were reported for many years, it was in the mid-1980's that the condition was first described as a syndrome with specific clinical and demographic features, a predictable clinical course, and a response to a particular form of treatment-namely light therapy. In contemplating the use of light therapy, several factors must be considered: How depressed is the patient? What is the time of year? What are the patient's daily habits, such as the time of sleep onset and waking, the amount of time in the morning before the patient has to leave home, and the patient's work set up? What is the patient's financial status (light fixtures can be quite costly)? When is the patient likely to be able to use the light box? For instance, if a patient presents in the autumn with mild symptoms of SAD, it may be appropriate to start with a short duration of light therapy (about 10-15 minutes in the morning) and gradually increase the duration as the season deepens. On the other hand, if a patient presents with severe symptoms in mid-winter, it may be best to start with much more light therapy (about 45 minutes in the morning and 20 minutes in the evening). Clinical experience suggests that the longer the duration of light therapy, the stronger the treatment effect. The most common short term side effects of light therapy are headache, eyestrain, nausea, and jumpiness or agitation.

Aerobic exercise has been shown to be useful for patients with SAD symptoms, alone or in combination with light therapy.

Because exercise appears to have antidepressant effects in other forms of depression, it is a safe bet to recommend it for SAD patients as well. It is easy to combine exercise with light therapy, for example, by using a stationary bicycle in front of a light ox or walking briskly outdoors.

Several other types of intervention show evidence of benefit. Preliminary evidence suggests that Vitamin D3 may be of some value in reversing winter depressive symptoms. Clinical impressions suggest that patients are greatly helped by treatment and that even when winter depressions do recur, they are milder and more quickly detected and successfully treated. Patients appear to benefit by recognizing the seasonal nature of their illness and learning about the available treatment approaches that can alleviate their symptoms. As with other forms of mood disorder, researchers have investigated neuroendocrine systems in SAD, particularly the hypothalamic-pituitary-adrenal axis and thyroid functioning. These observations suggest that untreated, SAD would continue to result in considerable morbidity year after year.

Chapter 9: Seasonal Affective Disorder
Examination Review

1. Treatment designed to prevent the return of the most recent mood episode

    A. Behavioral Therapy
    B. Cognitive Therapy
    C. Continuation Treatment
    D. Supportive Therapy

2. A return to the asymptomatic state, usually accompanied by a return to the usual level of psychosocial functioning.

    A. Remission
    B. Hypomania
    C. Intent-to-Treat Analysis
    D. Open trial

3. What syndrome serves as a bridge between dysthymic disorder and histrionic personality disorder?

    A. Completer Analysis
    B. Cyclothymic Disorder
    C. Hysteroid Dysphoria
    D. Somatization

4. Which seasonal variation occurs in most disorder?

    A. Unipolar depression is more likely to recur in the fall
    B. Bipolar depression is more likely to recur in the spring
    C. Reduced energy, downcast mood, excessive sleep, and weight gain occurs during the dark winter months
    D. Mania is more likely to recur during the fall

5. How does the seasonal affective disorder appear to resemble the depressed phase of bipolar illness?

    A. Hyperphagia
    B. Carbohydrate craving
    C. Hyper-somnia
    D. All of the above

6. What should be considered when contemplating the use of light therapy?

    A. How depressed is the patient?
    B. What is the time of year the patient have symptoms?
    C. What are the patient's daily habits, such as the time of sleep onset and waking?
    D. All of the above

7. If a patient presents in the autumn with mild symptoms of SAD, when is it appropriate to start light therapy?

    A. About 30-40 minutes in the evening
    B. About 10-15 minutes in the morning
    C. About 45 minutes in the morning and 30 minutes in the evening
    D. About 60 minutes in the morning

8. In what way does aerobic exercise has been shown to be a useful for patients with SSAD symptoms?

    A. In place of light therapy
    B. By using a stationery bicycle in front of a light box
    C. The longer the duration of light therapy, the stronger the treatment effect
    D. Equally in all of the above

9. When is bipolar depression more likely to recur?

    A. In the spring
    B. In the summer
    C. In the fall
    D. All of the above

10. What hormone secreted by the pineal gland serves as an important chemical regulator of sleep and seasonal behavior?

    A. Melatonin
    B. Serotonin
    C. Dopamine
    D. Norepinephrine

Chapter 9: SAD Examination Answers

1. C
2. A
3. C
4. C
5. D
6. D
7. B
8. B
9. C
10. A

Reference 2

Akiskal MS. Mood Disorders: Clinical features. In Sadock BJ, Sadock VA (eds): Comprehensive Textbook of Psychiatry. Philadelphia, Lippincott. Williams + Wilkins. 1999.

Akiskal HS. Dysthymic Disorder: Psychopathology of Proposed Chronic Depressive Subtypes. American Journal of Psychiatry 140: 11-20, 1983.

Akiskal HS. Dysthymia and Cyclothymia in psychiatric practice a century after Kraepelin. Journal of Affective Disorders: 62 (1-2): 17, 2001.

Akiskal HS, Kilzieh N, Maser JD, et al. The distinct temperament profiles of Bipolar I, Bipolar II and unipolar patients. Journal of Affective Disorder: 92 (1), 19-33. 2006.

Akiskal HS, Mendlowicz, Jean-Louis G, et al. Temps-A: Validation of a short version of a self-rated instrument designed to measure variations in temperament. Journal of Affective Disorders, 85 (1-2), 45-52, 2005.

Akiskal HS. Mood disorders: clinical features. In Sadock BJ, Sadock VA, eds. Kaplan + Sadock's Comprehensive Textbook of Psychiatry, 7th ed. Vol. 1. Baltimore: Lippincott Williams + Wilkins, 2000.

Allen MG, Cohen S, Pollin W, et al. Affective Illness in Veteran Twins: a Diagnostic Review. American Journal of Psychiatry 131: 1234-39, 1974.

Alexander FG, Selensnick ST. The History of Psychiatric Thought and Practice from Prehistoric Times to the Present. New York, Harper & Row, 1966.

American Psychiatric Association: Diagnostic and Statistical Manual of Medical Disorders, 4th Ed. Text Revision. Washington, DC. American Psychiatric Association, 2000.

Andreasen NC. Concepts, diagnosis and classification, in Handbook of Affective Disorders. Edited by Paykel ES. New York: Guilford, pp 24-44. 1982.

Arieti S. Affective Disorders: Manic Depressive psychosis and psychotic depression, In American Handbook of Psychiatry, 2nd E. Vol 3. New York: basic Books pp 449-490. 1974.

Baldessarini RJ. Treatment Research in Bipolar Disorder: Issues and Recommendation. CNS Drugs (16) 11: 721-729. 2002.

Barbini B, Di Molfetta D, Gasperini M, et al. Seasonal concordinace for recurrence in mood disorder patients. European Psychiatry. 10: 171-174. 1995.

Basco MR. The Bipolar Workbook: Tools for Controlling Your Mood Swings. The Guilford Press, 2006.

Basco MR and Rush AJ. Cognitive Behavioral Therapy for Bipolar Disorder 2nd Ed. New York: Guilford Press, 2007.

Baur MS, Kilbourne AM, Greenwald DE, etc. Overcoming Bipolar Disorder: A Comprehensive Workbook for Managing your Symptoms and Achieving Your Life Goals. New Harbinger Publications Inc., 2008.

Beck AT. Depressive Neurosis. American Handbook of Psychiatry, 2nd E. Vol. 3, New York: Basic Books, 61-90, 1974.

Birmaher B, Axelson D, Goldstein B, et al. Four-year longitudinal course of children and adolescents with bipolar spectrum disorders: The Course and Outcome of Bipolar Youth (COBY) Study. American Journal of Psychiatry, 166(7), 795-804, 2009.

Coryell W, Endicott J, and Keller M. Rapid Cycling Affective Disorder. Archives of General Psychiatry 49: 126-131, 1992.

Denicoff KD, Smith-Jackson EE, Disney ER, et al. Comparative prophylactic efficacy of lithium, carbamazepine, and the combination in bipolar Disorder. Journal of Clinical Psychiatry, 1997.

Eagles JM, Howie FL, Cameron IM, et al. Use of Health Care Services in Seasonal Affective Disorder. British Journal of Psychiatry. 180: 449-454. 002.

Eastman CL, Young MA, Fogg LF, et al.: Bright light treatment of winter depression: a placebo-controlled trial. Archives of General Psychiatry. 55: 883-889. 1998.

Faedola GL, Tondo L, Teicher MH, et al: Seasonal Mood Disorders: patterns of season recurrence in mania and depression. Archives of General Psychiatry. 50: 17-23. 1993.

Fawcett J, Golden B, and Rosenfeld N. New Hope For People worth Bipolar Disorder, Prima Publishing, 2000.

Fenichel O. Depression and Mania: the Psychoanalytic Theory of Neurosis. New York: Norton, 1945.

Fennell MJV. Depression, Low self-esteem, and mindfulness. Behavior Research and Therapy, 42 (9): 1053-67. 2004.

Frank E. Treating Bipolar Disorder: A Clinician's Guide to Interpersonal and Social Rhythm Therapy. New York: Guilford Press, 2007.

Frazer A, Ramsey TA, Swann A, et al. Plasma and erythrocyte electrolytes in affective disorders, Journal of Affect Disorder 5. 1983.

Gamble C, Brennan G. Working with Serious Mental Illness: A Manual for Clinical Practice: Elsevier, 2000.

Gillin JC, Duncan W, Pettigrew KD, et al. Successful separation of depressed, normal, and insomniac subjects by EEG sleep data. Archives of General Psychiatry 36: 85-90, 1979.

Golden RN, Gaynes BN, Ekstrom RD, et al: The efficacy of light therapy in the treatment of mood disorders: a review and meta-analysis of the evidence. American Journal of Psychiatry. 162: 656-662. 2005.

Goodwin F. and Jamison KR. Manic- Depressive Illness, 2nd Ed. New York: Oxford University Press, 2007.

Gotlib IH, Hammen CL. Handbook of Depression, The Guilford Press, 2002.

Hales RE, Yudofsky SC, and Talbott JA. Textbook of Psychiatry, 2nd Ed. Washington, DC: American Psychiatric Press, pp 465-494.1994.

Healy D. Mania: A Short History of Bipolar Disorder. The Johns Hopkins University Press, Baltimore. 2008.

Hegde AL, Woodson H: Prevalence of seasonal changes in mood and behavior during the winter months in central Texas. Psychiatry Research, 62: 265-271.1996.

Hellekson C. Phenomenology of Seasonal Affective Disorder: an Alaskan perspective in Seasonal Affect Disorders and Phototherapy. New York: Guilford, 1989.

Howland RH. Pharmacotherapy of Dysthymia: a Review. Journal of Clinic. Psychophramacol, 11: 83-92, 1991.

Ilfeld FW. Current Social Stressors and Symptoms of Depression. American Journal of Psychiatry 134: 161-166. 1988.

Jamison KR. Mood Disorders and Seasonal Patterns in British Writers and Artists. Psychiatry, 52: 125- 134. 1989.

Jackson SW. Melancholia and Depression: From Hippocratic Times to Modern Times, New Haven, CT. Yale University Press, 1986.

Johnson SL. Life Events in Bipolar Disorder: Towards More Specific Models. Clinical Psychology Review 25 (8): 1008-1027.

Jones- Webb RJ and Snowden LR. Symptoms of Depression Among Blacks and Whites. American Journal of Public Health; 83: 240-244. 1993.

Kaplan BJ, Crawford CJ, Field JSA, et al. Vitamins, Minerals, and Mood. Psychological Bulletin 133(5): 747-760. 2007.

Kasper S, Wehr TA, Bartko JJ, et al. Epidemiological findings of seasonal changes in mood and behavior. Archives of General Psychiatry. 46: 823-833. 1989.

Ketter TA, Post RM, Denicoff K, et al. Carbamazepine. In PJ Goodnick (Ed) Mania: Clinical and research perspectives. Washington, DC: American Psychiatric Press. 1998.

Klerman GL. Other Specific Affective Disorders, in Comprehensive Textbook of Psychiatry III, 3rd Ed., 1980.

Kochman FJ, Hantouche EG, Ferrari P, et al. Cyclothymic temperament as a prospective predictor of bipolarity and suicidality in children and adolescents with major depressive disorder. Journal of Affective Disorders. 85 (1-2) 2005.

Kraepelin E. Manic- Depressive Insanity and Paranoia. Edinburgh, E+S; Livingtone. 1921.

Lam RW, et al: Effects of light therapy on suicidal ideation in patients with winter depression. Journal of Clinical Psychiatry 61: 30. 2000.

Liebowitz MR, Klein DF. Hysteroid dysphoria. Psychiatric Clinical North American 2: 555-575, 1979.

Malhi GS, Adams D, and Berk M. Medicating Mood with maintenance in mind: Bipolar depression pharmacotherapy. Bipolar Disorders, II (Suppl. 2), 55-76, 2009.

Mc Neil GN. Depression, In Handbook of Psychiatric Differential Diagnosis. Edited by Soreff SM, McNeil GN. Littleton, MA. PSG Publishing pp 57-126. 1987.

Mc Intyre JS, Charles SC. Practice Guidelines for the Treatment of Psychiatric Disorders. American Psychiatric Association, 2006.

Meltzer HY, Arora RC, Baber R, et al. Serotonin uptake in blood platelets of psychiatric patients. Archives of General Psychiatry. 38. 1981.

Miklowitz DJ. The Bipolar Disorder Survival Guide: What You and Your Family Need to Know. 2nd ed. The Guilford Press, 2011.

Miklowitz DJ and Scott J. Psychosocial treatments for bipolar disorder: cost-effectiveness, medicating mechanisms, and future directions. Bipolar Disorders, 11 (Suppl 2) 110-122. 2009.

Miklowitz DJ, George EL, Richards JA, et al. A randomized study of family-focused psychoeducation and pharmacotherapy in the outpatient management of bipolar disorder. Archives of General Psychiatry: 60, 904-912. 2003.

Nierenberg A.A., Burt T, Mathews J, Weiss AP. Mania associated with St John's Wort. Biological Psychiatry: 46 (12). 1999.

Paykel ES. Cognitive therapy in relapse prevention in depression. International Jouranl of Neuro-psychopharmacology; 10(1): 131-136, 2006.

Partonen T, Leppamaki S, Hurme J, et al: Randomized trial of physical exercise alone or combined with bright light on mood and health-related quality of life. Psychol Med, 28: 1359-1364. 1998.

Pendse BP, Ojehagen A, Engstrom G, et al: Social characteristics of seasonal affective disorder patients: comparison with suicide attempts with non- seasonal major depression and other mood disorder patients. European Psychiatry, 18: 36-39. 2003.

Perris C. A study of Bipolar (manic- depressive) and Unipolar Recurrent Depressive Psychoses. Acta Psychiatry. Scand. 194: 1-18. 1966.

Potter WZ, Rudorfer MV, and Goodwin FK. Biological findings in bipolar disorders, In American Psychiatric Association Annual Review, Vol 6. American Psychiatric Press. pp 32-60. 1987.

Rosenthal NE. Sack DA, Gillin JC, et al. Seasonal Affective Disorder: a description of the syndrome and preliminary findings with light therapy. Archives of General Psychiatry 41: 72-80, 1984.

Rosenthal NE, Sack DA, Carpenter CJ, et al. Antidepresseant Effects of Light in Seasonal Affective Disorder. American Journal of Psychiatry; 142: 163-170. 1985.

Rosenthal, N. Winter Blues: Everything Your Need to Know to Beat Seasonal Affective Disorder. Revised Edition. New York: Guilford Press, 2006.

Sadock BJ and Sadock VA. Synopsis of psychiatry: Behavioral sciences? Clinical psychiatry, 9th Ed. Philadelphia: Lippincott Williams and Wilkins, 2003.

Shulman KI, Tohen M, and Kutcher SP (eds.). Mood Disorders Across the Lifespand. New York: John Wiley and Sons, 1996.

Stein DJ, Kupfer DJ, Schatzberg AF. Textbook of Mood Disorders. Washington, DC. American Psychiatric Publishing Inc, 2006.

Strosahl KD and Robinson PJ. The Mindfulness and Acceptance Workbook for Depression: Using Acceptance and Commitment Therapy to Move Through Depression and Create a Life Worth Living. New Harbinger Publications, Inc. 2008.

Tohen M. Outcome in Bipolar Disorder, PH. D Harvard University, 1988.

Tohen M, and Vieta E. Antipsychotic agents in the treatment of bipolar mania. Bipolar Disorders: 11 (2), 45-54. 2009.

Merk Manual of Diagnosis and Therapy. Mood Disorders. Retrieved March 14, 2007 from http://www.merck.com/

Wehr TA, Sack DA, Rosenthal NE, et al. Sleep and biological rhythms in bipolar illness, in American Psychiatric Association Annual Review, Vol 6. pp 61-80, 1987.

Wehr TA: Seasonal Affective Disorders: a historical overview, in Seasonal Affective Disorders and Phototherapy. Edited by Rosenthal NE, Blehar MC. New York: Guilford, 1989.

White RC and Preston JD. Bipolar 101: A Practical Guide to Identifying Triggers, Managing Medications, Coping with Symptoms, and more. New Harbinger Publications, Inc. 2009.

Whybrow PC. A Mood Apart: The Thinker's Guide to Emotion and Its Disorders. Harper Perennial, 1998.

Whybrow PC. A Mood Apart: The Thinker's Guide to Emotion and Its Disorders. Harper Perennial, 1997.

Woolis R. When Someone You Love has a Mental Illness: A Handbook for family, friends, and caregivers, 2003.

Wootton T. The Bipolar Advantage. www. Bipolar Advantage. com, 2005.

Wurtman JJ. Carbohydrate craving, mood changes, and obesity. Journal of Clinical Psychiatry 49 (No 8, Suppl): 37-39, 1988.

Yerevanian BI, Akiskal HS. Neurotic, Characterological, and Dysthymic Depressions. Psychiatry of Clinical North America 2: 595-617. 1979.

Section Three

Anxiety Disorders

> *We can live any way we want. People take vows of poverty, chastity, and obedience —even of silence- by choice. The thing is to stalk your calling in certain skilled and supple way, to locate the most tender and live spot and plug into that pulse. This is yielding, not fighting.*
>
> *Annie Dillard*
> *Living Like Weasels*

The symptoms in anxiety disorders reflect over activity of the cognitive, affective, and behavioral systems. This section focuses on disorders that are characterized by exaggerated and often disabling anxiety reactions. It is a feeling of dread accompanied hyperactive autonomic nervous system. In this text, anxiety can be distinguished form fear in several was. when the patient is afraid; fear is usually directed toward some concrete external object or situation. When the experience is anxiety, the focus is more internal than external. It seems to be a response to a vague, distant, or even unrecognized danger. Research has shown that anxiety disorders are the number one mental health problem among America women and are second only to alcohol and drug abuse among men.

Chapter 10

Panic Disorders with Agoraphobia

In the typical onset of a case of panic disorder, a person is engaged in some ordinary aspect of life when suddenly his heart begins to pound and he cannot catch his breath. The person feels dizzy, light-headed, and faint is convinced he is about to die.

Typically, during a panic attack, a patient will be engaged in a routine activity perhaps reading a book, eating in a restaurant, driving car, or attending a concert- when he or she will experience the sudden onset of overwhelming fear, terror, apprehension, and a sense of impending doom. Several of a group associated symptoms, mostly physical, are also experienced: dyspnea, palpitations, chest pains or discomfort, choking or smothering sensations, dizziness or unsteadiness, feelings of unreality, parethesis, hot and cold flashes, sweating, faintness, trembling and shaking, and a fear of dying, going crazy, or losing control of oneself.

The clinical picture in agoraphobia consists of multiple and varied fears and avoidance behaviors that center around three main themes: 1) fear of leaving home, 2) fear of being alone, and 3) fear of being away from home in situations in which one can feel trapped, embarrassed, or helpless. Agoraphobia without history of panic disorder is characterized by the presence of agoraphobia and panic-like symptoms without a history of unexpected panic attacks. Agoraphobia is anxiety about, or avoidance of, places or

Deborah Y. Liggan, MD

situations from which escape might be difficult (or embarrassing) or in which help may not be available in the event of having a Panic Attack or panic-like symptoms.

The idea of panic disorder may have its roots in the concept of irritable heart syndrome, which the physician Jacob Menders Da Costa (1833-1900) noted in soldiers in the American Civil War. Da Costa's syndrome included many psychological and somatic symptoms that have since been included among the diagnostic criteria for panic disorder. Sigmund Freud first noted the relation between panic attacks and agoraphobia. DSM-II (American Psychiatric Association, 1968) described an ill-defined condition of anxiety neurosis, a term first coined by Freud in 1895, which included any patient suffering from chronic tension, excessive worry, frequent headaches, or recurrent anxiety attacks. DSM-IV-TR (American Psychiatric Association, 2000) contains two diagnostic criteria for panic disorder, one without agoraphobia (Table 10-1) and the other with agoraphobia (Table 10-2) but both require the presence of panic attacks.

Table 10-1. DSM-IV-TR. Diagnostic Criteria for Panic Disorder without Agoraphobia.

A. Both (1) and (2):

(1) recurrent unexpected panic attacks
(2) at least one of the attacks has been followed by 1 month (or more) of one (or more) of the following:
a) persistent concern about having additional attacks
b) worry about the implications of the attack or its consequences
(e.g., losing control, having a heart attack, "going crazy")
c) a significant change in behavior related to the attacks

B. Absence of agoraphobia
C. Panic attacks are not due to the direct physiological effects of a substance (e.g. a drug abuse or medication) or a general medical condition (e.g. hyperthyroidism).

D. The panic attacks are not better accounted for by another mental disorder, such as social phobia (e.g., occurring exposure to feared social situation) specific phobia (e.g. on exposure to a specific phobic situation, obsessive-compulsive disorder (e.g., on exposure to dirt in someone with an obsession about contamination), post-traumatic stress disorder (e.g., in response to stimuli associated with a severe stressor), or separation anxiety disorder (e.g., in response to being away from home or close relatives.

Table 10-2. DSM-IV-TR. Diagnostic Criteria for Panic Disorder with Agoraphobia.

A. Both (1) and (2):

(1) recurrent unexpected panic attacks
(2) at least one of the attacks has been followed by 1 month (or more) of one (or more) of the following:
a) persistent concern about having additional attacks
b) worry about the implications of the attack or its consequences
(e.g., losing control, having a heart attack, "going crazy")
c) a significant change in behavior related to the attacks

B. Presence of agoraphobia
C. Panic attacks are not due to the direct physiological effects of a substance
(e.g. a drug abuse or medication) or a general medical condition (e.g. hyperthyroidism).

D. The panic attacks are not better accounted for by another mental disorder, such as social phobia (e.g., occurring exposure to feared social situation) specific phobia (e.g. on exposure to a specific phobic situation, obsessive-compulsive disorder (e.g., on exposure to dirt in someone with an obsession about contamination), posttraumatic stress disorder (e.g., in response to stimuli associated with a severe stressor), or separation anxiety disorder (e.g., in response to being away from home or close relatives.

Questions concerning the diagnosis of Agoraphobia:

The following questions, directed to the patient, may help reach or exclude a diagnosis of agoraphobia (Greist and Jefferson, (1988):

1. Are there specific situations or places you avoid? (The agoraphobic patient will often avoid crowded stores, open spaces, traveling on a bus or train, etc.)

2. What do you feel would happen if you would end up in one of those places or situations? (The agoraphobic will describe fear of having a panic attack, dying, of going crazy, or of being humiliated in public because of a panic attack.)

3. Do you think your fears are realistic or a little exaggerated? (The agoraphobic patient has intact reality testing and usually recognizes the fears as exaggerated or "silly." In contrast, the schizophrenic or paranoid individual will often have a rigidly held delusional belief justifying the fear).

4. If you must face the frightening situation or place, how do you handle it? (Agoraphobic individuals will usually describe anticipatory anxiety and the use of phobic partners to accompany them outside the home. Some will also give history of alcohol or substance abuse as a means to decrease anxiety.)

5. Have you ever noticed that your anxiety lessens if you ride out the frightening situation or are prevented from leaving it? (Many agoraphobic individuals will describe a reduction in anxiety in such fortuitous exposure therapy situations.)

Symptoms of agoraphobia include dizziness, abdominal pain, lack of control over thinking, involuntary trembling, paresthesia, depersonalization; some of these sensations may be attributable to hyperventilation, which may begin or increase during an attack. As symptoms start to mount, the patient begins to see them as signals of immediate danger such as: (1) mental and physical collapse; (2) heart attack or stroke; (3) loss of control of emotions (screaming, crying, weeping); (4) loss of control over behavior (hurting someone, attempting suicide, acting out sexually); (5) going crazy; and (6) other adversities (choking, epileptic fits, spontaneous termination of breathing).

The attack often begins with a 10 minute period of rapidly increasing symptoms. The major mental symptoms are extreme fear and a sense of impending death and doom. Patients usually cannot name the source of their fear; they may feel confused and have trouble concentrating. The attack generally lasts 20 to 30 minutes and rarely more than an hour, although they occur twice a week. Between attacks, patients may have anticipatory anxiety about having another attack.

Biological factors

Panic attacks are believed to be biological events related to excessive noradrenergic discharge from the locus ceruleus and the amygdala. First, it causes the adrenal glands to release large amounts of adrenaline. Then within seconds, the excess adrenaline causes 1) the heart to race, 2) respiration to become rapid and shallow, 3) profuse sweating, 4) trembling and shaking, and 5) cold hands and feet.

The amygdala, in turn, instigates panic by stimulating a variety of other structures, including 1) the locus coeruleus, which contributes to general behavioral and physiological arousal, 2) the hypothalamus, which regulates the release of adrenaline (via the pituitary gland, stimulating the adrenal glands), 3) the periaqueductal gray region, which stimulates defensive and avoidance behavior, and finally, 4) the parabrachial nucleus, which stimulates increased respiration.

With these caveats in mind, we can examine some of the leading biological hypotheses (Shear and Fyer, 1988).

- Central noradrenergic activation.
- Peripheral autonomic hyperactivity
- Respiratory dysfunction
- Metabolic imbalance

Central Noradrenergic activation. Clinical observation has long suggested that panic symptoms are related to surges in SNS activity- the venerable fight or flight response. The locus coeruleus, a noradrenergic center in the midbrain may be intimately involved in the production of panic attacks.

Peripheral autonomic hyperactivity. Some patients with panic like symptoms appear to have heightened sensitivity to (peripheral) beta-receptor agonists. These patients may get relief of their panic symptoms with beta-blocker medications. This fact has led to the logical notion that PD is a result of peripheral beta-receptor hypersensitivity.

Respiratory Dysfunction. You may recall the old saw that breathing into a paper bag is a good way to stop a panic attack. This observation led to various theories implicating carbon dioxide in the etiology of PD. Another related hypothesis (Carr and Sheehan 1984) is that CO_2 decreases the PH in brain stem neurons in turn stimulating central chemoreceptors and triggering panic in susceptible individuals.

Metabolic Imbalance. Patients with panic-like symptoms developed higher post exercise blood lactate levels than did normal control subjects implicating lactate hypersensitivity in PD. It is important to note that roughly a third of PD patients do not show a panic response to lactate infusion.

The following case illustrates the lifelong pattern of separation fears and dependency that develop into agoraphobia.

Vignette

A thirty-year-old woman had always had problems in being away from home. With the increase of anxiety, she experienced her first panic attack. From then on, it becomes increasingly more difficult for her to go out, and she finally became completely housebound. When she enters the department store, she is afraid of getting caught in the revolving door, of losing her balance on the escalator, of not being able to find the right counter, of not being able to select the items she wants, or of not being able to assert herself with the sales clerk. When she takes the elevator to the next landing, she feels faint andis afraid she may fall down. She decides to take the elevator down but is afraid that it may get stuck on the way. When she reaches the ground floor again, she feels crowded by the people scurrying around and begins to feel more and more breathless; she hyperventilates in order to get more air and then begins to feel pins and needles in her extremities. At this point, the woman interprets her shortness of breath, her weakness and the peculiar feeling in her extremities as signaling some terrible devastating disorder. She thinks that she may be dying right now.

Discussion. Certain features of agoraphobia seem too defy common sense or reason. The patient avoids spaces that are too narrow (crowds, closets, elevators) and too expansive (super markets, shopping centers, flat meadowland, or amphitheaters). Why should a woman who has progressed into her twenties, ostensibly with a minimum of psychological problems, suddenly develop a fear of going into public places, riding in cars, buses, trains, and elevators? Why should this person who is competent in many ways jeopardize a job or marriage or refuse to leave the house? Why should this person who is competent in many ways jeopardize a job or marriage or refuse to leave the house? Why should a woman who has engaged in numerous activities on her own in the past become so dependent that she will not travel without a companion (Beck and Emery, 1985)? Some authorities believe that agoraphobia results from a sudden panic attack away from home (Klein 1981). At some point in the progression of a specific panic attack, symptoms intensify beyond the person's capacity to discount them or to function effectively. A formal mental status examination during a panic attack may reveal rumination, difficulty speaking (e.g. stammering), and impaired memory. Some authorities believe that agoraphobia results from a sudden panic attack away from home (Klein, 1981). The panic attack severely undermines the patient's confidence that she can handle strips of this nature, and restricts her travel to places within easy access of home and to companions whom she can trust to help her if an attack should occur. Prior to entering a situation in which an attack has occurred, the patient may be primarily afraid of having the attack.

In the discussion literature, the result is that the individual perceives as increasingly vulnerable as he/she goes through each of these steps: (Liebowitz and Klein, 1982)

1. An unlimited number of opportunities is perceived to be immobilized, humiliated, crushed, suffocated, or attack (in crowds, elevators, buses, tunnels, streets). There is no reliable defense against these external dangers.

2. Automatic reflexive reactions produce symptoms suggestive of a serious internal disturbance (heart attack, stroke, fainting spell, attack of insanity). There is no way of warding off these internal attacks.

3. The patient experiences a sense of malfunctioning and decrement of competence. It is believed that the car cannot be kept on the road, maintain equilibrium while standing still, or communicate orally to other people without blocking or stuttering.

4. The loss of control over reaction to threat reinforces the notion that he/she is a victim of internal and external forces over which there is no control.

5. This loss of a sense of competence plus fears of the internal disturbance lead the patient to seek assistance form a caregiver.

6. The intense anxiety in the threatening situation (department store, supermarket) may escalate into a panic attack.

7. Home, or an equivalent haven, represents safety form the external danger. The patient experience a strong resistence to venturing out again and generally feel anxious if he/she does leave the house.

8. The multiple inhibitions, submissive tendencies, and negative appraisals of self-undermine self-confidence and thus lead to disequilibrium in relationships, further sense of inadequacy, and ultimately the sense of being trapped and dominated by other people.

Medical Causes for Panic Symptoms

Rule out possible medical causes for panic symptoms. Include a detailed physical examination; electrocardiogram (ECG); a complete chemistry profile, including electrolytes, calcium, and magnesium; thyroid function tests; a urine toxicology screen; a complete blood count and renal function tests.

An echocardiogram may help diagnose mitral valve prolapse. MVP

Obtain a detailed history of all the patient's medications and drugs, especially caffeine, alcohol, sedative- hypnotics, nicotine, and bronchodilators. Drug that are central nervous system (CNS) stimulants can precipitate panic attacks, as can withdrawal from drugs that are CNS depressants. Many panic disorder patients also self-medicate with alcohol or sedative-hypnotics.

Frankly it's difficult to sort out the different components of the patient's anxiety. That his panic attacks usually occur in the morning – after a drinking bout- suggest that withdrawal from the alcohol is the primary cause. The apparent visual and tactile hallucinations (formication) suggest full-blown delirium tremens (DTs). Panic attacks are found frequently in alcoholic individuals and may precede the excessive drinking (Jacob and Turner, 1988). Many patients who experience panic attacks report using alcohol as a form of self-medication. It is possible that subsequent alcohol withdrawal predisposes then to anxiety or panic attacks. Bottom-line: Have a high degree of suspicion for alcohol or substance abuse in patients complaining of panic attacks, particularly when they are evasive or defensive about their drinking and drug history.

- **Mitral Valve Prolapse.** This is a harmless condition that causes heart palpitations. It is caused by a slight defect in the valve separating the upper and lower chambers on the left side of the heart. It is present in about half of all patients with panic disorder. With mitral valve prolapse, the valve doesn't close completely and some of the blood can flow back form the lower to upper chamber, causing the heart to beat out of rhythm. Physical findings include a mid-systolic click and murmur. The resulting rhythm disturbance can be disconcerting enough to cause some people to panic, but it is not dangerous and does not cause heart attacks. Electrocardiograms (ECG) are also helpful I reassuring patients that they are not having a heart attack during the panic attack.
- **Premenstrual Syndrome (PMS).** In women it is important to observe whether panic reactions (or generalized anxiety) worsen around the time just before her period. Treatments usually involves improvements in diet and exercise, taking supplements such as vitamin B6 and in some cases taking natural progesterone.
- **Inner Ear Disturbances.** Panic attacks seem to be associated with a disturbance in balance caused by swelling of the inner ear (due to infection, allergy, meniere's syndrome, or other problems). Symptoms including dizziness, light-headiness are a prominent part of the problem manifesting anxiety or panic.

Medical Conditions that can cause panic attacks or generalized anxiety disorder

Sometimes panic reactions or anxiety can arise from medical conditions that are separate from recognized anxiety disorders.

Hyperthyroidism and hypoglycemia for example, can cause panic attacks that are by all appearances identical to those seen in panic disorder. A calcium or magnesium deficiency or an allergy to certain food additives can also produce panic anxiety. When these conditions re corrected the anxiety disappears. The following conditions are the ones most frequently seen:

- **Hyperventilation Syndrome.** Rapid, shallow breathing at the level of the chest can sometimes lead to excessive lowering of carbon dioxide in the bloodstream. This results in symptoms very similar to those of a panic attack, including light-headedness, dizziness, feelings of unreality, shortness of breath, trembling, and /or tingling in the hands, feet, or lips.

- **Hypo-glycemia.** When blood sugar levels fall to low as a result of improper diet or simply stress. When this happens, such people experience a variety of symptoms similar to panic reaction, including anxiety, shakiness, dizziness, weakness and disorientation.

- **Hyperthyroidism.** Excessive secretion of thyroid hormone can lead to heart palpitations (rapid heartbeat), sweating, and generalized anxiety. Other symptoms of hyperthyroidism include weight loss, elevated body temperature, insomnia, and bulging eyes.

Anxiety Treatments. Agroaphobia may be treated with cognitive behavioral therapy or a behavioral program "graded exposure" wherein the patient gradually and sequentially takes progressively greater steps toward and into the feared situation. The housebound patient may as a first step simply stand outside on the porch and then do that for a set amount of time everyday until the anxiety is minimal or absent. The next step would be to go to the end of the front walk, and then farther until the patient is walking around the block, then going to a local store, and so on. Such plans must be tailored to the patient's specific symptoms and the locale in which the plan is to be implemented. In some cases the presence of a therapist is required, and in others that of a friend or acquaintance, but the goal remains independent travel anywhere away from home. Most cases of agoraphobia are thought to be due to panic disorder is treated, the agoraphobia often improves with time.

Generally, panic attacks must be treated with medications before any psychotherapeutic techniques can be used. There are three old reliable in the pharmacotherapy of panic disorder: High-potency benzodiazepines, tricyclic antidepressants, and MAOI's. Benzodiazepines such as alprazolam (Xanax), clonazepam (Klonopin), and lorazepam (Ativan) are effective in stopping the panic attacks. Show the patient early that an effective treatment is available. Start with a low dosage every four hours, and increase the dosage as needed until it is clearly effective. Many patients carry benzodiazepine tablet with them and derive considerable relief from simply knowing that it is there, even if they never take it. Once the panic attacks are controlled with medication, the most effective psychotherapeutic approach is behavior therapy (desensitization or exposure). Family therapy, group therapy, hypnosis, relaxation techniques, and insight-oriented psychotherapy may also be helpful.

Chapter 10: Panic Disorder Examination Review

1. In a panic attack, the sympathetic nervous system sets aside feelings of dread or terror, racing heart, respiration that is rapid and shallow, profuse sweating, trembling and shaking after leading the patient to experience in the brain that initiate these physiological reactions

    a. Benzodiazepines
    b. Adrenaline
    c. Norepinephrine
    d. Serotonin

2. Which clinical picture consists of fear of leaving home; fear of being alone and fear of being away from home in situations in which one can feel trapped, embarrassed, or helpless?

    a. Generalized anxiety disorder (GAD)
    b. Posttraumatic stress disorder (PTSD)
    c. Agoraphobia
    d. Anorexia nervosa

3. What are reliable defenses against external dangers?

    a. Humiliated in elevators
    b. Suffocated in crowds
    c. Crushed in bus terminals
    d. All of the above

4. What happens to patient's body during a panic attack?

    a. Fight or flight response
    b. Respiration becomes rapid and shallow
    c. Trembling and shaking
    d. Cold hands and feet

5. What structure in the brain is thought to play a key role in instigating panic?

    a. Inner Ear Disturbances
    b. Amygdala
    c. Periaqueductal gray region
    d. Parabrachial nucleus

6. What are the most common antecedent stressors preceeding agoraphobia?

    a. Symptoms of hyperthyroidism
    b. Exposure to dirt in someone with an obsession about contamination
    c. Disruption of family relations
    d. Hyperactive center in temporal cerebral cortex

7. What are the most common symptoms experienced during a panic attack?

    a. Chest pain or discomfort
    b. Dyspnea
    c. Smothering sensations
    d. All of the above

8. Identify panic reactions that arise from medical conditions that are separate for recognized anxiety disorders.

    a. Excessive secretion of thyroid hormone
    b. Calcium deficiency
    c. Magnesium deficiency
    d. All of the above

9. What symptoms characterize the level of anxiety that the patient experiences in a panic attack?

    a. Ride out the frightening situation or are prevented from leaving it
    b. Avoid traveling on a bus or train
    c. Avoid toxic conditions in alcohol and drug withdrawal

    d.   History of rapid, deep respirations that respond to rebreathing in a paper bag

10. When does a patient meet the criteria for panic disorder with agoraphobia?

    a.   Fear of being in places or situations form which escape might be embarrassing

    b.   Patient restrict s travel or needs a companion when away from home

    c.   Common situations include being in a crowd standing in a line

    d.   All of the above

Chapter 10: Panic Disorders Examination   **Answers**

1. B
2. C
3. D
4. A
5. B
6. C
7. D
8. D
9. A
10. D

Chapter 11

Phobic Disorders

A phobia is a persistent and unreasonable fear of a specific object, activity, or situation that results in a compelling desire to avoid that dreaded object, activity, or situation. There are three characteristics that distinguish a phobia from ordinary, everyday fears. First, the patient is persistently afraid of the object or situation over a long period of time. Second, the fear is unreasonable, even though this recognition does not help to dispel it. Finally, what is most characteristic of a phobia is avoidance of the feared situation. The kind of objects and situations people fear, have changed during the course of history. The term "phobia" derives from the Greek phobos meaning "flight," "panic-fear," "terror," and from the diety phobos who could provoke fear and terror in one's enemies. The term phobia was not used in its own until 1801, and during the next seventy years, it slowly gained acceptance in the sense it has today. Namely, a persistent excessive fear attached to an object or a situation that objectively is not a significant source of danger (Marks, 1969). Being unreasonably afraid of something is not yet a phobia. The phobia begins when the person actually starts avoiding what is feared. What is avoided tends to vary among the different types if phobias. Invariably the person recognizes that his or her fear is excessive or unreasonable, but is powerless to change, even though the individual may occasionally endure the phobic stimulus when experiencing intense anxiety. Exposure to the phobic stimulus produces stimulus produces symptoms that include palpitations, sweating, dizziness and difficulty breathing. In fact, these symptoms may occur in response to the individual's merely thinking about the phobic stimulus. We have already alluded to the psychoanalytic formulation of phobic disorders. Despite much controversy over Freud's views, our modern understanding of social and specific phobias is influenced by psychoanalytic theory. What is avoided tends to vary among the different types of phobia. In this chapter we discuss two major phobic disorders, social phobia and specific phobias.

Social Phobia is an excessive fear of situations in which a person might do something embarrassing or be evaluated negatively by others. The individual has extreme concerns about being exposed to possible scrutiny by concerns about being exposed to passible scrutiny by others and fears social or performance situations in which embarrassment may occur. In some instances, the fear may be quite defined, such as the fear of speaking or eating in a public restroom, or fear or writing in the presence of others. In other cases, the social phobia may involve general social situations, such as saying things or answering questions I a manner that would provoke laughter on the part of others. Impairment interferes with social or occupational functioning, or causes marked distress. The DSM-IV-TR diagnostic criteria for social phobia are presented in Table 11-1.

Table 11-1. DSM-IV-TR. Diagnostic Criteria for Social Phobia

A. A marked and persistent fear of one or more social or performance situation in which the person is exposed to unfamiliar people or to possible scrutiny by others. The individual fears that he or she will act in a way (or show anxiety symptoms) that will be humiliating or embarrassing.

B. Exposure to the feared social situation almost invariably provoke anxiety, which may take form of a situationally bound or situationally predisposed panic attack.

C. The person recognizes that the fear is excessive or unreasonable.

D. The feared social or performance situations are avoided or else are endured with intense anxiety or distress.

E. The avoidance, anxious anticipation, or distress in the feared social situations interferes significantly with the person's normal routine, occupational (academic) functioning, or social activities or relationships, or there is marked distress about having the phobia.

F. In individuals under age 18 years, the duration is at least 6 months.

G. The fear or avoidance is not due to the direct physiological effects of a substance (e.g., panic disorder with or without agoraphobia, separation anxiety disorder, body dysmorphic disorder, pervasive developmental disorders, or schizoid personality disorder).

H. If a general medical condition or another mental disorder is present the fear in criterion A is unrelated to it, e.g., the fear is not of stuttering, trembling in Parkinson's disease, or exhibiting abnormal eating behavior in anorexia nervosa or bulimia nervosa.

Vignette

A 40 year old woman gave a 3 year history of avoiding social gathering of any kind. She had even given up going to her neighborhood church, where she had once been active participant in many church functions. Her fear of social or performance situations in which, she is exposed to possible scrutiny by others. She even fears that she will be humiliated or embarrassed. When asked about her reluctance to socialize, the patient gave this explanation: "Well, it's hard to explain, Doctor. I get embarrassed around people and a little scared. I don't think I trust them. "In the interview she recognizes that this fear is excessive or unreasonable. That is why in these situations, she constantly experiences symptoms of anxiety (e.g. palpitations, tremors, sweating, gastrointestinal discomfort, diarrhea, muscle tension, blushing, and confusion).

Discussion. A person who is phobic of certain social situations such as attending parties or giving lectures is less afraid of the situations themselves than of possible consequences of being in them. The social phobic is afraid, for example, that, in a social situation, she will make a fool of herself or ho out of control and embarrass herself. This person might feel jittery or shaky, sweat profusely, and experience any or all the uncomfortable affective and physiological symptoms of anxiety.

A phobia is a specific kind of fear. A it was first described by Hippocrates the condition is apparently quite common. A standard dictionary of psychological terms defines it as: the essential feature of this disorder is a marked, persistent, and excessive or unreasonable fear when in the presence of, or when anticipating an encounter with, a specific object or situation.

In the past it was fashionable to name the various specific phobias according to the feared object. The first characteristic is observed when an individual is forced to face an object or a situation about which he is phobic. He usually experiences an unpleasant degree of anxiety. He may experience the symptoms of a person in a medical emergency: pounding heart, racing pulse, dizziness, nausea, and faintness. His mouth may become dry, and he may start to sweat profusely.

The second characteristic is a powerful wish to escape or avoid contact with the object or situation of fear. Being unreasonably afraid of something is not yet a phobia; the phobia begins when the person actually starts avoiding what is feared. This restricts his life activities. If he is unable to avoid the situation, he either overcomes the phobia or develops chronic anxiety.

The third characteristic is the ability to recognize, when not in the phobic situation, that the fears are exaggerated but, despite such realization, the inability to eliminate the fears or reduce the avoidance.

Exposure to the phobic stimulus produces overwhelming symptoms of panic, including palpitations, sweating, dizziness, and difficulty breathing. In fact, these symptoms may occur in response to the individual's merely thinking about the phobic stimulus. The DSM-IV- TR diagnostic criteria for specific phobia are presented in Table 11-2.

Among the most common specific phobia are the following:

- Animal Phobias. These can include fear and avoidance of snakes, bats, rats, spiders, bees, dogs, and other creatures.
- Acrophobia (fear of heights). Patients tend to be afraid of high floors of buildings or of finding himself atop mountains, hills, or high-level bridges. In situations the person experiences 1) Vertigo (dizziness) or 2) and urge to jump, usually experienced as some external force drawing him to the edge.
- Elevator Phobia. This involves a fear that the cables will break and the elevator will crash or a fear that the elevator will get stuck and the patient will be trapped inside.
- Airplane Phobia. This most often involves a fear that the plane will crash or that the cabin will depressurize, causing the patients to asphyxiate.
- Doctor or Dentist phobias. This can begin as a fear of painful procedures (injections, having teeth filled) conducted in a doctor's or dentist's office.
- Disease Phobia (Hypochondria). Usually this phobia involves a fear of contracting or succumbing to a specific illness, such as a heart attack or cancer.

Table 11-2. DSM-IV-TR Diagnostic Criteria for Specific Phobia

A. Marked and persistent fear that is excessive or unreasonable, cued by the presence or anticipation of a specific object or situation (e.g. flying, heights, animals, receiving and injection, seeing blood).

B. Exposure to the phobic stimulus almost invariably provokes an immediate anxiety response, which may take the form of a situational bound or situational predisposed panic attack.

C. The person recognizes that the fear is excessive or unreasonable.

D. The phobic situation(s) is avoided or else is endured with intense anxiety or distress.

E. The avoidance, anxious anticipation, or distress in the feared situation(s) interferes significantly with the person's normal routine, occupational (or academic) functioning, or social activities ro relationships, or there is marked distress about having the phobia.

F. The anxiety, panic attacks, or phobic avoidance associated with the specific object or situation are not better accounted for by another mental disorder, such as obsessive-compulsive disorder (e.g. fear of dirt in someone with an obsession about contamination), posttraumatic stress disorder (e.g., avoidance of stimuli associated with a severe stressor), separation anxiety disorder (e.g. avoidance of school), social phobia (e.g. avoidance of social situations because of fear of embarrassment), panic disorder with agoraphobia, or agoraphobia without history of panic disorder.

Vignette

A 45 year old individual experiences a marked, persistent, and excessive or unreasonable fear when in the presence of, or when anticipating an encounter with, a specific object or situation. He fears air travel because of a concern about crashing and he fears driving because of concerns about being hit by other vehicles on the road. His phobias may also involve concerns about losing control, panicking, somatic manifestations of anxiety and fear (such as increased heart rate or shortness of breath) and fainting that might occur on exposure to the feared object.

Discussion. Most people fear various objects or situations to some degree, bit according to epidemiological reports for about 5 to 10 percent of the population those fears are severe enough to be labeled "phobia," making it the most common mental disorder it the United States. Although the patient in this case recognizes that the fear is unrealistic, the fear and the avoidance interfere with daily functioning. Depersonalization may also occur. This is when some patients may be able to steer themselves to this and stay nearby. But for the most part the fear is so great that they must escape no matter how humiliating or embarrassing such behavior might be to them.

Phobia Treatment

The primary treatment is behavior therapy (for example, systematic desensitization and imaginable or in vivo flooding), but such therapy requires considerable effort and a commitment by the patient. The patient must repeatedly encounter the phobic stimulus without the possibility of avoiding it and must learn to cope with the consequent anxiety. The treatment may begin by desensitizing the patient progressively to ever more anxiety-provoking stimuli. For example, patients who are phobic about elevator may start by imagining that they are in an elevator and slowly and repeatedly imagine that the elevator is going to higher and higher floors. The imagining is then replaced by actually getting into an elevator and then gradually going to higher and higher floors. Although the disorder is common among the general population, people seldom seek treatment unless the phobia interferes with ability to function. Flooding is in vivo exposure for a prolonged period of time with a highly feared stimulus. And implosion is prolonged period of time with a highly feared stimulus. And implosion is prolonged exposure to the highly feared stimulus through images or pictures. Practice Imagery desensitization for fifteen to twenty minutes each day. Begin each practice session not with a new step but with the last step you successfully negotiated. Then go on to a new step as in Table 11-3.

Table 11-3 Basic Procedures for Imagery Desensitization

Step 1.   Spend a few minutes getting relaxed. Use progressive muscle relaxation or any other relaxation technique that works well for you. (see chapter 28)

Step 2.   Visualize yourself in a peaceful scene. This is a relaxing place you can vividly picture in your mind. Above all, it is a place where you feel safe. Spend about one minute there.

Step 3.   Visualize yourself in the first scene of your phobia hierarchy. Stay there for thirty seconds to one minute, trying to picture everything with as much vividness and detail as possible, as if you were right there. Imagine yourself acting and feeling calm and confident. If you feel little or no anxiety, proceed to the next scene up in your hierarchy.

Step 4.   If you experience 4 mild to moderate anxiety, try to stay a full thirty seconds to one minute in the scene, allowing yourself to relax into it. You can do this by breathing away and anxious sensation in your body or by repeating a calming affirmation as, "I am calm and at ease." Picture yourself handling the situation in a calm and confident manner.

Step 5.   After up to a minute of exposure, retreat from the phobic scene to your peaceful scene. Spend about one minute in your peaceful scene or long enough to get fully relaxed. Then repeat your visualization of the same phobic scene as in step 4 for thirty seconds to one minute. Keep alternating between a given phobic scene until the phobic scene loses its capacity to elicit any anxiety. Then you are ready to proceed to the next step up in you hierarchy.

Step 6.   If visualizing a particular scene causes strong anxiety, especially if you feel you're approaching panic, do not spend more than ten seconds there. Retreat immediately to your peaceful scene and stay there until you're gradually to the more difficult scenes, alternating short intervals of exposure with retreat to your peaceful scene.

Step 7.   Continue progressing up your hierarchy step-by step. Generally, it will take a minimum of two exposures to a scene to reduce your anxiety to it. Keep in mind that it's important not to go on to a more advanced step until you're fully comfortable with the preceding step.

• Refer the patient to supportive psychotherapy and family therapy to help both the patient and the patient's family to cope with any impairments, related to the phobia. Consider hypnosis as an adjunct psychotherapy. In addition, refer the patient to group therapy, especially if the members of a group have a common phobia that they can help each other overcome together.

In dry treatment, benzodiazepines, tricyclic antidepressants, and monoamine oxidase inhibitors (MAOIs) are all helpful for phobic patients, although most of the available research is on the treatment of social phobia. The patient can also take B-blockers before encountering the phobic stimulus because they are helpful for social phobia (for example, stage fright).

Chapter 11: Phobia Examination Review

1. The process of unlearning the connection between anxiety and a particular situation is known as:

    a. Sensitization
    b. Desensitization
    c. Hierarchies
    d. Regression

2. When is it nest to avoid doing as a support person?

    a. Compare the phobic with other people, especially friends or family.
    b. Pressure the phobic to do activities that advance her/him to make her/him ready.
    c. Don't psychoanalyze. Offer encouragement and support, not to tell the phobic what you think is wrong with him/her
    d. Be flexible to change the plan for each given practice session.

3. Practice a technique called imagery desensitization before navigating a phobic situation in real life. What does this involve?

    a. Visualize the experience outlined in your hierarchy rather than confronting them in real life.
    b. Recognize that feeling worse indicates regression
    c. Exposure sessions are the same as the phobic situations the patients is forced into by circumstance
    d. Make your exposure practices only on good days.

4. What is most characteristic of a phobia?

    a. Avoidance of the feared situation
    b. Fear is unreasonable
    c. Everyday fears over a long period of time
    d. All of the above

5. For every phobia, there are usually on or more parameters the patient can use to vary the intensity of exposure. Common variables include

    a. Having a support person present
    b. Proximity of an exit or way out of the situation
    c. Duration of the exposure
    d. All of the above

6. What attitudes are particularly important in increasing the patient's ability to effectively face and overcome fears?

    a. Accept the permanent status of anxiety
    b. Try to deny or run away from fears
    c. Stay grounded in the present moment
    d. Stay grounded in breathing as a process that is centered in the body rather than the mind.

7. The most common form of phobia is

    a. Photophobia
    b. Acrophobia
    c. Agoraphobia
    d. Thanatophobia

8. Sigmund Freud postulated that the defense mechanisms necessary in phobias are

    a. Repression, displacement, and avoidance
    b. Regression, condensation, and projection
    c. Regression, repression, and isolation
    d. Repression, projection, and displacement

9. The anxiety, panic attacks, or phobic avoidance associated with the specific object or situation are better accounted for by another mental disorder, such as

    a. Obsessive-compulsive disorder (e.g. fear of dirt in someone with an obsession about contamination)

    b.   Posttraumatic Stress Disorder (e.g. avoidance of stimuli associated with a sever stressor)

    c.   Social Phobia (e.g. avoidance of social situations because of fear of embarrassment)

    d.   All of the above

10. Which of the following is true regarding flooding?

    a.   There is a systematic hierarchical progression from the least anxiety provoking stimulus to the most anxiety-provoking stimulus.

    b.   The patient is exposed by images or pictures to a highly feared stimulus for a prolonged period of time.

    c.   The patient is exposed to a highly feared stimulus for a prolonged period.

    d.   Patients initially observe the therapist as he or she makes contact with the feared stimulus.

Chapter 11: Phobic Disorder Examination Answers

1. B
2. C
3. A
4. A
5. D
6. D
7. C
8. A
9. D
10. B

Chapter 12

Generalized Anxiety Disorder

Anxiety is a feeling of dread accompanied by somatic signs indicative of a hyper-active autonomic nervous system. Generalized Anxiety disorder is the main diagnostic category for prominent and chronic anxiety in the absence of panic disorder. The essential feature of this syndrome, according to DSM-IV-TR (Table 12-1) is persistent anxiety lasting 6 months. In addition, the symptoms of this type of anxiety fall within two broad categories: 1) apprehensive expectation and worry and 2) physical symptoms. Patients with GAD are constantly worried over trivial; matters, fearful, and anticipating the worst. Muscle tension, restlessness or a keyed up feeling, difficulty concentrating, insomnia, irritability, ad fatigue are typical signs of generalized anxiety disorder. Motor tension and hyper-vigilance better differentiate GAD from other anxiety states than does autonomic hyperactivity (Marten et. al.1993).

A generalized anxiety d/o may derive from a reactivation or extension of developmental fears regarding a person's capability of mastering problems and his acceptability to other people, Thus, we often see the precipitation of the disorder when a person's life has shifted in the direction if increased demands and expectations; when there is a decrease in the amount of support from significant others; or when he undergoes experiences that sharply undermine self-confidence and sense of acceptability. A generalized anxiety disorder may derive from a reactivation or extension of developmental fears regarding a person's capability of mastering problems and his acceptability to other people.

The distinction of Generalized Anxiety Disorder (GAD) is discerned from formal anxiety by specifying that in GAD the worry must be clearly excessive, pervasive, difficult to control, and associated with marked distress or impairment. The diagnosis of GAD is excluded when the anxiety or worry occurs exclusively in relation to other major Axis I disorders. Given this multitude of conditions in Table 12-1 there are some general clues that might alert the clinician to an organic cause of generalized anxiety.

Table 12-1. DSM-IV-TR Diagnostic Criteria for Generalized Anxiety Disorder

A. Excessive anxiety and worry (apprehensive expectation), occurring more days than not for at least 6 months, about a number from events or activities (such as work or school performance).

B. The person finds it difficult to control the worry.

C. The anxiety and worry associated with three (or more) of the following six symptoms (with at least some symptoms present for more days than not for the past 6 months).
    1. restlessness or feeling keyed up or on edge
    2. being easily fatigued
    3. difficulty concentrating or mind going blank
    4. irritability
    5. muscle tension
    6. sleep disturbance (difficulty falling or staying asleep, or restless unsatisfying sleep)

D. The focus of the anxiety and worry is not confined to features of an Axis I disorder, e.g., the anxiety or worry is not about having a panic attack (as in panic disorder)

Being embarrassed in public (as in social phobia), being contaminated (as in obsessive-compulsive disorder), being away from home or close relatives (as in separation anxiety disorder), gaining weight (as in anorexia nervosa), having multiple physical complaints (as in somatization disorder), or having a serious illness (as in hypo-chondriasis), and the anxiety and worry do not occur exclusively during post-traumatic stress disorder.

E. The anxiety, worry, or physical symptoms cause clinically significant distress or impairment in social, occupational, or other important areas of functioning.

F. The disturbance is not due to the direct physiological effects of a substance (e.g., a drug of abuse, a medication) or a general medical condition (e.g., hyperthyroidism) and does not occur exclusively during a mood disorder, a psychotic disorder, or a pervasive developmental disorder.

Types of GAD:

1. There are two general types of cognitive content in GAD. In the first, there has been traumatic event, involving actual injury or threat of injury or a threat to an interpersonal relationship. The most dramatic expression of this type of disorder is the "combat neurosis", characterized by preservative ideation relevant to catastrophic events in battle.
2. The second from of GAD seems to be an extension- and aggravation- of fears that a person has experienced during his early development, and takes a more chronic form.

Organic Conditions. A multitude of organic disorders can present with symptoms of generalized anxiety. Table 12-2, is only a partial list of the many organic disorders presenting with symptoms of generalized anxiety. For example, a history of exercise intolerance may pint to a cardiovascular origin of the patient's anxiety; weight loss and heat intolerance to hyperthyroidism; and excess thirst and urination to diabetes and its possible insulin-related hypoglycemic reactions (McNeil 1987).

Table 12-2. Organic Causes of Generalized Anxiety

Cardiopulmonary Angina pectoris Arrythmias Congestive heart failure Acute asthma Pulmonary embolus Mitral valve prolapse Pneumothorax	**Metabolic** Hepatic failure Hypokalemia Hypoxia Acidoses (e.g. lactic acidosis)
Endocrine Hyperthyroidism Hypoglycemia Pheochromocytoma Carcinoid Syndrome	**Drug-related** Sympathomimetics (ephedrine, terbutaline) Xanthine derivatives (caffeine, aminophylline) Thyroid preperations
Neurological Degenerative diseases (Alzheimer's, Huntington's) Partial Complex (temporal lobe) seizures Transient ischemic attacks Meniere's disease	**Drug-related cont.** Insulin (via hypoglycemia) Psychotropics (e.g. fluoxetine, tricyclics) Sedative Withdrawal (alcohol, benzodiazepines)

Biological Theories

Recent work has focused on brain circuits underlying the neurobiology of fear in humans, and on how inherited and acquired vulnerabilities in these circuits might underlie a variety of anxiety disorders. It is speculated that alterations om the structure and function of the amygdala, which are central to fer-related behaviors, may be associated with generalized anxiety.

In addition, the frontal cortex and medical temporal lobe are involved in controlling fear and anxiety, and there is evidence for heightened cortical activity and decreased basal ganglia activity in GAD, possibly accounting for the observed arousal and hyper-vigilance.

Gamma-Amino-Butyric Acid (GABA). Neurons that are sensitive to the neurotransmitter gamma-aminobutyric acid (GABA for short) functions naturally in the brain as an inhibitory neurotransmitter. GABA tends to inhibit brain activity, particularly in the limbic system, which is the brain's center for emotions. That is why GABA tranquilizers tone sown anxiety, as well as any other form of emotional arousal. What is going on the GABA system in persons who are chronically anxious? Several hypothesis have been proposed. There may be a deficiency of GABA itself, resulting in less inhibitory activity of the GABA system. The situation is quite complicated because brain activation (hence anxiety) is controlled not only by the GABA system but by the serotonin and norepinephrine systems as well. The GABA system plays a major role in the neurobiological basis of generalized anxiety. Deficient activation of the GABA system results in insufficient inhibition of limbic system structures, such as the amygdala and locus coeruleus, which contributes to all forms of anxiety.

A multitude of organic disorders can present with symptoms of generalized anxiety. Before examining this daunting list, let's look at a clinical vignette.

Vignette

A 35 year-old male accountant with no prior psychiatric history, complained that for the past 7 months he had felt "incredibly uptight." His heart raced uncomfortably, like a bird fluttering in his chest. And he had both a lump in his throat and cold clammy skin evident upon a handshake. The patient noted two problems that were bothering him: the concern that he would screw up at work, and the worry that his wife might be having an affair.

After careful interview with both the patient and his wife, no objective evidence to substantiate either concern could be found. The patient conceded that his worries ere probably unrealistic. Nevertheless, he continued to experience muscle tension, restlessness and irritability, difficulty concentrating, difficulty performing simple calculations on the job, and occasional initial insomnia. He often complained of indigestion and cramping that was accented by constipation, flatulence, and frequent urination.

Physical examination and laboratory testing (including thyroid function) were unremarkable. The patient's caffeine intake was moderate, and there was no history of amphetamine or other substance abuse. A diagnose of GAD was made.

Discussion. Rollo May (1977) notes that until the coming of Freud, the problem of anxiety lay in the provinces or philosophy and religion. During his early work Freud understood anxiety as a manifestation of a physiologically induced tension state. In later studies Freud concluded that anxiety is a symptom of an unresolved unconscious conflict between the impulses for libidinal or aggressive gratification and the ego's recognition of the external danger that could result from that gratification.

The symptoms of generalized anxiety disorder are categorized under three general areas: (1) motor tension, (2) autonomic hyperactivity, (3) hyper-arousal. Motor tension manifests itself as shakiness and may have a fine tremor of the hands. There is also an inability to relax, restlessness, and fatigue; symptoms are frequently accompanied by back and neck pain. Headaches are common, mostly presenting as pressure or tension headaches. The signs of autonomic hyperactivity include shortness of breath, palpation, sweating, dizziness, hot and cold flashes, and frequent urination. Gastrointestinal symptoms may include upset stomach, nausea, heartburn, belching, and flatulence with occasional loose bowel movements. The signs of hyper arousal include vigilance and scanning. The patient is easily started and jumpy, and loud noises or sudden movements may be particularly alarming.

This vignette together a number of sociocultural factors associated with GAD: namely, familial issues, stressful life events, refugee status, and homelessness. Patients with GAD worry excessively about life circumstances, including their health, finances, social acceptance, job performance, and marital adjustment. This worry is central to the diagnosis of GAD.

There are many organic disorders that present with symptoms of generalized anxiety; particularly when there is no previous psychiatric history. For example, a history of exercise intolerance may pint to a cardiovascular origin of the patients' anxiety; weight loss and heat tolerance to hyperthyroidism; and excess thirst and urination to diabetes and its possible insulin-related hypoglycemic reaction. (McNeil, 1987).

Current Treatment. Behavioral approaches to GAD have focused on the somatic component of the disorder (e.g. muscle tension or tremulousness). Wilson (1989) concluded that overall treatment of GAD with biofeedback and relaxation procedures has yielded distinctly modest results. However, treatment featuring a combination of relaxation training and some form of cognitive restructuring has shown positive effects. Beck (1976) advocates a rigorous cognitive behavioral approach, arguing that "anxiety neurosis" is essentially a thinking disorder in which the patient repetitively alarms himself or herself with irrational or unrealistic cognitions. Therapy is directed as substituting more realistic cognitions. Therapy is directed as substituting more realistic cognitions and adaptive behaviors for the old ones. The definitive treatment of GAD includes psychotherapy, usually behavior and cognitive therapy.

In conclusion, although there are no specific phobias associated with generalized anxiety disorder, on views responded by Aaron Beck and Gary Emery suggests that the disorder is sustained by basic fears of a broader nature than specific phobias, such as,

- Fear of losing control
- Fear of not being able to cope
- Fear of failure

- Fear of rejection or abandonment
- Fear of death and disease

Generalized anxiety disorder can be aggravated by any stressful situation that elicits these fears, such as increased demands for performance, intensified marital conflict, physical illness, or any situation that heightens perception of danger or threat.

Chapter 12: GAD Examination Review

1. What philosopher spoke of anxiety as a desire for what one dreads, a sympathetic antipathy that one fears, but what one fears, one desires?

    a. Spinoza
    b. Pascal
    c. Kierkegaard
    d. Freud

2. Which term popularized by the Americans G.M. Beard, included symptoms of exhaustion and depression admixed with may autonomic signs of anxiety?

    a. Hypochondriasis
    b. Neurasthenia
    c. Inverse agonist
    d. Holding environment

3. What are the two general types of cognitive content in generalized anxiety disorder?

    a. A traumatic event and an extension of fears
    b. Fear of losing control or fear of failure
    c. Fear of rejection or fear of abandonment
    d. Difficulty concentrating or mind going blank

4. Patients with GAD exhibit all of the following symptoms except

    a. Hyper-vigilance
    b. Tachypnea
    c. Excessive worry
    d. Increased muscle tension

5. Which of the following personality disorders is found more frequently in patients with GAD?

    a. Avoidant Personality Disorder
    b. Dependent Personality Disorder
    c. Borderline personality Disorder
    d. None of the above.

6. A patient receives diazepam 5mg pot id for his GAD. Which of his symptoms is probably most relieved by this medication?

    a. Hypersensitivity to inter-personal relationships
    b. Hyper-vigilance
    c. Ruminations
    d. Catastrophization of daily events

7. What types of sleep disturbance is associated with GAD?

    a. difficulty falling asleep
    b. difficulty staying asleep
    c. restless unsatisfying sleep
    d. all of the above

8. What timeframe does excessive anxiety and worry suffer from with GAD?

    a. More days than not for at least 6 months
    b. Occasionally for 12 months
    c. Periodic every other day for 3 months
    d. More day than not for the past 3 months

9. Organic disorders that present with symptoms of generalized anxiety EXCEPT:

    a. Cardiovascular origin with exercise intolerance
    b. Heat intolerance with hyperthyroidism
    c. Abnormal eating behavior in anorexia nervosa
    d. Excess thirst and urination with diabetes

10. Patients with GAD exhibit all of the following symptoms EXCEPT:

    a. Hyper-vigilance
    b. Tachypnea
    c. Excessive worry
    d. Increased muscle tension

Chapter 12: GAD Examination Answers

1. C
2. B
3. A
4. B
5. D
6. B
7. D
8. A
9. C
10. B

Chapter 13

Obsessive-Compulsive Disorder (OCD)

The major anxiety disorders presented in this chapter are obsessive-compulsive disorder (OCD) because some people naturally tend to be more neat, tidy, and orderly than others. These traits can be useful in many situations, both at work and at home. However, they are carried to an extreme and disruptive degree. Obsessions are usually anxiety-provoking, whereas compulsions are usually anxiety-relieving.

Symptoms of obsession are intrusive and distressing thoughts that can include:

- Unwarranted fears about the family's safety, contamination, or neatness or symmetry
- Repetitive rituals and questions for no logical reason
- Unfounded fears about not paying bills or doing routine tasks
- Excessive concerns about blasphemous thoughts or morality
- Feat of having hurt someone or of acting out violent thoughts.

Compulsions are repeated behaviors in which they engage to rid themselves of the fears that their obsessive thought create:

- Constant washing
- Counting

- Checking of appliances or door lock
- Hoarding of useless articles
- Adjustment of household items to preserve symmetry
- Checking and rechecking of bank balances
- The need to touch or tap certain objects repeatedly or for a ritualized number of times.
- To look continually in the rear view mirror while driving to assuage anxiety about having hit somebody.

Psychoanalytical Theory. Psychoanalytical theorists propose that individuals with OCD have weak, under developed ego's for any of a variety of reasons: unsatisfactory parent-child relationship, conditional love, or provisional gratification. The psychoanalytical concept views clients with OCD as having regressed to earlier development stages of the infantile superego- the harsh exacting; punitive characteristics that now reappear as part of the psychopathology. Regression to the pre-Oedipal analsadistic phase, combined with use of specific ego defense mechanisms (isolation, undoing, displacement, reaction formation) produces the clinical symptoms of obsessions and compulsions (Sadock +Sadock, 2003).

Biological Factors. Recent brain research has identified an obsessive compulsive disorder neurocircuit in the brain involving three brain structures: the orbitofrontal cortex, thalamus, and caudate nucleus. There is now growing evidence that OCD involves some kind of dysregulation in the serotoergic function. When the patient worries, the orbitofrontal cortex sends a worry signal to the thalamus, which in turn sends the signal back (via the caudate) to the orbitofrontal cortex for interpretation.

Finally, there is some intriguing but preliminary evidence implicating hormonal factors in OCD (Rasmussen and Eisen, 1990). Thus, it is not uncommon to see OCD symptoms in late pregnancy or following childbirth. And about 60% of female OCD patients report that their symptoms worsen around their menstrual period. Interestingly, there has been at least one report that anti-androgen therapy in males improves OCD symptoms (Casas et al. 1986).

Table 13-1. DSM-IV-TR diagnostic criteria for obsessive compulsive disorder

A. Either obsessions or compulsions:

1. Recurrent and persistent thoughts, impulses, or images that are experienced, at some time during the disturbance, as intrusive and inappropriate and that cuse marked anxiety or distress
2. The thoughts, impulses, or images are not simply excessive worries about real-life problems
3. The person attempts to ignore or suppress such thoughts, impulses, images, or a to neutralize them with some other thought or action
4. The person recognizes that the obsession thoughts, impulses, or images are a product of his or her own mind (not imposed from without as n thought insertion)

Compulsions defined by (1) and (2):

1. Repetitive behaviors (e.g. hand washing, ordering, checking) or mental acts (e.g. praying, counting, repeating words silently) that the person feels driven to perform in response to an obsession, or accordance to rules that must be applied rigidly.
2. The behaviors or mental acts are aimed at preventing or reducing distress or preventing some dreaded event or situation; however, these behaviors or mental cts wither are not connected in a realistic way with what they are designed to neutralize or prevent or are clearly excessive.

B. At some point during the course of the disorder, the person has recognized that the obsessions or compulsion are excessive or unreasonable.
C. The obsessions or compulsions cause marked distress, are time consuming (take more than 1 hour a day), or significantly interfere with the person's normal routine, occupational (or academic) functioning, or usual social activities or relationships.

D. If another Axis I disorder is present, the content of the obsession or compulsions is not restricted to it (e.g. preoccupation with food in the presence of an eating disorder; hair pulling in the presence of trichotillomania; concern with appearance in the presence of body dysmorphic disorder; preoccupation with drugs in the presence of a substance use disorder; preoccupation with having a serious illness in the presence of hypochondriasis; preoccupation with sexual urges or fantasies int e presence of a paraphilia; or guilty ruminations in the presence of major depressive disorder).

E. The disturbance is not due to the direct physiological effects of a substance (e.g. a drug abuse, a medication) or a general medical condition.

Diagnosis. The DSM-IV-TR definition and criteria for OCD are presented in Table 13-1.

The differential diagnosis of OCD also includes the following conditions: (1) major depressive episode with "obsessive brooding"; (2) other anxiety disorders, in which rumination is common; (3) Tourette's disorder, in which "mental coprolalia" may be present (sudden, intrusive, senseless thoughts of obscene words that are not fought or suppressed); (4) various impulse control disorders such as kleptomania, pathological gambling, or trichotillomania; (5) eating disorders such as bulimia or anorexia nervosa in which rituals are common; and (6) idiosyncratic rituals/ habits that fall short of OCD criteria.

VIGNETTE

A 50 year old veteran presented with repetitive behaviors (e.g. hand washing, ordering and checking) and mental acts (e.g. Praying, counting, repeating words silently) the goal of which is to prevent r reduce anxiety of distress, not to provide pleasure gratification. He feels driven to perform the compulsion to reduce the distress that accompanies these obsessions or to prevent some dreaded event or situation. His obsessions about being contaminated reduce his mental distress by washing his hands until his skin is raw.

OCD appears to be more common in first-degree relatives of Tourette's patient's than in the general population. This patient usually shows multiple motor or vocal tics, such as grunts, sniffs, or coughs. His history demonstrates impulse control disorders such as pathological gambling or kleptomania, where there is a compulsive quality to his life. In the evaluation of an eating disorder the patient's history also relates peculiar preoccupations such as constantly thinking about food, cutting it up into tiny pieces and hoarding it.

Discussion. This case is fairly typical for OCD. He experienced recurrent, intrusive, illogical thoughts that he recognized as his own, and not broadcast to him from some external source. He felt compelled to act in order to neutralize these thoughts, and when unable to do so, he would experience intense discomfort. Nonetheless, he derived no real pleasure from the performance of his ritualized checking behavior. (Insel, 1990).

Discussion. In the history of OCD Insel (1990) describes four major symptom patterns. The most common pattern is an obsession of contamination, followed by washing or accompanied by compulsive avoidance of the presumably contaminated object. The feared object is often hard to avoid (e.g. feces, urine, dust, or germs). Patients may literally rub the skin off their hands but excessive hand washing or may be unable to leave their homes because of fear of germs. In addition, patients usually believe that the contamination is spread from object to object or person to person by the slightest contact.

The second most common pattern is an obsession of doubt, followed by a compulsion of checking. The obsession often implies some danger of violence (e.g. forgetting to turn off the stove or not locking a door). The checking may involve multiple trips back into the house to check the stove, for example.

In the third most common pattern there are intrusive obsessional thoughts of a sexual to aggressive act that is significant that patients with these thoughts may report themselves to police or confess to a priest. The fourth most common pattern is the need for symmetry or precision, which can lead to a compulsion of slowness. Patients can literally take hours to eat a meal or shave their face.

Treatment. Behavior Therapy is considered by many as the treatment of choice (Greist 1990). Exposure and response prevention are the main behavioral treatments. Patients are asked to make contact with or to imagine their anxiety or ritual-provoking stimuli. For example, a patient obsessed with being contaminated by germs might be instructed to touch a toilet seat (exposure). The patient is also instructed to forgo the usual ritual associated with exposure—in this case, for example, hand washing.

Obsession thoughts not associated with rituals may be more refractory to treatment. One technique, called saturation, requires the patient to focus exclusively on the obsessional thought for 10 to 15 minutes. This seems to result in diminished attention to the obsessional thought (Nemiah 1985). Thought stopping-a technique in which the patient learns to interrupt obsession thoughts by hearing the word "stop!"----May also be helpful in mild cases.

Behavior therapy is thought to be the treatment of choice for obsessive-compulsive disorder. It is successful in 60 to 75 percent of all patients. Possible behavioral therapeutic choices include in vivo exposure (flooding), desensitization, thought stopping, implosion therapy, and aversive conditioning. Behavior therapy requires considerable commitment by the patient. Often, the patient is forcibly prevented from carrying out the compulsive act and learns that the consequent anxiety or panic with eventually lessens. Some clinicians use insight- oriented psychotherapy for OCD bu usually in combination with medication. Clomipramine (Anafranil), fluvoxamine (Luvox), and fluoxetine (Prozac) are potent inhibitors of serotonin reuptake and are drugs of first choice. If the patient comes to the emergency room or doctor's office in an acutely anxious state, a benzodiazepine is administered every four hours as needed to reduce the acute anxiety.

Chapter 13 Obsessive- Compulsive Disorder (OCD) Self- Examination Review

1. Recent brain research has identified an OCD nuero-circuit in the brain involving which structures?

   a. Orbitofrontal cortex
   b. Thalamus
   c. Caudate nucleus
   d. All of the above

2. Which medications should be administered in the emergency room to help reduce the acute anxiety?

   a. Benzodiazepines
   b. Tricyclic antidepressants
   c. Beta-blockers
   d. Anticholinergic drugs

3. Some OCD patients are given this label because they are unable to throw anything out for fear that they might someday need something they discarded.

   a. Pyromania
   b. Hoarders
   c. Kleptomania
   d. Somnambulism

4. Recent brain research has identified an obsessive compulsive disorder neuro-circuit in the brain involving which brain structures?

   a. The orbitofrontal cortex
   b. The thalamus
   c. The caudate nucleus
   d. All of the above

5. Obsession are

   a. Intrusive thoughts or impulses
   b. Anxious thoughts
   c. Fears of heights
   d. Psychotic symptoms

6. Anxiety is a common symptom of all of the following illnesses except:

   a. Hypoglycemia
   b. Hyperparathyroidism
   c. Pheochromopcytoma
   d. Porphyria

7. A 35 year-old man with an obsessive- compulsive personality disorder is likely to exhibit all of the following symptoms except:

   a. Perfectionism that interferes with performance
   b. Compulsive checking behavior
   c. Preoccupation and concern for rules
   d. Stinginess with compliments

8. Which of the following disorders is thought to be especially related to obsessive-compulsive disorder?

   a. Somatization disorder
   b. Conversion disorder
   c. Body dysmorphic disorder
   d. Factitious disorder

9. In what way is ti important to remember that the obsessive –compulsive disorder is a different illness from the obsessive-compulsive personality disorder?

   a. They exhibit compulsive checking
   b. They exhibit excessive washing

c. Individuals with personality disorder have perfectionistic and inflexible personalities
d. Individuals with personality disorder are preoccupied by trivial details

10. What axis I disorder is present when the content of the obsessions or compulsion is not restricted to it?

    a. Preoccupation with food in the presence of an eating disorder
    b. Hair pulling in the presence of trichotillomania
    c. Concern with appearance in the presence of body dysmorphic disorder
    d. All of the above.

Chapter 13 OCD Answers

1. D
2. A
3. B
4. D
5. A
6. B
7. B
8. C
9. C
10. D

Chapter 14

Post-Traumatic Stress Disorder (PTSD)

This chapter is irate about the treatment of our soldiers who come home with a diagnosis of post-traumatic stress disorder, commonly referred to as PTSD. It is described by the DSM-5 as the development of characteristic symptoms following exposure to an extreme traumatic stressor involving a personal threat to physical integrity or to the physical integrity of others. The typical term before PTSD was "shell shock," and it was only considered as a weakness in soldiers.

Because of the presence of autonomic cardiac symptoms, "soldier's heart" was the name given by the Da Costa, during the U.S. Civil War to a syndrome similar to PTSD. In the 1900's the influence psycho-analysis was strong and clinicians applied the diagnosis of "traumatic neurosis" to the condition. In World War I, the syndrome was called "shell shock" and was hypothesized to result from chronic anxiety, nightmares, and flashbacks for weeks, months, or even years following combat. Later, during World War II veterans, survivors from Nazi concentration camps, and survivors of the atomic bombing had similar symptoms, sometimes called "combat neurosis," or "operational fatigue." In war time situations, for example, certain experiences are highly linked to the development of PTSD; witnessing atrocities or participating in atrocities.

Combat stress during World War II and in the post war period asked: What constituted a neurotic breakdown among WWII military? Perhaps the most clinical description of men who became victims is offered by Swank "1949"; who studied more than 4,000 cases of combat exhaustion was persistent fatigue. This was soon followed by the common symptoms of anxiety and tendency to exclusiveness and a fear of crowds. In some, combat veterans the mere site of an army jacket are capable of serving as the conditioned stimulus for panic type symptoms. That is why they avoided anything new or different; many feared the possibility of leaving or losing buddies. All patients exhibited emotional tension. Emotional displays of crying, laughing, pugnaciousness, or moodiness worry common appearing to act as a safety valve for the patient's tension.

Research in the 1970's shifted away from veterans of WWII to psychiatric casualties of Vietnam. The psychiatric morbidity associated with Vietnam Veterans finally brought the concept of PTSD as it is currently known as fruition. Post-traumatic stress disorder was therefore included in DSM-III as a separate diagnostic category. During this phase troops deployed to Afghanistan as part of Operation Enduring Freedom.

The diagnostic category of PTSD did not appear until the third edition of the Diagnostic and Statistical manual of Mental Disorders (DSM-III) in 1980' after a need was indicated by increasing numbers of problems with Vietnam veterans and victims of multiple disasters.

DSM-IV also stipulates that the person's response to the event involved intense fear helplessness, or horror. This based on Frued's postulated to broad responses to trauma: (1) attempts to remember of repeat the trauma and (2) attempts to avoid or fend off such memories and repetitions. Both mechanisms may be involved in the development of PTSD. Then Horrowitz(1985) pointed out that the response to trauma often occurs in phases. The immediate response to disaster is usually an outcry for help. There follows a denial phase which the individual may feel dazed, sometimes showing selective amnesia for the trauma. Then an intrusive phase ensues which the trauma victim may experience startle reactions, flashbacks, insomnia, and autonomic-hyperactivity. Finally, a process of working through the situations allows the victim to complete the phase of trauma.

Emotions such as fear play essential roles in our lives and are present as the deepest instinctual response to potential danger. These instinctual reactions are rooted deep inside the brain and serve to protect us. When a person senses fear, the brain reacts by activating two systems: the sympathetic system to alert the body and the parasympathetic system to restore and heal. When the sympathetic system is aroused, certain areas of the brain, called the amygdala and hypothalamus, become activated and biochemical, such as adrenaline and a stress hormone, cortisol, are released into the bloodstream.

Researchers believed that when a person experiences a threatening situation, the brain produces cortisol, a stress hormone that tells the victim to fight or run away. Over the years, researchers have studied PTSD to try to understand the underlying rain processes. Cortisol is known as the "fight or flight" hormone. Research has shown higher levels of cortisol may actually hurt the brain and be linked to PTSD symptoms.

In addition, fear triggers a rage response. Rage is a common reaction in those with PTSD, especially the soldiers because it is a behavior to defend oneself. Rage is an irrational attempt to relieve fear by attacking someone else or it can be effective in a battle situation.

The Science Behind PTSD

We now have evidence that PTSD is a complex medical condition, not just and emotional disorder. This new approach to PTSD results from advances in brain science. With the advent of new technology in the way of brain scans and micro-neural approaches, we now have unprecedented access to what is going on underneath our skulls. PTSD often includes biological damage along with the psychological trauma (Heim and Nemeroff, 2009).

For PTSD victim, the frontal lobes, which control the executive functioning of the brain (planning and organizing), and the temporal lobes, which handle memory and emotion, are both extremely inactive, almost asleep. Essentially, all these areas have shut down. This explains why a person with PTSD commonly experiences no joy and has a very short memory, little planning or executive power, and poor judgment. While the front of the brain is in slowest gear, the motor areas are going haywire. The motor areas of the brain are those associated with coordinating the active parts of our bodies (the limbs, the eyes, etc.). In this state, they are overly reactive. That explains why a person with PTSD might suddenly drop down on his belly or start running when he hears a loud sound similar to gunfire or an explosion. There is also no relaxation and usually no restoration stage in a brain showing the pattern. Many of those with PTSD have suffered brain damage. The most common form is called post-conclusive syndrome, which can be caused by direct blows to the head and even heavy sound blasts at a distance. This happens because a very loud noise can actually cause mild to moderate brain damage. The strong sound waves continue to cause inflammation in the brain and may cause the immune system to back fire, creating more damage as the signal of cell injury reverberate through the body.

Table 14-1. DSM-5- Diagnostic Criteria for PTSD

A. The person exposed to a traumatic event in which both of the following were present:

1. The person experienced, witnessed, or was confronted with an event or events that involved actual or threatened death or serious injury, a threat to the physical integrity of self to others.

2. The person's response involved intense fear, helplessness, or horror.

B. The traumatic event is persistently re-experiencing in one (or more) of the following ways:

1. Recurrent and intrusive distressing recollections of the event, including images, thoughts, or perceptions.
2. Recurrent distressing dreams of the event
3. Acting or feeling as if the traumatic event were recurring (includes a sense of reliving the experience, illusions, hallucinations, and dissociative flashback episodes, including those that occur on awakening or when intoxicated).
4. Intense psychological distress at exposure to internal or external cues that symbolize or resemble an aspect of the traumatic event.
5. Physiological reactivity on exposure to internal or external cues that symbolize or resemble an aspect of the traumatic event.

C. Persistent avoidance of stimuli associated with the trauma and numbing of general responsiveness (not present before the trauma), as indicated by three (or more) of the following:

1. Efforts to avoid thoughts, feelings, or conversations associated with trauma
2. Efforts to avoid activities, places, or people that arouse recollections of the trauma
3. Inability to recall an important aspect of the trauma
4. Markedly diminished interest or participation in significant activities
5. Feeling of detachment or estrangement from others
6. Restricted range of affect (e.g. unable to have loving feelings)

D. Persistent symptoms of increased arousal, as indicated by two (or more) of the following:

1. Difficulty falling asleep or staying asleep
2. Irritability concentrating
3. Difficulty concentrating
4. Hyper-vigilance
5. Exaggerated startle response

VIGNETTE

A 35 year old male, a Vietnam veteran presented in the ER with marked anxiety, agitation, and irritability. He gave a 15 year history of moderate anxiety and depression, sometimes accompanied by insomnia and feelings of estrangement from others. These symptoms followed a tour of duty in which the patient had seen "six of my buddies blown away." The patient said to the nurse, "I can't figure out why God took my buddies instead of me." Nighttime was the most difficult. Night after night his wife lay awake to the sound of the patient crying and calling out in a shrieking voice for whom she assumed were his war buddies. She suspected he was grieving over their deaths. She also heard shouting and screaming as the nightmares victimized his sleep. His wife was witnessing the destruction of her husband's mental capacities on a day-by-day basis. This was agonizing for both of them and was having a profound effect on their children as well. His wife was growing increasingly afraid for her children's lives and her own life. She had good reason. On six different occasions, he came into her room screaming with a knife in hand and plunged it into the mattress as she slept. Then he would awake from his nightmare to find his wife trembling under his hand. He would apologize and withdraw again to his space at the back of the house. Both of them feared that one night the blade would not miss her.

In psychotherapy, it was explained to him that the horrible events he lived through caused his problems, the memories did not match up with emotions. The problem with psychotherapy is that many people with PTSD are not ready to explore painful times again. The experience was so counter to everything he had ever coped with, and he could not create any psychological mechanism to understand it. The only wy to find relief was to withdraw and drink beer. He thus tried to block it from his mind and deny the experience, yet the emotional shame and terror remained.

Discussion. One psychosocial model that has become widely accepted seeks to explain why certain persons exposed to massive trauma develop PTSD and others do not. Variables include characteristics that relate to (1) the traumatic experience, (2) the individual, and (3) the recovery environment.

The traumatic experience. Specific characteristics relating to the trauma have been identified as crucial elements in the determination of an individual's long-term response to stress. They include:

- Severity and duration preparation for the stressor
- Degree of anticipatory preparation for the event
- Exposure to death
- Numbers affected by life threat
- Amount of control over recurrence
- Location where the trauma was experienced (e.g. familiar surroundings, at home, in a foreign country).

The individual. Variables that are considered important in determining an individual's response to trauma include:

- Degree of ego strength
- Effectiveness of coping resources
- Presence of pre-existing psychopathology
- Outcomes of previous experiences with stress/trauma
- Current psychosocial developmental stage
- Demographic factors (e.g. age, socioeconomic status, education)

The recovery environment. The quality of the environment in which the individual attempts to work through the traumatic experiences is correlated with the outcome. Environmental variables include:

- Availability of social supports
- The cohesiveness and protectiveness of family and friends
- The attitudes of society regarding the experience
- Cultural and subcultural influences

The Hyperbaric Experience

The hyperbaric chamber treatment can revitalize portions of the biologically damaged brain and is one of the most effective treatments for PTSD. It is a very powerful tool in regenerating damaged areas of the brain. The simplest way to explain what the hyperbaric chamber does for this victim is that is uses pressure to infuse a high concentration of oxygen into the body. With this high level of oxygenation, the healing rate is drastically increased. During the continuation of the hyperbaric chamber experience, there are usually a long series of deep sleep periods during which the patient is gaining huge strides toward a more complete biological and psychological health.

Exercise. Another method of reconnecting brain and taking control is through exercise. Research has shown that exercise can be just as therapeutic as psychotherapy. There are many good reasons why these results are true, including the improved breathing that comes from exerting effort every day. With exercise, breathing is more deeply and brain to coordinate healing mechanisms. Just as physical exercise generates strength in various parts of the body, mental exercises build strength in the exercised parts of the brain.

Clinical Features and Diagnosis

A mixture of the following symptoms are present initially:

- Marked anxiety
- Personality change with irritability and poor concentration
- An exaggerated startle response
- Insomnia and nightmares
- Intrusive thoughts of the event
- Relieving the feelings experienced at the time
- Avoidance of anything associated with the trauma
- Emotional blunting which can impair interpersonal relationships and day to day functioning.

The full symptoms picture must be present for more than 1 month and cause significant interference with social, occupational, and other areas of functioning. Symptoms may begin within the first 3 months after the trauma, or there may be a delay of several months or even years. Compare this with symptoms that have not been present for more than 1 month, when the diagnosis assigned is acute stress disorder (APA, 2013).

Treatment is a collaborative effort between client and therapist. Treatment options currently available for PTSD:

The most common effective treatment involves a combination of talk therapy and psychotropic medications, such as anti-anxiety and antidepressant medications. With information about CRF (corticotropin-releasing factor) and PTSD symptoms, researchers are trying to develop medications that incorporate these findings. Research involves taking an investigational drug intended to change CRF levels; thereby, reducing the severity of the symptoms of PTSD.

Cognitive therapy strives to assist the individual to reduce anxiety responses by altering cognitive distortions. Anxiety id described as being the result of exaggerated, automatic thinking. Cognitive therapy for anxiety is brief and time limited, usually lasting form 5 to 20 sessions. Brief therapy discourages the client's dependency on the therapist, which prevalent in anxiety disorders, and encourages the client's self-sufficiency. A sound therapeutic relationships is a necessary condition for effective cognitive therapy. The client must be able to talk openly about fears and feelings for the therapeutic process to occur. A major part of treatment consist of encouraging the client to face frightening situations to be able to view them realistically, and talking about them is one way of achieving this.

Cognitive therapy is very structured and orderly, which is important for the anxious client who is often confused and lacks self-assurance. The focus is on solving current problems. Rather than offering suggestions and explanations, the therapist uses questions to encourage the client to correct his or her anxiety-producing thoughts (see BOX 14-1). Together, the client and therapist work to identify and correct maladaptive thoughts and behaviors that maintain a problem and block its solution. The client is encouraged to become aware of the thoughts, examine them for cognitive distortions, substitute more balanced thoughts, and eventually develop new patterns of thinking.

BOX 14-1. Evaluation of the client with PTSD may be facilitated by gathering information using the following types of questions:

- Can the client discuss the traumatic event without experiencing pain anxiety?
- Does the client voluntarily discuss the traumatic event?
- Can't he client discuss changes that have occurred in his or her life because of the traumatic event?
- Does the client have flashbacks?
- Can the client sleep without medication?
- Does the client have nightmares?
- Has the client learned strategies for assistance with recovery?
- Can the client demonstrate successful use of these new coping strategies in times of stress?
- Can the client verbalize stages of grief and the normal behaviors associated with each?
- Can the client recognize his or her own position in the grieving process?
- Is guilt being alleviated?
- Has the client maintained or regained satisfactory relationships with significant others?
- Can the client look to the future with optimism?
- Does the client attend a regular support group for victims of similar traumatic experiences?
- Does the client have a plan of action for dealing with symptoms, if they return?

Behavior Therapy. Two common forms of behavior therapy include systematic desensitization and implosion therapy (flooding). They are commonly used to treat clients with phobic disorders and to modify stereotyped behavior of clients with PTSD.

In systematic desensitization the client is gradually exposed to the phobic stimulus, either in a real or imagined situation. The concept was introduced by Joseph Wolpe in 1958, and is based on behavioral conditioning principles. It involves two main elements:

1. Training in relaxation techniques
2. Progressive exposure to a hierarchy of fear stimuli while in the relaxed state.

The individual is instructed in the art of relaxation using techniques most effective for him or her (e.g. progressive relaxation, mental imagery, tense and relax, meditation). When the individual has mastered the relaxation technique, exposure to the phobic stimulus is initiated. He or she is asked to present a hierarchal arrangement of situations pertaining to the phobic stimulus in order ranging from most to least disturbing.

Implosion therapy, or flooding, is a therapeutic process in which the client must imagine situations or participate in real-life situations that he or she finds extremely frightening, for a prolonged period of time. Relaxation training is not a part of this technique. In flooding, the therapist floods the client with information concerning situations that trigger anxiety in him or her. The therapist describes anxiety-provoking situations in vivid detail and is guided by the client's response. The more anxiety provoked, the more expedient is the therapeutic endeavor.

With continuous and regular contact with an interested, sympathetic, and encouraging professional person, patients may eb able to function by virtue of this help, without which their symptoms would incapacitate them. Psycho-therapeutic approaches in post-traumatic stress disorder includes: cognitive therapy, behavior therapy, all within an emphasis on short-term treatment.

Psychoactive Agents. Start drug treatment only in the context of an ongoing therapeutic relationship. Although these medications have been approved by the FDA for treatment of PTSD, many believe they are contributing to the problem rather than helping it. The labels of these medications warn of s significant risk of suicide. Should we then be surprised that two out of every five veterans who commit suicide were taking these medications? The bottom line: in some cases medication is not the answer.

Antihypertensive Drugs. Several studies have called attention to the effectiveness of beta-blockers and alpha 2 –receptor agonists in the amelioration of anxiety symptoms. The beta-blockers have been tried with success in clients experiencing anticipatory performance anxiety or stage fright. This type of phobic response produces symptoms such as sweaty palms, racing pulse, trembling hands, dry mouth, labored breathing, nausea, and memory loss. The beta-blockers appear to be quite effective in reducing t these symptoms in some individuals. The beta-blockers have been successful in alleviating some of the symptoms associated with PTSD. In clinical trials, marked reductions in nightmares, intrusive recollections, hyper vigilance, insomnia, startle responses, and angry outburst were reported with the use of these drugs. They suggest that these drugs should be reserved for the short-term control of severe aggression and agitation.

Anxiolytics. The benzodiazepines have been successful in the treatment of social phobia. Controlled studies have shown their efficacy in reducing symptoms of social anxiety. They are well tolerated and have a rapid onset of action. However, because of their potential are not considered first-line choice of treatment for social phobia.

Drugs
Opioids, including endogenous opioid peptides, have the following psychoactive properties:
- Tranquilizing action
- Reduction of rage/aggression
- Reduction of feelings of inadequacy

- Antidepressant action

These studies suggest that physiological arousal initiated by re-exposure to trauma-like situations enhances production of endogenous opioid peptides and results in increased feelings of comfort and control. When the stressor terminates, the individual may experience opioid withdrawal, the symptoms of which bear strong resemblance to those of PTSD.

Gum

An extremely simple exercise we are encouraged to consider is chewing gum for a few minutes before bedtime. It may sound like a basic action, but believe it or not, the research done on chewing gum to relieve stress is pretty impressive. The act of chewing gum pumps healing blood into the frontal lobe, whre executive functions are controlled, and into the temporal lobe, where stressful emotions are found. There is clear evidence that stress is reduced by as much as 50 percent by chewing gum, and the patient may gain some IQ points during the process.

Researchers at the Michael E. Debakey VA Medical Center (MEDVAMC) an Baylor College of Medicine are currently looking for female Veterans with Post-traumatic Stress Disorder (PTSD) who are interested in participating in a study examining the role a neuropeptide called corticotropin-releasing factor (CRF) plays in causing PTSD symptoms. Researchers believed that when a person experiences a threatening situation, the brain produces cortisol, a stress hormone that tells the victim to fight or run away. These studies have shown higher levels of cortisol may actually hurt the brain and be linked to PRSD symptoms.

We hope that everyone who treats the victims of PTSD- the war wounded, military veterans, patients who have been assaulted or injured, and those who have lived through a natural or personal disaster- will read this chapter and put it to use in their lives. There are daunting number of veterans with PTSD in this nation, with more than eight hundred thousand diagnosed and countless others who have not sought help as thousands of soldiers continue to return home from war.

Chapter 14: Post-Traumatic Stress Disorder (PTSD) Examination Review

1. Identify a therapeutic process in which the client must imagine situations or participate in real-life situations that he or she finds extremely frightening for a prolonged period of time.

    a. Cognitive therapy
    b. Implosion therapy (flooding)
    c. Reciprocal Inhibition
    d. Systematic desensitization

2. In what form of behavior therapy is the client gradually exposed to the phobic stimulus, either in a real or imagined situation?

    a. Cognitive therapy
    b. Hypnosis
    c. Systematic desensitization
    d. Biofeedback

3. Which of the following statements are true regarding pharmacotherapy in the treatment of PTSD?

    a. pharmacotherapy should be instituted immediately
    b. Pharmacotherapy alone is sufficient treatment of PTSD
    c. A 4-week trial of tricyclic antidepressant or SSRI therapy is required to assess the effectiveness of treatment
    d. Pharmacotherapy may be continued for years

4. What techniques repracticed when a therapist or support person helps the patient confront fearful situations that should be avoided because they trigger strong anxiety?

    a. Relaxation training
    b. Exposure therapy
    c. Cognitive therapy
    d. Hypnotherapy

5. Which of the following therapy regimens are most appropriate for a patient with PTSD?

    a. Paroxetine and group therapy
    b. Diazepam and implosion therapy
    c. Alprazolam and behavior therapy
    d. Carbamazepine and cognitive therapy

6. When is acute stress disorder distinguished form PTSD?

    a. When it occurs to a duration of 3 days to 1 month following exposure to the traumatic event
    b. When the symptom pattern is restricted to 6 months following the traumatic event
    c. When symptoms of PTSD are absent
    d. When flashbacks in PTSD can distinguished from acute stress disorder

7. What distinguished flashbacks in PTSD form illusions and hallucinations or other psychotic disorders?

    a. Intrusive recollections in PTSD are distinguished form depressive rumination in that they apply only to involuntary and intrusive distressing memories
    b. Recurrent memories occur in schizophrenia but not in PTSD
    c. Dissociative states that last form a few seconds to several hours in PTSD but not in brief psychotic disorder
    d. Negative alterations in cognitions or mood associated with the event exposure to the event occur in bipolar disorder but not in PTSD

8. What techniques are helpful in enabling PTSD victims to retrieve and work through memories for the original traumatic incident?

    a. Cognitive therapy
    b. Eye-movement desensitization and reprocessing
    c. Relaxation training
    d. Exposure therapy

9. What percentage of the general population exhibit the full symptomatology pattern of post-traumatic stress disorder (PTSD)?

   a. 1%
   b. 5%
   c. 9%
   d. 15%

10. If alcohol or drug abuse is suspected, what drugs should be avoided in the treatment of PTSD?

    a. Benzodiazepines and MAOIs
    b. Tricyclic antidepressants
    c. SSRI medications
    d. Heterocyclic compounds

Chapter 14: PTSD Examination Answers

1. B
2. C
3. D
4. B
5. A
6. A
7. A
8. B
9. C
10. A

Reference Section-3

American Psychiatric Association: Diagnostic and Statistical Manual of Mental Disorders, 4th Edition. Washington, DC, American Psychiatric Association, 2000.

Amies PL, Gelder MG, and Shaw PM. Social Phobia: A comparative Clinical Study, British Journal of Psychiatry 142:174-79, 1983.

Andreasen NC, Black DW. Introductory Textbook of Psychiatry, 4th Edition. American Psychiatric Publishing, 2006.

Andreasen NC. Posttraumatic Stress Disorder, in Comprehensive Textbook of Psychiatry/ III, 3rd Edition, Vol 2, 1980.

Barlow D and Craske M. Mastery of Your Anxiety and Panic: Workbook Fourth Edition. New York: Oxford University Press, 2007.

Barlow, David H. Anxiety and It's Disorders: The Nature and Treatment of Anxiety and Panic. The Guildford Press, 2002.

Barlow DH. Current models of panic disorder and a view from emotion theory, in American Psychiatric Press Review of Psychiatry, Vol. 7. Edited by Frances AJ, Hales RE. Washington DC: American Psychiatric Press, 1988.

Beck A. and Emery g. Anxiety Disorders and Phobias: A Cognitive Perspective. Basic Books, 1985.

Beck AT. And Emery G. Cognitive Therapy of Anxiety and Phobic Disorders. Philadelphia: Center for Cognitive Therapy, 1979.

Beck AT. Cognitive Therapy and the Emotional Disorders. New York, International Universities Press, 1976.

Blanchard EB, Kolb LC, Gerardi RJ, et al. Cardiac response to relevant stimuli as an adjunctive tool for diagnosing posttraumatic stress disorder in Vietnam Veterans. Behavior Therapy 17: 592-606, 1986.

Blazer D, Hughes D, Georder LK. Stressful life events and the onset of Generalized Anxiety Syndrome. American Journal of Psychiatry 144: 1178-1183, 1987.

Bourne EJ. The Anxiety & Phobia Workbook, 5th Edition. New Harbinger Publications, Inc. 2010.

Bourne EJ. Overcoming Specific Phobia: Therapist and Client Protocols. Oakland, CA: New Harbinger Publications, 1998.

Bourne EJ. The Anxiety and Phobia Workbook: A Step-by-Step Program for Curing Yourself of Extreme Anxiety, Panic Attacks, and Phobias. Revised Second Edition. MJF Books, New York, 1995.

Carr DB, Sheehan DV. Panic Anxiety: a New Biologic Model. Journal of Clinical Psychiatry 45: 323-330, 1984.

Charney DS, Dutch AY, Krystal JH, et al. Psychobiologic Mechanisms of post-traumatic stress disorder. Archives of General Psychiatry 50: 294-305,1993.

Coupland NJ. Social Phobia: Etiology, neurobiology, and treatment. Journal of Clinical Psychiatry: 62 (Suppl): 25, 2001.

Department of Veteran Affairs HSE & D. The Assessment and Treatment of Individuals with History of Traumatic Brain Injury and Posttraumatic Stress Disorder: A systematic Review of the Evidence. August 2009.

Dobbs D and Wilson WP. Observations on persistence of war neurosis. Disease of the Nervous System 21: 686-691, 1980.

Ehlers A, Clark DM: A cognitive Model of Post-traumatic stress disorder. Behavior Research Therapy 38: 319-345, 2000.

England D. The Post-traumatic Stress Disorder Relationship. Avaon, MA: Adams Media, 2009.

First M, Frrances A, and Pincuye HA. DSM-IV Handbook of Differential Diagnosis. Washington, DC: American Psychiatric Press, 1995.

Fishman GS. Psychoanalytic psychotherapy (of anxiety disorder), In Treatments of Psychiatric of Psychiatric Disorders, Vol. 3. Washington, DC, American Psychiatric Association, 1989.

Foa EB, Keanse TM, Friedman MJ. Effective Treatments for PTSD: Practice Guidelinnes from the International Society for Traumatic Stress Studies. The Guilford Press, 2000.

Freud S (1915-1917). Introductory Lectures on Psychoanalysisis, in the Standard Edition, Vol 16. J. Strachey, trans. London: Hogarth Press, 1963.

Freud S. On the grounds for detaching a particular syndrome form neurasthenia under the description anxiety neurosis. In The Standard edition of the complete psychological works of Sigmund Freud (Vol. 3) London: Hogarth Press, 1959.

Freud S: Inhibitions, symptoms and anxiety. In Standard Edition of the Complete Psychological Works of Sigmund Freud, Vol 20. Pp. 77 Hogarth Press, London, 1966.

Fyer AJ, Mannuzzas, Gallops MS, et. Al: Familial transmission of simple phobia and fears: a preliminary report. Archives of GeneralPsychiatry 47, 1990.

Gold MS. The Good News about Panic, Anxiety and Phobias. New York: Villard Books, 1989.

Goodwin DW. Anxiety. New York: Oxford University Press, 1986.

Gorman JM, section ed. Anxiety Disorders. In: Sadock BJ, Sadock VA, eds. Kaplan+ Sadock's Comprehensive Textbook of Psychiatry, 7th ed. Vol 1. Baltimore: Lippincott Williams + Wilkins: 14-41, 2000.

Greist JH and Jefferson JW. Anxiety Disorders, in Review of General Psychiatry, 2nd Edition. Edited by Goldman HH, Norwalk CT, Appeton +Lange, 1988.

Hiem C and Nemerroff CB. Neurobiology of Post-traumatic Stress Disorder. The International Journal of Neuropsychiatric Medicine. 14(1):13-24, 2009.

Hoge CW, McGurk D, Thomas JL, et al. Mild Traumatic Brain Injury in U.S. Soldiers Returning from Iraq. The New England Journal of Medicine. 358: 453-463, 2009.

Hollifield M, Katon W, Skipper B, et al. Panic disorder and quality of life: variables predictive of functional impairment. American Journal of Psychiatry; 154: 766, 1997.

Horowitz MJ. Post-traumatic Stress Disorder, in Treatments of Psychiatric Disorders, Vol 3. Washington DC, American Psychiatric Association, 1989.

Horowitz M. Disasters and psychological responses to stress. Psychiatric Annals 15: 135-142, 1985.

Hyman BM andd Dufrene T. Coping with OCD: Practical Strategies for Living Well with Obsessive-Compulsive Disorder. Oakland, CA: New Harbinger Publications, 2008.

Insel TR. Phenomenology of obsessive Compulsive Disorder. Journal of Clinical Psychiatry 51 (No Suppl); 4-8, 1990.

Jacob RG, Turer SM: Panic Disorder: diagnosis and assessment, in American Psychiatric Press Review of Psychiatry, Vol 7. Edited by Frances AJ, Hales RE. Washington DC, American Psychiatric Press, 1988.

Jackson SW. Melancholia and Depression: From Hippocratic Times to Modern Times. New Haven, CT, Yale University Press 1986

Klein DF. Anxiety conceptualized, in D.F. Klein and J.G. Rabkin, ends, Anxiety: New Research andd changing Concepts. New York: Raven Press, 1981.

Levitt EE. A brief commentary on the psychiatric breakthrough with emphasis

Kraepelin E (1907). Clinical Psychiatry. A.R. Defender, trans. New York: Macmillan. Reprint, Delmar, NY: Scholars' Facsimiles and Reprints, 1981.

Lawlis F. The PTSD Breakthrough: The Revolutionary, Science-Based Compass Reset Program. Sourcebooks, 2010.

Lawlis F. Retraining your bran. Plume: New York, 2009.

Levitt EE. A brief commentary on the psychiatric breakthrough with emphasis on the hematology of anxiety, C. Spielberger, ed. Anxiety: Current Trends in Theory and Research, Vol. 1. New York: Academic Press, 1972.

Liebowitz MR, and Klein DF. Agoraphobia: Clinical features, pathophysiology, and treatment, in Agoraphobia: Multiple Perspectives on Theory ad Treatment, pp 153-81. New York: John Wiley, 1982.

Macklin ML, Metzger LJ, Lasko NB, et al: Five-Year follow-up study of eye movement desensitization and reprocessing therapy for combat- related post-traumatic stress disorder. Comprehensive Psychiatry. 41: 24-27, 2000.

Malloy PF, Fairbank JA, Keane TM. Validation of a multi-method assessment of post-traumatic stress disorders in Vietnam Veterans. Journal. Consultation Clinical Psychology 51: 488-494, 1983.

Manu P, Suarez RE, Barnett BJ. Handbook of Medicine in Psychiatry. American Psychiatric Publishing Inc., 2006.

Marks IM. Fears and Phobias. New York: Academic Press, 1969.

McNeil GN. Anxiety, In Handbook of Psychiatric Differential Diagnosis. Edited by Soreff SM, McNeil GM. Littleton MA, PSG Publishing, 1987.

Nestadt G, Samuels J, Riddle M, et al: A family study of obsessive-compulsive disorder. Archives General Psychiatry 57: 358- 363, 2000.

Pits FN Jr. The biochemistry of anxiety. Scientific American 220, 1969.

Rosenbaun JF and Pollack MH. Panic Disorder and Its Treatment, Marcel Dekker, Inc., 1998.

Roth M. The phobic anxiety depersonalization syndrome. Proc Royal Soc Med, 1959.

Ruskin PE, Talbott JA. Aging and Post-traumatic Stress Disorder. American Psychiatric Press, 1996.

Schiraldi G. The Post-traumatic Stress Disorder Sourcebook: A Guide to Healing, Recovery, and Growth. Second edition. New York: McGraw-Hill, 2009.

Shear MK, Fyer MF. Biological and Psychologic findings in panic disorder, In American Psychiatric Press Review of Psychiatry, Vol 7., 1988.

Snell B: The Discovery of the Mind. New York, Dover. 1982.

Swank RL. Combat Exhaustion. Journal. Nervous Mental Disorder, 109: 475-08, 1949.

Tanielian, T and Lisa Jaycox L, Invisible Wounds of War: Psychological and Cognitive Injuries, Their Consequences, and Services to Assist Recovery. Center for Military Health Policy Research, 2008.

Terhune W.B. The phobic syndrome: A study of eighty-six patients with phobic reactions. Archives of Neurological Psychiatry, 62, 1949.

Thorpe GL, and Burns LE. The Agoraphobic Syndrome. New York: John Wiley, 1983.

Uhde AT, Roy-Byrne P, Gillin JC, et al. The sleep of patients with panic disorder: a preliminary report. Psychiatry Research. 12: 251-259, 1984.

Veterans and Agent Orange: Committee to Review the Health Effects in Vietnam Veterans of Exposure to Herbicides. The National Academics Press, 2007.

Wilson JP, Keane TM. Assessing Psychological Trauma and PTSD, 2nd Edition, the Guilford Press, 2004.

Wilson T. Behavior Therapy, in Treatments of Psychiatric Disorders, Vol 3. Washington, DC, American Psychiatric Association, 1989.

Zuercher-White, E. The Agoraphobia Workbook. Oakland, CA: New Harbinger Publications, 2003.

Section Four

Psychotic Disorders

> *It is a peculiar sensation, this double- consciousness, this sense of always looking at one's self through the eyes of others, of measuring one's soul by the tape of a words that looks on in the amused contempt and pitty. —an American, a Negro; two souls, two thoughts, two unreconciled striving; two warring ideals in one dark body, whose dogged strength alone keeps it from being alone keeps it from being torn asunder.*
>
> *W.E.B. Du Bois (1868-1963)*
> *Of Our Spiritual Strivings*

The term psychotic disorders are an insidious and pervasive disturbance of thought content and process, they affect social function, and overall behavior. In characterizing the development of psychotic disorders, three phases may be identified. The active phase of the illness is usually preceded by a prodromal phase, in which there is increasing social withdrawal, impairment in role functioning, peculiar behavior, poor hygiene, blunted or inappropriate affect, bizarre ideation (not yet reaching delusional proportions), and disturbed communication. During the active phase – which may follow a major stressor – psychotic symptoms such as frank delusions, hallucinations, and grossly incoherent thinking are prominent. A residual phase usually follows the active phase of the mental illness which consists of predominantly negative symptoms (i.e. social isolation, blunted affect, and marked lack of energy and initiative). In the time between psychotic episodes, a residual phase takes place where the patient is in touch with reality.

Chapter 15

Schizophrenia

Schizophrenia is a disorder of unknown etiology, which is characterized by psycho tic symptoms that significantly impair functioning and that involve disturbances in feeling, thinking, and behavior. The disorder is chronic and generally has a prodromal phase, an active phase with delusions, hallucinations, or both, and a residual phase in which the disorder may be in remission.

Taken together with the work of Shenton et al, these data suggest that schizophrenia is a neurodevelopmental disorder. In his land mark work on schizophrenia, Silvano Arieti (1974) named Kraepelin, Bleuer, Myere, Freud, Jung, and Sullivan as the workers most fundamentally responsible for developing our modern concept of schizophrenia. Perhaps Arieti himself is most helpful I summarizing the psychodynamics felt by some to predispose toward schizophrenia.

The concept of schizophrenia was initially formulated by two European psychiatrists, Emil Kraeplin and Eugen Bleuler. Emil Kraepelin (1856-1926), the German psychiatrist whose descriptions of dementia praecox, the early term for schizophrenia. Kraepelin brought together the previously described phenomena of catatonia, hebephrenia, and paranoia under the rubic dementia praecox. Eugen Bleuler (1857-1939), the swiss psychiatrist who contributed importantly to our conceptions of schizophrenia and coined the term. The word was derived from the Greek "Skhizo" (split) and "phren" (mind). The pioneering efforts of Kraepelin and Bleuler led to two views of schizophrenia.

In describing schizophrenia, Bleuler broke with Kraepelin on two major points, for he believed that the disorder in question did not necessarily have an early onset and that it did not inevitability progress toward dementia. This Bleuler was much less attentive to the course of the disorder than was Kraeplin, and the label dementia praecox was no longer considered appropriate. In 1908 Bleuler proposed his own term, schizophrenia to capture what he viewed as the essential nature of the condition.

Adolf Meyer (1866-1950) was skeptical of Kaepelin's disease model of schizophrenia instead the adaptive use of fantasy- as opposed to action – in the illness. Meyere Stressed the longitudinal, psychodynamic development of schizophrenia, arguing that the preschizophrenia individual begins with trivial and harmless subterfuges, such as daydreaming or rumination, which eventually progresses to frank delusions, hallucinations and thought blocking.

Although Sigmund Freud (1856-1939) is best known for his work on the "neuroses," he contributed some fundamental ideas in the area of paranoid psychoses and schizophrenia. Essentially, Freud regarded schizophrenia as a regression to a primitive narcisstic state- one which libido is withdrawn form objects (i.e. other people), and directed into the self. Clinically, Freud's hypothesis seems to fir the very regressed, uncommunicative schizophrenic patient, who spends all day rocking, muttering, and responding to internal stimuli.

While we often associate Carl Jung (1875-1961) with the archetypal psychology. Jung was the first author to suggest a psychosomatic mechanism in schizophrenia. He hypothesized that a primary emotional disturbance in dementia praecox engendered some form of abnormal brain metabolism. This consistent with more recent theories, in which stress is thought to induce changes in dopamine metabolism, perhaps precipitating a psychotic relapse in the chronic schizophrenic patient. Harry

Stack Sullivan (1892-1949) contributed significantly to our understanding of schizophrenia as an interpersonal phenomenon.

Origins of Schizophrenia

Our understanding of the origins of schizophrenia; which characterized by disordered thinking: hallucinations, delusions, and a tendency to withdraw from reality, are light —years ahead of what it was just a decade ago.

Abnormalities within the brain. There is evidence that the normally occurring, fluid-filled spaces in the brain (called ventricles) are enlarged in schizophrenia patients. Why should the size of the ventricles be significant? Scientists believe that the larger the space, the smaller the total tissue in the brain; with noticeable less gray matter. This has been confirmed by MRI scans. An area of the frontal lobes just over the eyes, called the prefrontal cortex, has also been implicated in schizophrenia. This is the seat of what is called the working memory- our ability to hold new bits of information and interrelate them with what we already know, and to release information we no longer need. People with schizophrenia experience a malfunction in this area. They have difficulty clearing their working memory of irrelevant information and keeping visual images in mind after they have disappeared from sight. (Andreasen,1994). Another interesting area of inquiry relates to the fact that the brains of people with schizophrenia have too much dopamine (the neurotransmitter), which regulates movement and influences mood and motivation. New medications seemed to work because they block the dopamine receptors. (see chapter 23)

The Dopamine Hypothesis. This theory suggests that schizophrenia (or schizophrenia-like symptoms) may be caused by an excess of dopamine-dependent neuronal activity in the brain. This excess activity may be related to increased production or release of dopamine at nerve terminal, increased receptor sensitivity, too many dopamine receptors, or a combination of these mechanisms.

Pharmacological support for this hypotheses exists. Amphetamines, which increase levels of dopamine, induce psychotomimetic symptoms. The neuroleptics (e.g. chlorpromazine and haloperidol) lower brain levels of dopamine by blocking dopamine receptors, thus reducing the schizophrenic symptoms. This suggests that an increased dopamine response may not be important in all schizophrenic clients. It is possible that more than one biological factor is at work and that different subgroups of schizophrenia have different biochemical etiologies in which dopamine is not the only neurotransmitter implicated in schizophrenia. Studies hypothesized that NMDA receptors which are activated by the excitatory neurotransmitters, aspartate and glutamate which play a critical role in schizophrenia.

Other Biochemical Hypothesis. Various other biochemical have been implicated in the predisposition to schizophrenia. Can family interaction patterns cause schizophrenia? The answer is most probably not. Researchers are now focusing their studies more interns of schizophrenia as a brain disorder. Abnormalities in the neurotransmitters norepinephrine, serotonin, acetylcholine, and gamma-aminobutyric acid. With the use of neuroimaging technologies, structural brain abnormalities have been observed in individuals with schizophrenia. Ventricular enlargement is the most consistent finding; however, sulci enlargement and cerebellar atrophy are also reported. Magnetic resonance imaging (MRI) provides a greater ability to image in multiple planes. Studies with MRI have been revealed a possible decrease in cerebral and intracranial size in clients with schizophrenia. Studies have also revealed a decrease in frontal lobe size. MRI has been used to explore possible abnormalities in specific sub-regions such as the amygdala, hippocampus, temporal lobes, and basal ganglia in the brains of people with schizophrenia.

Symptoms

A more neuro-biologic approach to the phenomenology of schizophrenia, by isolating the many persistent mental and behavioral features and subjecting them to factor analysis, discloses three clustering's of symptoms, or syndromes:

1. Diminished psychomotor activity (poverty of speech and spontaneous movement, flatness of affect);
2. A disorganization syndrome, or thought disorder (fragmentation of ideas, loosening of associations, tangentially, and inappropriate emotional expression); and
3. Reality distortion, compromising special types of hallucinations and delusions.

The essential features of schizophrenia are a mixture of characteristic sign and symptoms, both positive and negative.

Early in the illness, negative symptoms may be prominent, appearing primarily as prodromal features. Subsequently, positive symptoms appear. Because these positive symptoms are particularly responsive to treatment, they typically diminish, but in many individuals, negative symptoms persist between episodes of positive symptoms.

TABLE 15-1

TYPE I (positive schizophrenia)	TYPE II (negative schizophrenia)
Delusions, hallucinations, and thought process disorder prominent	Less prominent
Relatively acute onset	Insidious onset
Good premorbid functioning	Poor premorbid functioning
Exacerbations/ Remissions	Deteriorating Course
Normal CT scan	Ventricular Enlargement Common
Good response to anti-psychotics	More refractory to meditation
Normal Cognitive Function	Cognitive Impairment

Dementia. It is important clinically to rule out dementias of all three common types, which include Alzheimer's Disease, Vascular Dementia, and dementia with Lewy Body's. They can all present with psychotic symptoms.

Mood Disorders with Psychotic features. Delusions tend to be grandiose or nihilistic.

Delusional Disorders. The delusions are non bizarre and can have different themes. Like persecution, infection, love, or infidelity, Persecutor delusions are most commonly seen. The characteristic symptoms include dysfunctions in nearly every capacity of which the human brain is capable-perception, inferential thinking, language, memory, and executive functions. The symptoms are sometimes divided into two groups: positive and negative.

Positive, Type I. Eugen Bleuer conceived of schizophrenia as characterized by fundamental symptoms fo the four A's- disturbances of association and affect, and symptoms of autism and ambivalence- to be invariable and fundamental symptoms. These symptoms "e.g. hearing voices" are characterized by the presence of something that should be absent.

Negative, Type II. Symptoms that are characterized by the absence of something that should be present. For example, alogia is characteristic by a diminution, in the amount of spontaneous speech or a tendency to produce speech that is empty or impoverished in content, when that amount is adequate. Affective flattening or blunting is a reduced intensity of emotional expression, decreased spontaneous movements, poverty of expressive gestures, poor eye contact, lack of voice inflections, and slowed speech. Avolition is loss of the ability to initiate goal directed behavior and carry it through to completion. Patients seem to have lost their will or drive. **Anhedonia** is the inability to experience pleasure. Many patients describe themselves as feeling emotionally empty. They are no longer able to enjoy activities that previously gave them pleasure, such as playing sports, or seeing family or friends.

In the 20th century psychiatry has seen the elaboration of four major psycho-dynamic models of schizophrenia: psychoanalytic, family transaction, vulnerability-stress, and parallel-distributed processing. All have provided useful description of this mysterious disease.

The classical psychoanalytic model of Sigmund Freud postulates the existence of three functional entities in the mind: the id is the wellspring of sexual and aggressive drives and wishes. The superego or conscience and ego-ideal is the warehouse of rules and various learned symptoms from parents and society during development. It is also largely unconscious but makes its presence known through the affects of guilt and shame. And the ego is a group of psychological functions that mediate adaption between the person and the environment (for example, reality testing) and among conflicting psychological forces within the person. The family transaction models of schizophrenia represent attempts to understand and explain the syndrome as the transmission of aberrant interactions from the family to the patient. Family transaction models emerged after World War II from the families of schizophrenic patients. In the vulnerability-stress model schizophrenia is viewed as a product of interacting forces, some genetic of biological and some psychological, some innate or constitutional, and some learned through experience. This model of regards nature as important a suggested by genetic studies and the efficacy of biological treatments. Parallel- distributed processing model. The latest, neuro-dynamic model of schizophrenia hypothesizes with specificity the neuronanatomical nature of vulnerability to schizophrenia and its biophysical contribution to symptom formation. The model is built on postulates that most human mentation arises form neuronal networks organized in parallel distributed processing systems. Furthermore, the systems can, under certain physiological condition generate thoughts for feelings in ways in which the normal processes by which psychology in generated.

Five subtypes of schizophrenia are recognized in DSM-IV-TR (APA, 2000);

Paranoid. This subtype involves preoccupation with one or more systematized delusions or frequently auditory hallucinations. Compared with patients who have the disorganized subbtype, paranoid patients tend to be an older age at onset and are more likely to be married, to have children particularly with regard to occupational functioning and capacity for independent living.

Disorganized. This subtype is characterized by disorganized speech and behavior, and flat or inappropriate affect. Onset occurs at an early age with the development of negative symptoms. These patients often seem silly and childlike an occasionally, grimace, giggle inappropriately, and appear self-absorbed. Facial grimaces and bizarre mannerisms are common, an communication is consistently in coherent. Personal appearance is genereally neglected, and social impairment is extreme.

Catatonic. This subtype is characterized by extreme psychomotor retardation. The individual exhibits a pronounced decrease in spontaneous movements and activity. Mutism (i.e. absence of speech) is common, and negativism (i.e. an apparently motiveless resistance to all instructions or attempts to be moved) may be evident.

Catatonic excitement is manifested by a state of extreme psychomotor agitation. The movements are frenzied and purposeless, and are usually accompanied by continuous incoherent verbalizations and shouting. Clients require physical and medical control because they are often destructive and violent to others, and their excitement may cause them to injure them selves or to collapse from complete exhaustion.

Undifferentiated. Tis subtype is a residual category for patients meeting criteria for schizophrenia but not criteria for the paranoid, disorganized, or catatonic subtypes. However, the behavior is clearly psychotic. Diagnostic, there is evidence of delusions, hallucinations, incoherence, and bizarre behavior.

Residual. This diagnostic category is used when the individual who has chronic form of the disease and is the stage that follows and acute episode (prominent delusions, hallucinations, incoherence, bizarre behavior, and violence). Residual symptoms may include social isolation, eccentric behavior, impairment in person hygiene and grooming, blunted or inappropriate affect, poverty of or overly elaborate speech, illogical thinking or apathy.

Table 15-2 Diagnostic Criteria for Schizophrenia

A. Characteristic Symptoms: Two (or more) of the following, each present for significant portion of time during a 1-month period (or less if successfully treated):

1. Delusions
2. Hallucinations
3. Disorganized speech (e.g. frequent derailment or incoherence)
4. Grossly disorganized or catatonic behavior
5. Negative symptoms (i.e. affective flattening, alogia, or avolition)

NOTE: Only one Criterion A symptom is required if delusions are bizarre or hallucinations consist of a voice keeping up a running commentary on the person's behavior or thoughts, or two or more voices conversing with each other.

B. Social/ Occupational dysfunction: For a significant portion of the time since the onset of the disturbance, one or more major areas of functioning such as work, interpersonal relations, or self-care are markedly below the level achieved prior to the onset.
C. Duration: Continuous signs of the disturbance persist for a t least 6 months. This 6-month period must include at least 1 month of symptoms that meet Criterion A and may include periods of prodromal or residual symptoms.
D. Schizoaffective and Mood Disorder exclusion: Schizoaffective Disorder and Mood Disorder with Psychotic Features have been ruled out because either (1) no major Depressive,

Manic, or Mixed Episodes have occurred concurrently with the active phase symptoms; or (2) if mood episodes have occurred during active0 phase symptoms, their total duration has been brief relative to the duration of the active and residual periods.

E. Substance/General medical condition exclusion: The disturbance is not due to the direct physiological effects of a substance is not due to the direct physiological effects of a substance (e.g. a drug of abuse, a medication) or a general medical condition.

F. Relationship to a Pervasive Developmental Disorder: if there is a history of Autistic Disorder or another Pervasive Developmental Disorder, the additional diagnosis is made only if prominent delusions or hallucinations are also present for at least a month.

What distinguishes schizophrenia is the course: at least 6 months of continuous signs of the disturbance, failure to return to the previous level of functioning, and continuing vulnerability to stress. Patients are frightened by the confusion of their thought process; there bizarre, alien thoughts; novel perceptual disturbances and either a welter of emotions or deadening of emotional responses. Patients may explicitly wonder if they are losing their minds. Let's begin our examination of schizophrenia with the following vignette:

VIGNETTE

A fifty year old veteran reported 6 months of persecution and control in which he believed others are spying on him, spreading false rumors about him, planning to harm him, trying to control his thoughts or actions, or reading his mind. He believes that he is the victim of conspiracies by the FBI.

His most common hallucinations are auditory. They may involve solitary or multiple voices. The voices may seem to come from within his body or from outside sources, such as radios or walls. The voices may criticize, ridicule, or threaten; often they urge the patient to do something that he believes is wrong. His chief complaints of hearing voices telling him to kill himself and others. Visual hallucinations are also frequent. They may vary form frightening vague forms to images of dead or absent relatives, or scenes of violence or hell. Olfactory hallucinations, which are frequent, usually consist of unpleasant smells arising from the patient's own body. Tactile hallucinations, also infrequent, consistent of feelings that his genitals are being manipulated, that there are animals inside his body and that there are insects crawling over his skin. There was no previous psychiatric history, and according to the patient's family, he had been well until 6 months ago, when he began to do and say strange things. For example, he started saying that the FBI had been looking into his window. He described recently filing a lawsuit against the police for discrimination and he now believes hat they were taking revenge. He also noticed that a lock on the door of his apartment was broken a few weeks before and that since then his food has tasted different. On mental status examination, the patient was alert and oriented to month and year, but not the date. He appeared disheveled and malodorous. His speech was halting with many interruptions. His thought process was circumstantial ad over inclusive of details. And thought process content was disturbed by clear paranoid delusions about the police poisoning his food. His affect was guarded and suspicious thought most of the interview.

Discussion. Premorbid personality often indicates social maladjustment or schizoid or other personality disturbances (Ho, Black & Andresen, 2003). This premorbid behavior is often a predictor in the pattern of development of schizophrenia, which can be viewed in four phases.

Phase I: The Schizoid Personality. The DSM-IV-TR (APA, 2000) describes individuals in this phase as indifferent to social relationships and having a very limited range of emotional experience and expression. They do not enjoy close relationships and prefer to be loners. That is why they appear cold and aloof. Not all individuals who demonstrate the characteristics of

Deborah Y. Liggan, MD

schizoid personality will progress to schizophrenia. However, many individuals with schizophrenia show evidence of having had these characteristics in the premorbid condition.

Phase II. The Prodromal Phase. Characteristics of this phase include social withdrawal; impairment in role functioning; behavior that is peculiar or eccentric; neglect of personal hygiene and grooming; blunted or inappropriate affect; disturbances in communication; and lack of initiative, interests, or energy. The length of this phase is highly variable, and may last for many years before deteriorating to the schizophrenic state.

Phase III. Schizophrenia. In the active phase of the disorder, psychotic symptoms are prominent. Following are the DSM-V,2013 diagnostic criteria for schizophrenia:

- Characteristic Symptoms: Two (or more) of the following each present for a significant portion of time during a 1 month period.
  - ➢ Delusions
  - ➢ Hallucinations
  - ➢ Disorganized speech (e.g. frequent derailment or incoherence)
  - ➢ Grossly disorganized or catatonic behavior
  - ➢ Negative Symptoms (i.e. affective flattening, alogia, or avolition)
- Social/Occupational Dysfunction: For a significant portion of the time sinces the onset of the disturbance, one or more major areas of functioning-Such as work, interpersonal relationships, or self-care- are markedly below the level achieved before the onset, failure to achieve expected level of interpersonal academic, or occupational achievement.
- Duration: Continuous signs of the disturbance persist for at least 6 month

Phase IV. Residual Phase. Schizophrenia is characterized by periods of remission and exacerbation. A residual phase usually follows an active phase of the illness. Symptoms during the residual phase are similar to those of the prodromal phase, with flat affect and impairment in role functioning being prominent. Residual impairment often increases between episodes of active psychosis.

Diagnostic Issues. Schizophrenia has been found in every racial and social group studied. Cultural and socioeconomic factors must be considered, particularly when the individual and the clinician and socioeconomic background. In some cultures, visual or auditory hallucinations with a religious content (e.g. hearing God's voice) are a normal part of religious experience. A number of features distinguish the clinical expression of schizophrenia in the female and males. The general incidence of schizophrenia tends to be slightly lower in females. The age are onset is later in females, with a second mid-life peak as described earlier. Symptoms tend to be more affect laden among females, and there are more psychotic symptoms, as well as a greater propensity for psychotic symptoms to worsen in later life.

Suicide Risk. Potential for suicide is a major concern among patients with schizophrenia. Cases with a gradual or incidous onset may present because of school failure, social withdrawal, or bizarre behavior. Some patients despite the best f care, follow a downhill course, become totally and permanently disacled, and require custodial care to maintain the basic hygiene. As the illness progresses and the psychosocial consequences mount, secondary depression may result in suicidal ideation.

Radomsky and associates (1999) report that suicide is the primary cause of premature death among individuals with the disorder. They estimated that approximately 10 percent of patients with schizophrenia die by suicide (Addington, 2006).

Summary

A striking feature of these cases described by Kirby is that they showed a complete recovery. The onset was generally acute and not of the insidious type associated with schizophrenia. The premorbid personality, moreover, was not of the schizoid type usually associated with patients developing schizophrenia. He concluded that the catatonic syndrome could be broken down into two main types:

(1) Cases with an insidious onset and poor prognosis allied to dementia praecox; and
(2) Cases with an acute onset and good prognosis allied to manic-depressive psychosis.

Chapter 15: Schizophrenia Examination Review

Match the schizophrenia subtype with the clinical presentation:

1. Paranoid Type   A. Disorganized speech and flat affect
2. Disorganized Type   B. Continuing Evidence of Negative Symptoms
3. Catatonic Type   C. Psychomotor disturbance with motoric immobility
4. Residual Type   D. Prominent delusions or auditory hallucinations

5. This diagnostic category is used when the individual has a history of at least one previous episode of schizophrenia with prominent psychotic symptoms:

   A. Residual schizophrenia
   B. Paranoid Schizophrenia
   C. Undifferentiated Schizophrenia
   D. Schizoaffective Disorder

6. Sometimes clients with schizophrenic symptoms do not meet the criteria for any of the subtype. The behavior of these patients is clearly psychotic; that is there is evidence of delusions, hallucinations, incoherence, and bizarre behavior.

   A. Disorganized Schizophrenia
   B. Undifferentiated Schizophrenia
   C. Paranoid Schizophrenia
   D. Brief Psychotic Disorder

7. Which diagnostic criteria for schizophrenia are characterized by prominent negative symptoms?

   A. Delusions, hallucinations, and thought process disorder prominent
   B. Normal CT scan
   C. Normal Cognitive function
   D. Emotional blunting and social withdrawal

8. Which associate was the first author with archetypal psychology to point out that a psychomatic mechanism in schizophrenia?

   A. Sigmund Freud
   B. Carl Jung
   C. Adolf Meyer
   D. Harry Sullivan

9. Which symptom is the most common predictor of non-adherence to treatment, and its predicts higher relapse rates, increased number of involuntary treatment, poorer psycho-school functioning, aggression, and a poorer course of illness?

   A. Anosognosia
   B. Hostility and aggression
   C. Catatonia
   D. Disorganized speech

10. What symptoms occur when patients misinterpret external events, as directly related to themselves?

    A. Grandiose delusions
    B. Neologisms with aphasia
    C. Ideas of Reference
    D. Stupor alternating with excitement

Chapter 15: Schizophrenia Examination Answers

1. D
2. A
3. C
4. B
5. A
6. B
7. D
8. B
9. A
10. C

Chapter 16

Schizoaffective Disorder

Schizoaffective Disorder is a major psychiatric disorder that is quite similar to schizophrenia. Schizoaffective disorder is defined as a disorder with concurrent features of both schizophrenia and a mood disorder that cannot be diagnosed as wither one separately. Schizoaffective patients have a better prognosis than schizophrenic ones and a worse prognosis than mood disorder patients. The disorder can affect all aspects of daily living, including work, social relationships, and self-care skills (such as grooming and hygiene). People with schizoaffective disorder can have a wide variety of symptoms, including problems with their contact with reality (hallucinations and delusions), mood (such as marked depression), low motivation, inability to experience pleasure, and poor attention.

Diagnosis. Schizoaffective disorder can only be diagnosed by a clinical interview. The disorder cannot be diagnosed with a blood test, an x-ray, a CAT scan, or any other laboratory test. The purpose of the interview is to determine whether the client has experienced specific symptoms of the disorder, and whether these symptoms have been presented long enough to merit the diagnosis. In addition to conducting the interview, the diagnostician must also check to make sure the client is not experiencing any physical problems that could cause symptoms similar to schizoaffective disorder, such as a brain tumor or alcohol or drug abuse.

Table 16-1. DSM-5 Diagnostic Criteria for Schizoaffective Disorder

A. An uninterrupted period of illness during which there is a major mood episode (major depressive or manic) concurrent with Criterion A of schizophrenia

B. Delusions or hallucinations for 2 weeks or more weeks in the absence of a major mood episode (depressive or manic) during the lifetime duration of the illness.

C. Symptoms that meet criteria for a major mood episode are present for the majority of the total duration of the active and residual portions of the illness.

D. The disturbance is not attributable to the effects of a substance (e.g. a drug of abuse, a medication) or another medical condition. Specify whether this subtype (bipolar) applies if a manic episode is part of the presentation. Major depressive episodes may also occur. Depressive subtype applies if only major depressive episodes are part of the presentation. Specify whether this refers to the criteria for catatonia associated with another mental disorder.

The historical clinical observation that schizoaffective disorder is an overlap of schizophrenia and mood disorders is explained by genes for both illnesses being present in individuals with schizoaffective disorder. Schizoaffective disorder was included as a subtype of schizophrenia in DSM-I and DSM-II. Then DSM-III-R placed schizoaffective disorder in "psychotic Disorders Not Otherwise specified." DSM-IV and DSM-IV-TR (published in 2000) criteria for schizoaffective disorder were poorly defined and poorly operationalized. DSM-IV and DSM-IV-YTR (published in 2000) are there the presence of either a depressive or manic episode concurrent with symptoms characteristic of schizophrenia, such as bizarre delusions, flight of ideas, distractibility, impulsivity and intrusiveness that can compromise the examination. DSM-5 schizoaffective disorder workgroup analyzed all of the available research evidence on schizoaffective disorder, and concluded that "presenting symptoms of psychosis have little validity in determining diagnosis, prognosis, or treatment response.

Box 16-1. History of Schizoaffective Psychosis

A review of the older literature indicates that historical mainstreams converged ot produce the current concept of schizoaffective reactions.

- Jacob Kasanin in 1933 described an episodic psychotic illness with predominant affective symptoms, that was thought at the time to be a good-prognosis schizophrenia.
- Kasinin's concept of the illness was influenced by the psychoanalytic teachings of Adolf Meyer. German psychiatrist Adolf Meyer postulated that schizoaffective psychosis was caused by emotional conflicts.
- In 1863, German psychiatrist Karl Kahlbaum described schizoaffective disorders as a separate group in his vesania typical circularis.
- In 1920, psychiatrist Emil Kraepelin, the founder of contemporary scientific psychiatry, observed a great number of cases that had characteristics of both groups such as dementia praecox (now called schizophrenia) and manic depressive insanity (now called bipolar disorders).
- In 1959, psychiatrist Kurt Schnieder began to further refine conceptualizations of the different forms that schizoaffective disorders can take since he observed concurrent and sequential types.
- As Clark and Mallet (1963) have pointed out, a large proportion of psychotic patients show an admixture of schizophrenic and affective features, and it is difficult to decide whether a given case should be regarded as "Schizophrenia with affective features," or as "affective disorder with schizophrenia."

Biological Factors. The cause of schizoaffective disorders is not known, but current theories suggest that an imbalance in brain chemicals (specifically, dopamine) may be at the root of these two disorders (schizoaffective and schizophrenia).

The leading biochemical hypothesis holds that schizophrenia involves a disorder of dopamine function. Historically, it was attributed to excessive dopamine in the limbic system. As suggested above, dopamine is not the only neurotransmitter implicated in schizophrenia, which are activated by the excitatory neurotransmitters aspartate and glutamate. About half of clients with schizoaffective disorder use drugs or alcohol excessively. Amphetamine, cocaine, and to a lesser extent alcohol, can result in psychosis that presents clinically like psychosis in schizoaffective disorder.

Symptoms. The diagnosis of schizoaffective disorder requires that the client experience some decline in social functioning for at least a six-month period, such as problems with school or work, social relationships, or self-care. The symptoms of schizoaffective disorder can be divided into five broad classes: positive symptoms, negative symptoms, and symptoms of mania, symptoms of depression, and other symptoms.

Positive Symptoms refer to thoughts, perceptions, and behaviors that are ordinarily absent in people in the general population, but are present in persons with schizoaffective disorder. Hallucinations are false perceptions such as hearing, seeing, feeling, or smelling things that are not actually there; the most common type of hallucinations. Delusions are false beliefs that is, a belief that others can clearly see is not true. For example, some clients have paranoid delusions, believing that others want to hurt them. In delusions of reference the client believes that something in the environment is referring to him or her when it is not (such as the television talking to the client). In summary, the client talks in a manner that is difficult to follow by jumping form one topic to the next, stop in the middle of the sentience, make up new words, or simply be difficult to understand.

Negative Symptoms are the opposite of positive symptoms. They are the absence of thoughts, perceptions, or behaviors that are ordinarily present in people in the general population. These symptoms are often stable throughout much of the client's life. N the presence of a blunted affect, the expressiveness of the client's face, voice toe, and gestures is diminished or restricted. However, this does not mean that the person is not reacting to his or her environment or having feelings. The client may feel lethargic or sleepy and does not feel motivated to pursue goals and activities. Anhedonia is the experience of little or no pleasure form activities that he or she used to enjoy. The client says very little due to poverty of speech or content of speech. Within attention the client has difficulty attending and is easily distracted.

Symptoms of Mania involve an excess in behavioral activity, mood states (in particular, irritability or positive feelings), and self –esteem and confidence. When the client's mood is abnormally elevated, he or she is extremely happy or excited (euphoria). The client is extremely self-confident and may be unrealistic about his or her abilities (grandiosity). The client talks excessively and may be difficult to interrupt. This is achieved by jumping quickly from one topic to another (called flight of ideas). The thoughts come so rapidly that the client finds it hard to keep up with them or express them. In distractibility, the client's attention is easily drawn to irrelevant stimuli, such as the sound of a car honking outside on the street. Increased goal-directed activity results in a great deal of time spending specific goals, at work, school, or sexually.

Symptoms of Depression reflect the opposite end of the continuum of mood form manic symptoms, with a low mood and behavioral inactivity as the major features. Mood is low most of the time and the client has few interests and gets little pleasure from anything, including activities previously found enjoyable. There is a change in sleep pattern such as difficulty falling asleep or staying asleep, or may wake early in the morning and not be able to get back to sleep. Alternatively, the client may sleep excessively (such as over twelve hours per night), spending much of the day in bed. There is also a change in activity level is reflected by slowness and lethargy, in t terms of both the client's behavior and his/ her thought processes. Then the client experiences fatigue throughout the day, or there is a chronic feeling of loss of energy. In depression, the client may feel they are worthlessness, hopelessness, or helplessness. Inappropriate guilt may be present about events that the client did not even cause, such as a catastrophe, a crime, or an illness. Significant decreases in the ability to concentrate make it difficult for the client to pay attention to others or may make decisions.

Other Symptoms. Clients may use alcohol and drugs excessively either because of their disturbing symptoms, to experience pleasure, or when socializing pleasure, or when socializing with others.

Let's consider another vignette.

VIGNETTE

A 25 year old single male was brought to the psychiatric ER by his mother. She reported that for the past 3 months the patient, had been increasingly seclusive, sometimes remaining in his room for days at a time. His hygiene and diet had been very poor, such that (according to his mother) the patient "smells horrible ... I don't think he's showered in two weeks, and he's probably lost 15 pounds in the last couple of months." At times, the patient would be heard laughing or talking of himself from within his room. This prompted his mother and older brother to break in through a window and forcibly bring the patient in for assessment.

There was no previous psychiatric history, and according to the patient's family, he had been well until approximately 1 year ago, when he began to say and do strange things. For example, he started saying that the neighbors were "poisoning our lawn with Agent Orange."

On mental status examination, the patient was alert and oriented to month and year, but not the date. He appeared disheveled and malodorous. His speech was halting with many interruptions. His affect was guarded and suspicious through most of the interview.

Despite denied auditory or visual hallucinations, the patient was admitted involuntarily to the inpatient psychiatric unit.

Physical examination and laboratory testing disclosed no abnormalities, except mild dehydration. The patient attended group therapy on the unit three times per week, during which a supportive reality-centered approach was used, with minimal confrontation or interpretation of unconsciousness impulses. He also met twice weekly with a psychiatric resident who knew he could work with him after discharge form the unit.

Discussion. Schizoaffective disorder is less common that either schizophrenia or mood disorders. Manic energy, irritably, and a reduced need for sleep may coexist with bizarre ideation or behavior and constricted or in appropriate affects. It is apparent form the review of the pertinent literature that the presence of affective factors significantly increases the probability of improvement in cases of schizophrenia. This finding was reported in a recent study of the schizo-affective of schizophrenia. The improvement in this type of schizophrenia is greater that in the other types at all levels. These observation could be expressed graphically by viewing the cases of functional mental illness in terms of a spectrum: at one end are the pure manic-depressive cases with good prognosis; and at the other are the pure schizophrenic cases with a poor prognosis. In between are varying blends of these disorders (the schizoid-affective cases) with a fair prognosis. The cases at either end of the spectrum represent one of these variables – either the schizophrenic or the affective. The cases between the poles contain both variables, and the resultant prognosis depends on the relative strength of each.

TREATMENT

Many of the same methods used to treat schizophrenia are also effective for schizoaffective disorder. Antipsychotic medications are an effective treatment for schizoaffective disorder. These drugs are not a cure for the disorder, but they can reduce symptoms and prevent relapses among the majority of people with the disorder.

Deborah Y. Liggan, MD

Antidepressant medications and mood stabilizing medications are occasionally used to treat affective symptoms (depressive or manic symptoms) in schizoaffective disorder. Other important treatments include social-skills training, vocational rehabilitation and supported employment, and intensive case management. Family therapy helps reduce stress in the family and teaches family members how to monitor the disorder. In addition, individual supportive counseling can help the person with the disorder learn to manage the disorder more successfully and obtain emotional support in coping with the distress resulting from the disorder.

During the illness, hallucinations or delusions must be present for two weeks or more, in the absence of prominent mood symptoms. Consequently, there are two subtypes: the bipolar type marked by a current or previous manic syndrome, and the depressive type marked by the absence of any manic syndromes. The major treatment modalities for schizoaffective disorder are hospitalization, medication, and psychosocial interventions.

Chapter 16: Schizoaffective Reaction
Examination Review

1. What symptom consisted of marked stiffening of the body with scowling, swearing, or striking?

    A. Catalepsy
    B. Negativism
    C. Complete affectlessness
    D. Mentation

2. The term schizoaffective disorder has been understood in various ways:

    A. It may be a type of either schizophrenia or a mood disorder
    B. It may be a combination of both schizophrenia and a mood disorder
    C. It may be completely a distinct form wither of those disorders
    D. It may comprise a group of disorders that include all three possibilities

3. During the illness, how long must hallucinations or delusions be present for in the absence of prominent mood symptoms?

    A. Two weeks or more
    B. One month or more
    C. Six weeks or more
    D. Three-to-four months

4. During what negative symptoms does the client not feel motivated to pursue goals and activities because there is little sense of purpose in their lives?

    A. Blunted affect
    B. Anhedonia
    C. Apathy
    D. Euphoria

5. In which stage of cooperation is a personality disorder preceded by diagnosis:

    A. Schizoid Personality disorder: intimacy avoidance, social withdrawal, and lack of emotional expression
    B. Schizotypal Personality Disorder: Suspiciousness, bearing grudges, and feeling victimized.
    C. Paranoid Personality Disorder: Majority are nonviolent, but overall, like any psychotic disorder, and there is an above average risk of physical violence
    D. Borderline Personality Disorder: eccentricity, odd beliefs and perceptual distortions.

6. What diagnostic feature characterizes an individual has a psychosis which partly overlaps with a major mood episode. Then the individual typifies schizoaffective disorder?

    A. Compared to schizophrenia, insight is better, and there are less negative symptoms.
    B. The individual has a major mood episode concurrent with criterion A (psychotic symptoms of schizophrenia.
    C. The incidence is higher in males than females (due to increased incidence of the depressive-type in males).
    D. The incidence is synopsis compared with schizophrenia, Bipolar Disorder, or Major Depressiveness Disorder.

7. Effective psychological treatments: Schizoaffective Disorder in

    A. Assertive community treatment
    B. Skills improved adherence to care
    C. Mood stabilizer medications and antidepressants used in combination with antipsychotic medication
    D. The typical age or onset is late (geriatric) care.

8. What is the difference in aged type of schizoaffective Disorder?

    A. Bipolar (manic) type of schizoaffective Disorder is more common in aged patients.

    B. The Depressive Type is more common in younger patients.

    C. Individuals with Schizoaffective Disorder have less than a better prognosis

    D. For individuals with Schizoaffective Disorder who refuse to take their antipsychotic medication, response is to treat them with injections of long-lasting antipsychotic medication (that can last one month).

9. During the period of mood disturbance and increased energy or activity, three (or more) of the following symptoms have persisted (four if the mood is only irritable)

    A. Inflated self-esteem or grandiosity

    B. Decreased need for sleep (e.g. feels rested after only 3 hours of sleep).

    C. Flight of ideas or subjective experienced that thoughts are racing

    D. All of the above

10. What form of thought is characterized in schizoaffective disorder?

    A. Tangentially-literal interpretations represent a regression to an earlier level of cognitive development.

    B. Neologisms- the psychotic person invents new words

    C. Word salad- an individual's inability or refusal to speak

    D. Mutism- a group of words that are put together randomly, without any logical connection

Chapter 16: Schizoaffective Disorders
Examination Answers

1. B
2. D
3. A
4. C
5. A
6. A
7. C
8. D
9. D
10. B

Chapter 17

Schizophreniform Disorder

The essential features of this disorder are identical to those of schizophrenia, with the exception that the duration, including prodromal, active, and residual phases, is at least 1 month but less than 6 months (APA, 2000 and Strakowski, 1994).

The onset is characterized by a more or less lengthy prodromal, marked by peculiar behavior or a change in personality, after which psychotic symptom appear. Patients seem to differ from schizophrenic patients in several important ways:

1. Symptoms begin and end more abruptly
2. Symptoms are usually more turbulent and acute
3. There is good premorbid adjustment and higher functioning after recovery
4. There is only a slightly increased prevalence of schizophrenia in the family. There may be a higher prevalence of affective disorder.

Psychotic Symptoms include hallucinations, delusions, loosening of associations, bizarre behavior or catatonia. In some cases, these psycho tic symptoms may be accompanied by considerable confusion or perplexity, or by flattening or blunting of affect. This six month period encompasses not only the time during which the patient had psychotic symptoms, but also any produce before that, and any residuals afterward, or if the premorbid social and occupational functioning was satisfactory.

At the end of this six month period, patients are said to be fully restored to health, without psychotic symptoms, residual peculiarities or any impairment at all. Above all, when considering the diagnosis of schizophreniform disorder it must be borne in mind that the diagnosis cannot be made with confidence until after one has observed a full, complete and spontaneous remission within six months (Benazzi, 1998).

Table 17-1. DSM-5. Diagnostic Criteria for Schizophreniform Disorder

A. Two (or more) of the following, each present for a significant portion of time during a 1 month period. At least one of these must be (1), (2), or (3):

1. Delusions
2. Hallucinations
3. Disorganized Speech (e.g. frequent derailment or incoherence)
4. Grossly disorganized or catatonic behavior
5. Negative symptoms (i.e. diminished emotion expression or avolition)

B. An episode of the disorder lasts a t least 1 month but less than 6 months. When the diagnosis must be made without waiting for recovery, it should be qualified as "provisional."

C. Schizoaffective disorder and depressive or bipolar disorder with psychotic features have been ruled out because either 1)no major depressive or manic episodes have occurred concurrently with the active-phase symptoms, 2) they have been present for a minority of the total duration of the active residual periods of the illness.

D. The disturbance is not attributable to the physiological effects of a substance (e.g. a drug of abuse, a medication) or another medical condition.

Specify if:

- <u>With good prognostic feature:</u> This specified requires the presence of a t least two of the following features: onset of prominent psychotic symptoms within 4 weeks of the first noticeable change in usual behavior or functioning; confusion or perplexity; good premorbid social and occupational functioning; and absence of blunted or flat affect.
- <u>Without good prognostic features:</u> This specifier is applied if two or more of the above features have not been present.
- <u>With Catatonia.</u> The specifier is defined by the presence of three or more of 12 psychomotor features in the diagnostic criteria for catatonia associated with another mental disorder and catatonic disorder due to another medical condition.

Let's begin out examination of schizophreniform with the following vignette.

VIGNETTE

A 25 year old black male who moved from a southern state to the Northeast 5 years prior to evalutation. His older brother, who accompanied him to the ER, gave the following history: His symptoms were of decreased sleep and racing thoughts that state, "The spirit of Martin Luther King has infiltrated my metabolism. He also stated that God's voice was instructing him to "minister to the needs of all the world's people." One month prior to evaluation, the brother talked of being "posed by the spirit of black godliness." He had no psychiatric problems until 2 months prior to evaluation, at which time he began to experience intense anxiety surrounding the people in the trees. He stated that he heard these tree people discussing him in racially derogatory terms. On examination, the patient showed intense anxiety, confusion, disorientation to day and date, and loosening of associations. This is significant because physical and laboratory testing were completely normal.

Discussion. The development of schizophreiform disorder is similar to that of schizophrenia. About one-third of individuals with an initial diagnosis of schizophreniform disorder (provisional) recover within the 6- month period and schizophreinform disorder is their final diagnosis. This case presents us with another illness whose precise nature still eludes us: namely, schizophreniform disorder. The majority of the remaining two-thirds of individuals eventually receive a diagnosis of schizophrenia or schizoffective disorder. Schizophreniform disorder meets criterion A of schizophrenia, does not fit the criteria for schizoaffective disorder or mood disorder with psychotic features, and has duration of at least 1 month but less than 6 months. Typically, schizophreniform disorder presents with more emotional turmoil, anxiety, confusion, and hallucinatory symptoms than does schizophrenia.

Medical Condition- The many medical conditions that may present with schizophreniform features are summarized in Table 17-2. In general, the mental status and physical examinations are the key to differential diagnosis.

Table 17-2. Medical conditions sometimes presenting with schizophreniform features:

Neurological: head trauma, tumors, infarcts, CNS infection, dementia

Endocrine: hyper/ hypothyroidism, hyper/hypoparathyroidism, pituitary, adrenal disorders

Metabolic: Cardiac, hepatic, renal, respiratory failure; Na+/ K+ imbalance

Deficiencies: thiamine, pyridoxine, niacin, cobalamine

Intoxication-withdrawal: alcohol, barbiturate, amphetamines, PCP

Iatrogenic: antidepressants, anti-cholinergics, anti-hypertensive, L-dopa

---

Prognosis. The prognosis varies depending upon the nature, the variety, and duration of the symptoms, but abut two-thirds of individuals diagnosed with schizophreniform disorder go on to develop schizophrenia. The following specifiers for schizophreniform disorder may be used to indicate the presence or absence of features that may be associated with a better prognosis:

- With good Prognostic Features at least two of the following features are present:
  o Onset of prominent psychotic symptoms within 4 weeks of the first noticeable change in usual behavior or functioning
  o Confusion or perplexity at the height or the psychotic episode
  o Good premorbid social and occupational functioning,
  o absence of blunted or flat affect

Without Good Prognostic Features, used if two or more of the above features have not been present.
  o The presence of negative symptoms and poor eye contact both appear to be prognostic of a poor outcome.

Treatment

Various modalities of treatment including pharmacology, psychotherapy and various others psychosocial and education interventions, are used in the treatment of schizophreniform disorder. Pharmocotherapy is the most commonly used treatment modality as psychiatric medications can act quickly to both reduce the severity of symptoms and shorten their duration. Antipsychotic medication should be used to treat psychotic symptoms, but should be withdrawn after 3 to 6 months. Along with a variety of social support, is critical in helping patients to understand and deal with their psychotic experiences. As improvement progresses during treatment, help with coping skills, problem-solving techniques, psycho-educational approaches, and eventually occupational therapy and vocational assessments are often very helpful for patients and their families. Virtually all types of individual psychotherapy are used in the treatment of schizophreniform disorder, except for insight-oriented therapies as patients often have limited insight as a symptom of their illness.

Chapter 17: Schizophreniform Examination Review

1. What qualifies the schizophreniform disorder as provisional?

   A. The diagnosis is symptomatic for more than 2 years
   B. The diagnosis is symptomatic for less than 6 months
   C. The diagnosis is changed to schizophrenia when it persists beyond 2 years
   D. The diagnosis is changed to schizophrenia when residual phases last for a t least 1 week.

2. In what way does schizophreniform disorder differ from brief psychotic disorder?

   A. In both cases, psychotic symptoms include hallucinations, delusions, or loosening of associations
   B. In both cases, considerable confusion or perplexity, or by flattening or blunting affect
   C. Duration of active symptoms is 1-6 months as opposed to remission within 1 month
   D. All of the Above

3. In what way does the clinical picture dominated by t him following symptoms?

   A. Stupor-i.e. slight, even resistance to positioning by examiner
   B. Waxy flexibility-I.e. no psychomotor activity; not actively relating to environment
   C. Negativism-i.e. opposition or not response to instructions or external stimuli
   D. Catalepsy- i.e. mimicking another's movements

4. Under what conditions is the diagnosis of schizophreniform disorder made?

   A. When an episode of illness lasts between 1 and 6 months
   B. When the disturbance persists beyond 1 year

C. The total duration of the illness, including prodromal, active, and residual phases, is at least 1 year but less than 6 months

D. When and individual is symptomatic for less than 1 year duration

5. What diagnostic features persist if the disturbance lasts beyond 6 months?

A. The diagnosis should be changed to schizophrenia

B. Symptoms which lasts more than 1 week and remits by 6 months

C. The presentation of negative symptoms for a significant portion of time during a 6 month period

D. Onset of prominent psychotic symptoms within 6 months of the first noticeable change in usual behavior or functioning.

6. What good prognostic features are included in schizophreniform disorder?

A. absence of blunted or flat affect

B. Good premorbid functioning

C. Confusion and disorientation at the height of the psychotic episode

D. All of the above

7. What course defines treatment for schizophreniform?

A. Poor prognosis associated with positive family history of schizophrenia

B. Antipsychotic mediations should be used to treat psychotic symptoms, but should be withdrawn after 3 to 7 months.

C. If medication is required, use as low dose as possible and discontinue as soon as possible

D. Antidepressant or anti-manic treatments should always be attempted, and antipsychotic medication should be used to control acute psychotic symptoms.

8. What symptoms produce good prognostic features of schizophreniform disorder?

   A. Absence of blunted or flat affect
   B. good premorbid functioning
   C. Confusion and disorientation fat the height of the psychotic episode
   D. All of t he above

9. What definition characterizes schizophreniform disorder?

   A. A disorder with concurrent features of both features of both schizophrenia and a mood disorder that cannot be diagnosis as either one separately.
   B. Symptom presentation identical to schizophrenia except that symptoms resolve within 6 months and there is a return to normal functioning
   C. Disorder in which the primary manifestation is a delusion that is fixed and unshakeable
   D. Symptoms are of less than 1 month's duration and following an obvious stress in the patient's life.

10. How does schizophreniform disorder differ in duration in from brief psychotic disorder?

    A. Symptoms are greater than 6 month's duration and follow an obvious stress in the patient's life.
    B. If the disturbance persists beyond 1 year, the diagnosis would be changed to schizophrenia
    C. Schizophreniform disorder differs in duration form brief psychotic disorder, which has a duration of less than 1 month
    D. Symptoms are of less than 1 month's duration and follow an obvious stress in the patient's life.

Chapter 17: Schizophreniform Examination Answers

1. B
2. D
3. C
4. A
5. A
6. D
7. B
8. D
9. B
10. C

Chapter 18

Brief Psychotic Disorder

In the past, this was known as "brief reactive psychosis" in deference to the belief that brief psychosocial stressors played a prominent role in its onset. The word "reactive" was dropped from the name in order widen the diagnostic concept to include cases that occur in the absence of significant stressors (Beighley et al, 1992).

Good prognostic indicators of brief reactive psychosis include a severe precipitating stressor (usually followed within hours by the psychosis), confusion and lability during the episode, good premorbid history, negative family history for schizophrenia, and short duration of symptoms (may last a few hours to days). This condition describes those patients who experience an acute psychotic episode lasting longer than 1 day but less than 1 month; in response to some identifiable stressor.

The illness comes a surprise. There is usually no forewarning that the person is likely to breakdown, although this disorder is more common in people with a preexisting personality disorder (particularly histrionic and borderline types).

Table 18-1. DSM-5. Diagnostic Criteria for
Brief Psychotic Disorder

A. Presence of one (or more) of the following symptoms:

1. Delusions
2. Hallucinations
3. Disorganized speech (e.g. frequent derailment or incoherence)
4. Grossly disorganized or catatonic behavior

   NOTE: Do not include a symptom if it is a culturally sanctioned if it is a culturally sanctioned response pattern.

B. Duration of an episode of the disturbance is at least 1 day but less than 1 month, with eventual full return to premorbid level of functioning.
C. The disturbance is not better accounted for by a mood disorder with psychotic features, schizoaffective disorder, or schizophrenia and is not due to the direct physiological effects of a substance (e.g. a drug of abuse, a medication) or general medical condition.

Specify if: With marked stressor(s) (Brief Reactive Psychosis): if symptoms occur shortly after and apparently in response to events that, singly or together, would be markedly stressful to almost anyone in similar circumstances in the person's culture.

Without marked stressor(s): IF psychotic symptoms do not occur shortly after, or are not apparently in response to events that, singly or together, would be markedly stressful to almost anyone in similar circumstances in the person's culture.

With Postpartum onset: if onset within 4 weeks postpartum

The psychosis is typically very turbulent and f=dramatic with marked emotional lability, bizarre behavior, confused and incoherent speech, transient disorientation and memory loss, and /or brief but striking hallucinations and delusions. Generally in the setting of profound confusion emotional turmoil and intense and labile affect occur.

Symptoms. It is a long-standing clinical observation that otherwise well-functioning people may develop psychotic symptoms when confronted wit overwhelming stress. Symptoms are often dramatic and florid and are often thematically related to precipitating circumstances. Presence of at least one of the following symptoms indicating impaired reality testing:

1. Incoherence or marked loosening or associations
2. Delusions
3. Hallucinations
4. Catatonic or disorganized behavior

Brief Psychotic disorders may be preceded by a stressful event or series of events such as automobile accidents, divorces or separations, and financial setbacks. The onset of symptoms is abrupt, without the gradually developing prodrome often seen in schizophreniform disorder or schizophrenia. Instead, there is emotional turmoil with rapid shifts form one intense affect too another. Most importantly, there is an eventual full return to the premorbid level of functioning.

Table 18-2. Good Prognostic Features for Brief Psychotic Disorder

- Good premorbid adjustment
- Few premorbid schizoid traits
- Severe precipitating stressor
- Sudden onset of symptoms
- Affective symptoms
- Confusion a perplexity during psychosis
- Little affective blunting
- Short duration of symptoms
- Absence of schizophrenic relatives

Patients with brief psychotic disorder generally have good prognoses, and European studies have indicated that 50 to 80 percent of all patients have no further major psychiatric problems.

Always carefully rule out medical conditions. For example, the patient's thyroid function should be evaluated: both hyperthyroidism and hypothyroidism can cause psychosis.

VIGNETTE

A 60 year-old widower was admitted to the urology service for evaluation of acute onset of inability to void. While a physician was explaining the nature of a planned procedure, bright re blood appeared in the catheter bag in full view of the patient. He became extremely frightened and developed the conviction that he would ot survive the upcoming procedure. When a psychiatric consultant visited him several hours later, he was sobbing uncontrollably and was unable to lye still. He overheard messengers form God telling him he would be dead soon, and he saw visions of his deceased wife, who promised him a reunion.

The patient's psychiatric history dated rom World War II, when he had experienced two episodes of psychogenic amnesia nd had traveled long distances before finding himself in strange cities. Since then, he had had periods of anxiety, particularly in crowded public situations, and he had finally stopped working at 50 years of age. After 2 days of treatment and frequent reassurance form the medical staff, his symptoms disappeared almost as dramatically as they had begun.

Discussion. Psychological factors may be more important in brief psychotic disorder than in schizophreniform or schizoaffective disorders. When a person is confronted with a stressful situation, the natural response is to use familiar problem-solving behavior patterns either to achieve a resolution or to maintain psychological equilibrium until external events change. Psychotic symptoms may emerge within the patient's psychological defenses are completely overwhelmed. For some patients, only chaotic events such as natural disasters or combat experiences are severe enough to upset the equilibrium. Other people may be overwhelmed by divorce, physical illness, or financial disaster. Some patients with character defects (i.e., personality disorder) may be unable to cope with transitions or disappointments that most other people would be able to tolerate, even though they might find them unsettling.

Postpartum cases may be influenced by endocrine changes as well as psychological stress. In cases without associated stressors, there may be as yet undetermined biological causes. Such discussion offers the patient a model for dealing with crises in the future.

Some clinicians have observed that labile mood, confusion, and impaired attention may be more common at the onset of brief psychotic disorder than the onset of eventually chronic disorders. Characteristic symptoms in brief psychotic disorder include emotional volatility, strange or bizarre behavior, screaming or muteness, and impaired memory for recent events. Some of the symptoms suggest a diagnosis of delirium and warrant a medical workup, especially to rule out adverse reactions to drugs.

Postpartum Psychosis. Patients with postpartum onset generally develop symptoms within 1-2 weeks after delivery. Symptoms include disorganized speech, misperceptions, labile mood, confusion, and hallucinations. Obsessions are common and often focus on an impulse to hurt or kill the infant. Features suggesting a good prognosis are similar to those for schizophrenia: a severe stressor sudden onset prominent mood symptoms, good premorbid functioning, the absence of schizoid traits, the absence of a family history of schizophrenia, symptoms that cause subjective distress and little blunting of affect.

The most severe postpartum disorder is an agitated, highly changeable psychosis that develops usually between the 3rd and 14th day postpartum.

The disorder should be distinguished from postpartum blues, which occurs in up to 80% of new mothers, lasts for a few days after delivery, and is considered normal. Postpartum blues is self-limited, last only a few days, and is characterized by tearfulness, fatigue, anxiety, and irritability that begins shortly after childbirth and lessens in severity over the course of a week.

Treatment. Brief Psychotic disorder is associated with an increased incidence of suicide compared within the general population. That is why the first step in treatment of a patient with this disorder is containment in a safe and secure environment, which does not, however, necessarily imply an inpatient psychiatric unit. Educating and strengthening the patient's support system are also critical. Interviewing the family and significant others in the patient's life is important in gaining historical information concerning the patient and in determining what factors could be precipitating the psychosis.

The two classes of drugs to be considered are the dopamine receptor antagonist antipsychotic drugs and the benzodiazepines. Antipsychotics may be helpful early on, especially when the patient is highly agitated or experiencing great emotional turmoil. Although these drugs have limited usefulness in the long-term treatment of psychotic disorders, they can be effective for a short time and are associated with gewer side effects than are the antipsychotics.

Psychotherapy is of use in providing an opportunity to discuss the stressors and the psychotic episode. Associated issues include helping patients deal with the loss of self-esteem and to regain self-confidence. Exploration and development of coping strategies are the major topics in psychotherapy. After the patient has sufficiently recovered the clinician can help him or her explore the meaning of the psychotic reaction and of the triggering stressor.

Psychological treatment may take several forms. Simply being removed form the crisis and being cared for by the hospital staff may allay the patient's anxiety enough to permit constructive discussion and problem solving. Enlisitng the aid of family members may also be important for the same reason. Encouraging the patient to recount the events that led to the breakdown and to discuss their impact and meaning will facilitate recovery. An individualized treatment strategy based on increasing problem solving skills while strengthening the ego structure through psychotherapy appears to be the most efficacious.

Chapter 18: Brief Psychotic Disorder
Examination Review

1. What features suggest a good prognosis that are similar to those for schizophrenia?

    A. Good premorbid functioning
    B. Absence of a family history of schizophrenia
    C. Prominent mood symptoms
    D. All of the above

2. What time frame is responsible for a diagnosis for patients who experience psychotic symptoms?

    A. Less than one month in response to some identifiable stressor
    B. Greater than six months in response to some stressor
    C. As much as two years of interrupted stressor
    D. No association between stressor and psychotic symptoms

3. How does one explore the patient's experience of the psychotic symptoms without confronting the unreality of the symptoms?

    A. By adhering t a rigid interview structure
    B. By indicating that the medication can help them feel calm and think clearly
    C. Interview the patient with detailed questions and phrases
    D. By confronting the reality of the symptoms

4. What premorbid personality disorders often are diagnostic of brief psychotic disorder?

    A. Borderline Personality Disorder
    B. Narcissistic Personality Disorder
    C. Paranoid Personality Disorder
    D. All of the above

5. When di patients with postpartum onset develop symptoms of brief psychotic disorder?

    A. Within 1-2 weeks after delivery
    B. 6 months after delivery
    C. 6 months during pregnancy
    D. During second month of pregnancy

6. True statements concerning brief psychotic disorder include all of the following EXCEPT

    A. The stressor must be sufficient severity to cause significant stress to any person in the same socioeconomic and cultural class.
    B. Many patients may also have pre-existing personality disorders
    C. Prodromal symptoms appear before the onset of the precipitating stressor
    D. Good prognostic features include a severe precipitating stressor, acute onset, and confusion or perplexity during psychosis

7. What class of drugs is therapeutic in the treatment of brief psychotic disorder?

    A. Antipsychotic drugs and benzodiazepines
    B. Antidepressant drugs and SSRIs
    C. Anticonvulsant drugs and TCAs
    D. Anesthetic drugs and sedatives

8. What characteristics of postpartum onset of brief psychotic disorder features a good prognosis?

    A. Symptoms occur within 6 months postpartum
    B. Good premorbid functioning
    C. The presence of schizoid traits
    D. The presence of a family history of schizophrenia

9. What symptoms characterize the postpartum blues?

   A. Begins shortly after childbirth and lessens in severity over the course of a weel

   B. Obsessions focus on an impulse to hurt or to kill the infant

   C. Tearfulness, anxiety, and irritability

   D. All of the above

10. Why was the word "reactive" dropped form the name of brief psychotic disorder?

    A. To widen the diagnostic concept in the absence of significant stressors

    B. No forewarning that the person is likely to breakdown

    C. If grossly disorganized or catatonic behavior

    D. Do not include a symptom if it is a culturally sanctioned response pattern

Chapter 18: Brief Psychotic Disorder Examination Answers

1. D
2. A
3. B
4. D
5. A
6. C
7. A
8. B
9. D
10. A

Chapter 19

Shared Psychotic Disorder

The first description of shared psychotic disorder is commonly attributed to Ernest Charles Lasegue and Jules Falret, who described the condition in 1877 and gave it the name of folie a` deux. In the past, these rare cases were called folie a` deux, a French term meaning "double insanity." In folie a` deux, a patient, usually dependent and impressionable, having fallen under the influence of a dominant person who has a psychosis, comes to adopt and believe in the delusions expressed by the dominant person. Although it may occur at any time form late childhood to old age, the average of onset is the late forties. It may be slightly more common in females than in males. Old age, low intelligence, sensory impairment, cerebrovascular disease, and alcohol abuse are among the factors associated with this peculiar form of psychotic disorder.

Shared psychotic disorder is characterized by the presence of a delusion in an individual who is influence by someone else who has a longer-standing delusion with similar content. The diagnosis of Shared Psychotic Disorder is made only when the delusion is not due to the direct psychological effects of a substance or a general medical condition. It occurs when an otherwise healthy person (secondary partner) begins believing the delusions of someone with whom they have a close relationship (primary partner) who is already suffering from a psychotic disorder with prominent delusions (Silveira and Seeman, 1995).

Clinical observation suggests that separation may result in rapid improvement of the submissive person. These imposed false beliefs of the patient with folie a` deux are not to be considered delusions, because the patient gradually loses belief in them if separated from the dominant partner.

In DSM-IV-TR, shared psychotic disorder involves the presence of a delusion that develops in the context of a close relationship with another person, who already has an established delusion. (Table 19-1).

Diagnostic Features

The essential feature of a Shared Psychotic Disorder (Folie a` Deux) is a delusion that develops in an individual who is involved in a close relationship with another person (sometimes termed the primary case) who already has a psychotic disorder with prominent delusions (Criterion A). The individual comes to share the delusional beliefs of the primary case in whole or in part (Criterion B). The delusion is not better accounted for by another psychotic disorder (e.g. schizophrenia) or a mood disorder with psychotic features and is not due to the direct physiological effects of a substance (Criterion C).

Table 19-1 DSM-IV-TR Diagnostic Criteria for Shared Psychotic Disorder

A. A delusion develops in an individual in the context of a close relationship with another person(s), who has an already established-delusion.
B. The delusion is similar in content to that of the person who already has the established delusion
C. The disturbance is not better accounted for by another psychotic disorder (e.g. schizophrenia) or a mood disorder with psychotic features and is not due to the direct physiological effects of a substance (e.g. a drug abuse, a medication) or a general medical condition.

Family Issues. Most of the time, this disorder occurs in a nuclear family. Shared Psychotic disorder usually occurs only in long-term relationships in which one person is dominant and the other is passive. In fact, more than 95% of the cases reported involved people in the same family, most commonly siblings, a parent and child, or a husband and wife. Family therapy might focus on increasing exposure to outside activities and interests as well as the development of social supports to decrease isolation, encourage medication adherence, and help prevent relapse. Family Therapy also might help to improve communication and family dynamics.

The dominant person is possessed by a persecutory delusion that often evolves from some past experience that the dominant person and the patient went through together. Occasionally a grandiose delusion may be shared. Having heard the delusion expressed over and over, the patient, often impressionable and dependent and perhaps suffering from some other disorder such as depression, dementia, or mental retardation, gradually comes to believe in it.

Although two people are most commonly involved (folie a` deux), cases have been reported involving three or more and in some instances an entire family. The patients are usually relatives or persons who have lived in intimate contact for a long time.

VIGNETTE

A 50-year-old married female and her 48 year old husband with multiple sclerosis and who believed that they were being harassed and watched by the Irish Republican Army. This course is determined by the longevity of the relationship between the patient and the dominant person, and as this tends to be long lasting, folie a` deux likewise tends to be chronic. Both of the couple received psychiatric care for predominantly negative symptoms (i.e. social isolation, blunted affect, and marked lack of energy and initiative). On examination, the patients showed intense anxiety, confusion, disorientation to day and date, and loosening of associations.

Discussions. In this case, persons with a psychotic disorder believes aliens are spying on him and her. The delusions are induced in the secondary case and usually disappear when the people are separated. Aside from the delusions, the thoughts and behaviors of the secondary case usually are fairly normal. Impairment is often less severe in the individual with shared psychotic disorder than in the primary case, with separation form the primary case, the individual's delusional beliefs disappear, sometimes quickly and sometimes quite slowly. A clinical interview is required to diagnose shared psychotic disorder. There are basically three symptoms required for the determination of the existence of this disorder:

- An otherwise healthy person, in a close relationship with someone who already has an established delusion, develops a delusion himself/herself.
- The content of the shared delusion follows exactly or closely resembles that of the established delusion,
- Some other psychotic disorder, such as schizophrenia, is not in place and cannot better accounts for the delusion manifested by the secondary partner.

With treatment, a person with shared psychotic disorder has a good chance for recovery. Treatment options for the person with shared psychotic disorder might include the following:

- **Psychotherapy.** A type of counseling, psychotherapy can help the person with shared psychotic disorder recognize the delusion and correct the underlying thinking that has become distorted.
- **Family therapy.** Focus on increasing exposure to outside activities and interests as well as the development of social supports to decrease isolation, encourage medication adherence, and help prevent relapse. Family therapy also might help to improve communication and family dynamics.
- **Medication.** Short-term treatment with anti-psychotic medication might be used if the delusions do not resolve after separation from the primary case. In addition,

tranquilizers or sedative agents can help alleviate intense symptoms that might be associated with the disorder.

Separation from the dominant person and immersion into normal social interaction is generally sufficient to effect disappearance of the patient's false belief. Should separation not be possible, successful treatment of the dominant person's psychotic illness with antipsychotics may also be helpful.

Chapter 19: Shared Psychotic Disorder
Examination Review

1. The main defense mechanism used in shared Psychotic Disorder is

    A. Identification with the aggressor
    B. Projection
    C. Regression
    D. Reaction Formation

2. Shared Psychotic Disorder occurs most frequently among

    A. Women
    B. Low socioeconomic groups
    C. Members of the same family
    D. All of the above

3. What characterizes shared Psychotic Disorder?

    A. A pattern avoid of dominance and submission
    B. Acceptance by one person of the delusional belies of another
    C. The presence of schizophrenia or another psychosis in the submissive partner
    D. Two members of the same family not related, especially siblings, parent and child, or husband and wife.

4. What describes a patient with an established folie a` deux symptoms?

    A. A passive relationship that is cut off from the rest of society
    B. Resisting any outside efforts to separate the dominant person from the submissive partner
    C. Influence of a dominant person not subject to psychosis
    D. Symptoms tend to be of short duration

5. The final diagnosis in cases where paranoid features are prominent should be made only following:

    A. A complete medical and psychiatric history with special attention to alcohol and drugs of abuse
    B. A thorough physical examination, including neurological and mental status examinations
    C. Appropriate laboratory studies, particularly serological, toxicological, endocrine, and microbiological studies
    D. All of the above

6. The major treatment methods used for shred psychotic disorder are all the following except

    A. Short-term treatment with anti-psychotic medication
    B. Tranquilizers or sedative agents
    C. Without separation from the primary case, delusional beliefs disappear.
    D. Psychotherapy can help recognize the delusion and correct the underlying thinking that has become distorted.

7. The main defense mechanism used in shared psychotic disorder is

    A. Projection
    B. Regression
    C. Identification with aggressor
    D. Reaction formation

8. True statements concerning the treatment of shared psychotic disorder include

    A. Separation of the submissive person form the dominant person is the primary Intervention
    B. The submissive person often requires treatment with antipsychotic drugs
    C. The submissive person and the dominant person usually move back together after treatment
    D. All of the above

9. When is folie à deux typically of gradual onset

   A. It may occur at any time form late childhood ot old age
   B. The average age of onset is in the late sixties
   C. The average age of onset is in the early twenties
   D. It may be slightly more common in males than females

10. A clinical interview is required to diagnose shared psychotic disorder. What symptoms are required for determination of the existence of this disorder?

   A. An otherwise healthy person, in a close relationship with someone who already has an established delusion, develops a delusion himself/herself
   B. The content of the shared delusion follows exactly or closely resembles that of the established delusion.
   C. Some other psychotic disorder that is not in place and cannot better account for the delusion manifested by the secondary partner.
   D. All of the above.

Chapter 19: Shared Psychotic Disorder
Examination Answers

1. A
2. D
3. B
4. B
5. D
6. C
7. C
8. D
9. A
10. D

Chapter 20

Delusional Disorders

Delusions are false personal beliefs that are inconsistent with the person's intelligence or cultural background. The individual continues to have the belief in spite of obvious proof that it is false or irrational. A person with delusional disorder may be high functioning in daily life, and this disorder bears no relation to one's IQ. The traditional name for this disorder and the name originally bestowed on it by the German psychiatrist Emil Kraeplin is paranoia. Although the most common type of delusion seen in paranoia is that of persecution, other themes may be prominent: erotomanic, grandiosity, jealousy, and somatic may all occur. These patients do not display the pervasive disturbances of mood and thought in other psychotic conditions. In addition to social and occupational dysfunction, when it occurs, usually is in direct response to their delusions.

Table 20-1. DSM-5. Diagnostic Criteria
Delusional Disorder

A. The presence of one (or more) delusions with a duration of 1 month or longer.

B. Criterion A for schizophrenia has never been met
    NOTE: Hallucinations, if present, are not prominent and are related to the delusional theme(e.g. the sensation of being infested with insects associated with delusions of infestations.

C. Apart from the impact of the delusion(s) or its ramifications, functioning is not markedly impaired, and behavior is not obviously bizarre or odd.

D. If manic or major depressive episodes have occurred, these have been brief relative to the duration of the delusional periods.

E. The disturbance is not attributable to the physiological effects of a substance or another medical condition and is not better explained by another mental disorder, such as body dysmorphic disorder or obsessive-compulsive disorder.

Culture- Related Diagnostic Issues

An individual's cultural and religious background must be taken into account in evaluating the possible presence of delusional disorder. The social role is useful for cultural psychology because it designates a historically specific set of norms, rights, responsibilities, and qualifications.

Culture-Vygotsky outlined the foregoing pints about culture and psychology. He made scattered, general comments about the importance of culture, activity, social environment, social system, social role, social relationships, social class, social conditions, tools, and ideology if forming psychological phenomena.

Current-Culture is a system of enduring behavioral and thinking patterns that are created, adopted, and promulgated by a number of individuals. Studying cultural processes in order to understand psychology is a daunting task. The content of delusions also varies across cultural contexts. It requires a specific, comprehensive conceptualization of what culture is and how it encompasses human psychology.

African Americans do not benefit as much in current psychology because they remain segregated form many of the institutional resources. The fact that an individual occupies different roles in different activities makes one's social experience diverse. This is an important example of how social influences of psychology are modulated by specific positions (occupied by ethnic groups and genders) within activities.

Culture/Religious Beliefs.

The two predominant religious doctrines-Evangelicalism and Unitarianism-were adopted by two distinctive social classes. Evangelicals espoused traditional Calvinist ideals-including the omnipotence of God, reliance on the literal truth of scripture, and saving people from sin. Unitarians, in contrast, gave greater value to developing ethical principles on the basis of reason. Unitarians conceived God to be a benevolent figure rather than a punishing one.

Cultural/Buddhists. A great deal of research demonstrates that the quality of emotions is significantly structured by cultural concepts. For example, the Buddhist concept of suffering and sorrow with a distinctive quality. Buddhists accept suffering and sorrow as everyone's common fate. They are usual, expected, understandable, and shared. Accepting this state of affairs defines one as a good person. Striving to avoid or alter one's fateful position is a manifestation of hubris. As a result of this concept, sadness is enobling and, paradoxically, pleasurable. It testifies to one's strength of character and to one's commonality with other people.

McAllister (1992) gives us several other pointers, as summarized in Table 20-2.

TABLE 20-2. Central Nervous System Disorders and Associated Delusions

Condition	Comment
Cerebrovascular Disorders	More common with right posterior infarcts; subcortical atrophy may predispose.
Degenerative Disorders	In around 40% of the cases, delusions, usually of the simple persecutory type, will occur at some point
Extrapyramidal Disorders	Delusions are often complex and tightly held.
Epilepsy	Delusions are more common with temporal lobe focl; left temporal lobe focl are associated with first- rank schizophrenic symptoms.

Subtypes. The following Diagnostic and Statistical Manual of Mental Disorders (DSM) -5 subtypes are based on the following predominant delusional themes:

- **Erotomanic type:** In this subtype (also known as de-Cierambault's Syndrome), patients come to believe that they are loved by someone else, someone of very high social situation. This imagined lover maybe mayors, governors, singers, or movie stars are frequent candidates.
- **Grandiose type:** This subtype applies when the central theme of the delusion is the conviction of having some great (but recognized) talent or insight or having made some important discovery.
- **Jealous type:** This subtype applies when the central theme of the individual's delusion is that his or her spouse or lover is unfaithful.

- **Persecutory type:** This subtype applies when the central theme of the delusion involves the individual's belief that he or she is being conspired against, cheated, spied on, followed, poisoned or drugged, maliciously maligned, harassed, or obstructed in the pursuit of long-term goals.
- **Somatic type:** This subtype applies when the central theme of the delusion involves bodily functions or sensations.

The DSM-5 identifies the most common types of somatic delusions as those in which the individual believes that he or she:

- Emits a foul odor form the skin, mouth, rectum, or vagina
- Has an infestation of insects in or on the skin
- As an internal parasite
- Has misshapen and ugly body parts
- Has dysfunctional body parts

Let's begin our examination of delusional disorder with the following vignette.

Vignette

A 30 year old male veteran came into treatment because he was coerced by family members to suffer from the impossible delusions that his belief that he was controlled by green Martians, lasting for at least one month. In addition, he believes that he is being poisoned by the KGB and that a computer has been implanted into his brain, He feels overwhelmed by other aspects of his environment or isolated and lonely. During the interview, his self-care deficit was related to withdrawal, regression, panic anxiety, perceptual or cognitive impairment, inability to trust, evidenced by difficulty carrying out tasks associated with hygiene, dressing, grooming, eating, and toileting.

His family was receptive for hallucinations that are most commonly auditory. They often entailed the perception of the two voices commenting on the suffer in a threatening or derogatory.

Discussion. Paranoid Schizophrenia is characterized mainly by the presence of delusions of persecution or grandeur and auditory hallucinations related to a single theme. The individual is often tense, suspicious, and guarded, and may be argumentative, hostile, and aggressive. Onset of symptoms is usually later (perhaps in the late 20's or 30's), and less regression of mental faculties, emotional response, ad behavior is seen than in the other subtypes of delusional disorder.

In persecutory delusions, which are the most common type, individuals believe they are being malevolently treated in some way. Frequent themes include being conspired against, cheated, spied on, followed, poisoned or drugged, maliciously maligned, harassed, or obstructed in the pursuit of long-term goals. (APA, 2013). The individual may obsess about and exaggerate a slight rebuff (either real or imagined) until it becomes the focus of a delusional system. Repeated complaints may be directed at legal authorities, lack of satisfaction form which may result in violence toward the object of the delusion.

In this case, the patient suffers from delusion persecution. The individual feels threatened and believes that others intend harm or persecution toward him in some way (e.g. the FBI has bugged my room and intends to kill me: I can't take a shower in this bathroom; the nurses have put a camera in there so that they can watch everything I do). Delusions are deemed bizarre if they are clearly implausible, not understandable, and not derived from ordinary life experiences (e.g. an individual's belief that a stranger has removed his or her internal organs and replaced them with someone else's organs without any wounds or scars).

The more acute the psychosis, the more likely the delusion is to be disorganized and non-systematized. Consider in delusions of influence the patient believes that he can control events though telepathy. In delusions of reference the patient's convinced that there are meanings behind events and people's actions which are directed specifically toward himself. In delusions of thought broad-casting the belief is that others can hear the patient's thoughts.

Treatment

A challenge in the treatment of delusional disorders is that most patients have limited insight, and do not acknowledge that there is a problem. Most patients are treated as out- patients, although hospitalization may be required in some cases if there is a risk of harm to self or others.

Individual psychotherapy is a recommended rather than group psychotherapy, as patients are often quite suspicious and sensitive. Consider psychotherapy for patients with delusional disorder can include cognitive therapy. This therapy has been mostly studied in patients with the persecutory type. Psychotherapy has been said to be the most useful form of treatment because of the trust formed in a patient and therapist relationship. During the process, the therapist can ask hypothetical questions in a form of therapeutic Socratic questioning.

Supportive therapy has also been shown to be helpful. Its goal is to facilitate treatment adherence and provide education about the illness and its treatment. Furthermore, providing social skills training has helped many persons. It can promote interpersonal competence as well as confidence and comfort when interacting with those individuals perceived as a threat.

Insight –oriented therapy is rarely indicated or contraindicated: yet there are reports of successful treatment. Its goals are to develop therapeutic alliance, containment of projected feelings of hatred, impotence, and badness: measured interpretation as well as the development of a sense of creative doubt in the internal perception of the world

Deborah Y. Liggan, MD

Chapter 20: Delusional Disorder Examination Review

1. With this type of delusion, what does the individual believe that someone, usually of a higher status, is in love with him or her.

   A. Jealous Type
   B. Somatic Type
   C. Eroto-manic Type
   D. Grandiose Type

2. Individuals with somatic delusions believe they have some physical defects, disorder, or disease. The DSM-IV-TR (APA 2000) identifies the most common types of somatic delusions as those in which the individual believes that he or she:

   A. Emits a foul odor form the skin, mouth, rectum, or vagina
   B. Has an internal parasite
   C. Has dysfunctional body parts
   D. All of the above

3. In persecutory delusions, which are the most common subtype of delusional disorder?

   A. Individuals have irrational ideas regarding their own worth, talent, knowledge, or power
   B. Individuals believe they are being malevolently treated in some way
   C. Individuals believe that someone, usually of a higher status is in love with him or her.
   D. Individuals believe he/she has an internal parasite

4. With this type of delusion, the individual believes certain objects or persons have control over his/her behavior (e.g. the dentist put a filling I my tooth; I now receive transmission through the filling that control what I think and do).

   A. Delusion of Reference
   B. Delusion of Control or Influence

C. Delusion of Grandeur

D. Somatic Delusion

5. What conditions are defined by abnormalities limited to one domain of psychosis?

   A. Symptoms that characterize at least 1 month of delusions but no other psychotic symptoms

   B. Brief psychotic disorder that lasts more than 1 day and remits by 6 months

   C. The diagnosis of a schizophrenia spectrum disorder

   D. Psychotic symptoms that last for 1 year without termination

6. Delusional disorder has a significant familial relationship with what conditions?

   A. Schizoaffective disorder with catatonic features

   B. Schizophrenia and schizotypal personality disorder

   C. Schizophreniform disorder with provisional character

   D. Schizophrenia with autism spectrum disorder

7. This behavior is deficiency of energy. The individual with schizophrenia may lack sufficient energy to carry out activities of daily living or to interact with others

   A. Anergia

   B. Anhedonia

   C. Regression

   D. Waxy Flexibility

8. What term describes the inability to experience pleasure. This is a particularly distressing symptom that compels some clients to attempt suicide?

   A. Posturing

   B. Anhedonia

   C. Regression

   D. Echopraxia

9. What term describes the condition created by the person with schizophrenia who focuses inward on a fantasy world while distorting or excluding the external environment?

   A. Alogia
   B. Loose associations
   C. Autism
   D. Anergia

10. In this content of thought the individual feels threatened and believes that others intend harm or persecution toward him or her in some way.

   A. Somatic delusion
   B. Delusion of Reference
   C. Nihilistic delusion
   D. Delusion of Persecution

Chapter 20: Delusional Disorder Examination Answers

1. C
2. D
3. B
4. B
5. A
6. B
7. A
8. B
9. C
10. D

Reference Section 4

Addington, DE. Reducing suicide risk in patients with schizophrenia. Medscape Psychiatry & Mental Health, 2006.

Adebimpe VR. Overview: White Norms and Psychiatric Diagnosis of Black Patients. American Journal of Psychiatry. 138: 279-285. 1981.

American Psychiatric Association (APA). Diagnostic and Statistical Manual of Mental Disorders 4th Ed. Text revision, Washington, DC. 2000.

Andreasen NC and Black DW. Introductory Textbook of Psychiatry 4th Edition. Washington, DC: American Psychiatric of Publishing, 2006.

Andreasen NC, Flashman L et al. Regional Brain Abnormalities in Schizophrenia Measured with Magnetic Resonance Imaging. Journal of the American Medical Association 272: 1763- 1769; 1994.

Andreasen NC. Affective flattening and the criteria for schizophrenia. American Journal of Psychiatry 136: 944-947, 1979.

Arieti S. Interpretation of Schizophrenia 2nd Edition, New York. Basic Books, 1974.

Beighley PS, Brown GR, Thompson JW, et al. DSM-III-R Brief Reactive Psychosis Among Air Force recruits. The Journal of Psychiatry, 53: 283-288, 1992.

Benabarre A, Vieta E, Colom F, et al. Bipolar disorder, schizoaffective disorder and schizophrenia: epidemiologic, clinical and prognostic differences. European Psychiatry, 16: 167-172. 2001.

Benazzi F. DSM III-R- Schizophreniform disorder with good prognostic features: a six-year follow-up. Canadian Journal of Psychiatry; 43: 180-182. 1998.

Benazzi F, Mazzoli M, and Rossi E. A follow-up and family study of DSM-III-R Schizophreniform disorder with good prognostic features. European Archives of Psychiatry Clinical Neurosis, 1992.

Bleuler E. Dementia Praecox or the Group of Schizophrenias, Zinkin J (trans). New York, International Universities Press, 1950.

Breier A, Schreiber JL, Dyer J, et al. National Institute of Mental Health longitudinal study of chronic schizophrenia. Archives of General Psychiatry 48: 239-246, 1991.

Brockington IF, Meltzer HY. The nosology of schizoaffective psychosis. Psychiatry Development 1: 317-338, 1983.

Crow TJ. The Biology of Schizophrenia. Experiential. 38: 1275-1282. 1982.

Dearth N, Labenski BJ, Mott MF et al. Families Helping Families: Living with Schizophrenia. New York: Norton, 1986.

Frackowiak RS., Friston KJ, and Frith CD. e.g. Human Brain Function, Elsevier Academic Press, 2004.

Goff D. Psychosis. MerckMedicus, 2002.

Gotttesman II, Schizophrenia Genesis: The Orgins of Madness. New York: W.H. Freeman and Company, 1991.

Guiness EA. Brief reactive psychosis and the major functional psychoses: Descriptive case studies in Africa. British Journal of Psychiatry. Supple: 24. 1992.

Gur RE, Resnick SM, Alavi A, et al. Regional brain function in schizophrenia I: a positron emission tomography study. Archives of General of Psychiatry. 44:119-125. 1987.

Kaplan HI, Sadock BJ. Synopsis of Psychiatry, 5th Editon. Baltimore, MD. Williams + Wilkins, 1988.

Keefe RSF and Harvey PD. Understanding Schizophrenia. New York: Free Press, 1994.

Kendler KS, McGruire M, Gruenberg AM, et al. Examining the validity of DSM-III-R schizoaffective disorder and its putative subtypes in the Roscommon Family Study. American Journal of Psychiatry 152: 755-764. 1995.

Kraepelin RM. Dementia Praecox and Paraphrenia (1907). Translated by Barclay RM, Roberts GM. New York. Robert E. Kreiger, 1971.

Levinson DF, Levitt MEM. Schizoaffective mania reconsidered. American Journal of Psychiatry. 144:415-425. 1987.

Levitt JJ, Tsuang MT. The Heterogeneity of Schizoaffective Disorder: Implications for Treatment. American Journal of Psychiatry; 145: 926-936, 1988.

Maj M, Pirozzi R, Formicola AM, et al. Reliability and validity of the DSM- IV diagnostic category of schizoaffective disorder: preliminary data. Journal of Affective Disorder 57: 95-98. 2000.

Manschreck TC. Delusional disorder: The cognition and management of paranoia. Journal of Clinical Psychiatry 57(Supple 3): 32-38, 1996.

Mathes B, Wood SJ, Profitt TM, et al. Early processing deficits in object working memory in first episode schizophreniform psychosis and established schizophrenia. Psychology of Medicine. July, 2005.

Mc Allister TW. Neuropsychiatric aspects of delusions. Psychiatric Annals, 22: 269-277, 1992.

Munoz RA, Amado H, Hyatt S. Brief Reactive Psychosis. Journal of Clinical Psychiatry 48: 324-327, 1987.

Mendlewicz J. Current genetic concepts on schizoaffective psychosis in Genetic Aspects of Affective Illness. Edited by Mendlewicz J, Shopsin B. New York, SP Medical and Scientific Books, 1970., Inc. 1979.

Mueser KT and Gingeric SL. Coping with Schizophrenia: A Guide for Families. Oakland, CA: New Harbinger, 1994.

Munoz RA, Amado H, Hyat S. Brief Reactive Psychosis. Journal Clinical of Psychiatry 48:324-327, 1987.

Pies, R.W. Clinical Manual of Psychiatric Diagnosis and Treatment: A Biopsychosocial Approach, American Psychiatric Press, Inc. 1994.

Radomsky ED, Haas GL, Mann JJ, and Sweeny JA. Suicidal Behavior in Patients with Schizophrenia and other psychotic disorders. American Journal of Psychiatry. 156 (10). 1999.

Ratner C. Cultural Psychology: Theory and Method. Kluwer Academic/Plenum Publishers, 2002.

Sautter F, McDermott B, and Garver D. The course of DSM-III-R schizophreniform disorder. Journal of Clinical Psychology. May, 1993.

Shenton ME, Kikinis R, Jolesz FA. Abnormalities of the left Temporal Lobe and Thought Disorder in Schizophrenia. New Engand Journal of Medicine. 327: 604-612, 1992.

Siegel A. and Sapru HN. Essential Neuroscience, ippincott Williams + Wilkins, 2006.

Silveira JM, Seeman MV. Shared psychotic disorder: a critical review of the literature. Candian Journal of Psychiatry, 40: 389-395. 1995.

Strakowski SM. Diagnostic validity of Schizophreniform Disorder. The American Journal of Psychiatry, 151: 815- 824. 1994.

Strauss JS, Carpenter WT. Schizophrenia. New York, Plenum; 1981.

Tomb DA. Psychiatry, 5th Edition. Williams+ Wilkins, 1995.

Torrey EF. Surviving Schizophrenia: A Manual for Families, Consumers, and Providers 3rd Edition. New York: Harper and Row, 1995.

Trois A, Pasini A, Bersani G, et al. Negative symptoms and visual behavior in DSM-III-R prognostic subtypes of schizophreniform disorder. Acta Psychiatry Scand. May, 1991.

Vygotsky LS. Collected works Vol. 6. New York: Plenum, 1999.

Waitzkin H. Doctor-patient Communication: Clinical Implications of Social Scientific Research. JAMA 252: 2441-2446. 1984.

Zarate CA, Tohen M, Land ML. First-episode schizophreniform disorder: comparisons with first- episode schizophrenia. Schizophrenia Research, 46: 31-34, 2000.

Section Five

Disorders of Cognition

> *Thou ill-formed offspring of my feeble brain,*
> *Who after birth did'st by my side remain.*
> *Till snatched from thence by friends,*
> *less wise than true,*
> *Who thee abroad exposed to public view;*
> *Made thee in rags, halting, to the press to trudge.*
> *Where errors were not lessened all may Judge,*
> *At thy return my blushing was not small.*
> *My rambling brat (in print) should mother call,*
> *I cast thee by as one unfit for light,*
> *Thy visage was so irksome in my sight.*
>
> *Anne Bradstreet (1612-1672)*
> *The Author to Her Book*

Cognition encompasses the realms of memory, attention, language, visuospatial ability, conceptual, and general intelligence. I cognitive disorders, disturbances of memory are common but alteration in the other spheres of cognition are often present and may even dominant the clinical picture. A systematic approach to evaluating the various cognitive faculties is therefore key distinguishing among the three major classes of cognitive disorder described in the Diagnostic and Statistical manual of mental disorders, fifth edition (DSM-5): delirium, dementia, and amnestic disorder. Delirium is a global decline in cognitive function, accompanied by alterations in consciousness and attention. Dementia is characterized by a chronic decline in multiple functions occurring in clear consciousness. And amnestic disorder is a disability in learning new information or recalling previously learned information in the absence of other intellectual deficits. These disorders represent a significant change from a previous level of functioning.

Chapter 21

Delirium and Acute Confusional States

Delirium is an acute, potentially reversible brain dysfunction manifested by a syndromal array of neuropsychiatric symptoms. Delirium is a psychiatric syndrome characterized by a transient disorganization of a wide range of cognitive functions due to widespread derangement of cerebral metabolism. Lipowski (1983, 1987) characterized delirium as a disorder of attention, wakefulness, cognition, and motor behavior. This disruption of attention is often considered the core symptom. Patients struggle to sustain attentional focus, are easily distracted and often vary in their level of alertness. Sleep and wake cycles are disrupted as well. The delirious patient commonly naps or sleeps during daytime hours and is awake all night long. Nocturnal insomnia, bewilderment, and restlessness are often striking parts of a prodromal pattern. It is significant that patients with global cognitive impairment are at their best after a good sleep. Deficits can occur in perception, memory, language, processing speed, and executive functioning.

The term delirium is synonymous with the acute confusional states, although it describes a clinically distinct variety of acute confusional state characterized by periods of agitation, heightened mental activity, increased wakefulness, marked intrusive visual hallucinations, motor hyperactivity, and autonomic stimulation. Impairment of attention, essential to the acute confusional state, is present despite the apparent arousal.

The hallmark of delirium expressed in Box 21-2 depicts a fluctuating level of consciousness, a condition that is not usually seen in dementia until quite late in the disease process. The delirious patient, for example, may "nod off" every few minutes or show a marked inability to attend to interview questions for more than a few minutes.

TABLE 21-1 DSM-5 Diagnostic Criteria for Delirium

A. A disturbance in attention (i.e. reduced ability to direct, focus, sustain, and shift attention) and awareness (reduced orientation to the environment).

B. The disturbance develops over a short period of time (usually hours to a few days), represents a change from baseline attention an awareness, and tends to fluctuate in severity during the course of a day.

C. An addition disturbance in cognition (e.g. memory deficit, disorientation, language, visuospatial ability, or perception).

D. The disturbance in Criteria A and C are not better explained by another preexisting, established, or evolving neurocognitive disorder and do not occur in the context of a severely reduced level of arousal, such as coma

E. There is evidence from the history, physical examination, or laboratory findings that the disturbance is a direct physiological consequence of another medical condition, substance intoxication or withdrawal (i.e. due to a drug of abuse or to a medication), or exposure to a toxin, or is due to multiple etiologies.

Diagnostic Features

The essential feature of delirium is a disturbance of attention or awareness that is accompanied by a change in the baseline cognition that cannot be better explained by a pre-existing or evolving neurocognitive disorder. The individual with delirium may exhibit emotional disturbances, such as anxiety, fear, depression, irritability, anger, euphoria, and apathy. There may be rapid and unpredictable shifts from one emotional state to another. The disturbed emotional state may also be evident in calling out, screaming, cursing, muttering, moaning, or making other sounds. These behaviors are especially prevalent at night and under conditions in which stimulation and environmental cues are lacking. The prevailing mood may have a profound influence on all aspects of cognition, especially at the extremes of the continuum of mood. Hypomania may be accompanied by illusions, flight of ideas, and extreme motor and verbal output sometimes mimicking delirium. The disturbance develops over a short period of time, usually hours to a few days, and tends to fluctuate during the curse of the day, often with worsening in the evening and night when external orienting stimuli decrease. The duration of delirium is usually brief (e.g. 1 week; rarely more than 1 month) and, on recovery from the underlying determinant, symptoms usually diminish over a 3 to 7 day period, but in some instances may take as long as 2 weeks.

The first step diagnosis is to recognize that the patient is confused. This is obvious in most cases, nut the mildest forms of confusion, particularly when some other acute alteration of personality is prominent may ne overlooked. In these mild forms, a careful analsis of the pateitn's thought processes as details of the history of the illness and the patient's personal life are obtained will usually receal an incoherence. Digit span and serial subtraction of 3s and 7s form 100 are useful bedside tests of the patient's capacity for sustained mental activity. The mental task of crossing out all certain letters on a printed page over a period of a few minutes is a useful measure of attention. Another is the efficiency in performing dual tasks such as tapping alternately with each hand while reading aloud.

Psychomotor changes are common. In most patients, spontaneous motor activity is depressed, but hyperactivity y and restlessness characterize delirium. Repetitive stereotyped motor behavior, such as plucking at the bed clothes or tossing from side to side, is frequent. Involuntary movements, including irregular tremor, asterixis, and myoclonus, are usually seen in drug withdrawal or metabolic encephalopathy. Specifiers include switching between hyperactive and hypoactive states. Liptzin and Levkoff (1992) characterized delirious patients with restlessness, hyper-vigilance, rapid speech, irritability, and combativeness as hyperactive, where as those showing slowed speech and kinetics, apathy, and reduced alertness were designated hypoactive. Hypoactive patients tend to have more severe cognitive disturbances (Koponen et al, 1989) and a poorer prognosis.

Renal and cardiac symptoms are common. The cardiovascular disorder that most often presents with psychiatric symptoms is hypertensive encephalopathy. It usually presents with a diastolic blood pressure

of greater than 130 mmHg which causes a medical emergency. TH e goal of treatment is a diastolic blood pressure of 90 to 100 mg Hg.

There is an accompanying change in at least one other area that may include memory and learning (particularly recent memory), disorientation (particularly to time and place), alteration in language, or perceptual distortion or a perceptual-motor disturbance. Delirium may be increase in the context of functional impairment, immobility, a history of falls, low levels of activity, and use of psychoactive properties (particularly alcohol and anti-cholinergic). Delirium is often associated with a disturbance in the sleep-wake cycle. This disturbance can include daytime sleepiness, night time agitation, and difficulty falling asleep, excessive sleepiness throughout the night. Delirium may progress to stupor, coma, seizures, or death, particularly if the underlying cause remains untreated.

Causes of Delirium

The first step after diagnosis of delirium should be the determination and correction of the underlying causes. Many medical conditions and other problems can lead to delirium. Remember this helpful hint Table 21-2. the letters in the word "DELIRIUM" stand for the common reasons for this condition.

Table 21-2

D rugs: Many medications, recently started or stopped, changes in dosages, over-the counter medications, herbals, and alcohol

E lectrolyte imbalance: especially form dehydration

L ack of drugs: stopping certain medications, alcohol withdrawal

I nfection: such as urinary or respiratory tract infections; blood or wound infection after an injury or surgery

R educed sensory input: such as poor or uncorrected vision and hearing

I ntracranial: such as from a stroke

U rinary or fecal problems: such as inability to empty bladder or bowel

M yocardial (heart) and lungs: heart attack, pneumonia, or other condition causing lack of oxygen in the blood and the brain.

- • Psychiatric causes
- • Evaluation of psychological and cognitive symptoms
- • Psychotherapy in later life

Evaluating confused patients for the following signs and symptoms may assist in diagnosing depression: a) tearfulness, depressed appearance; b) social withdrawal, decreased talkativeness; c) brooding, self-pity, pessimism; and d) lacked activity.

Some have proposed a single question to screen for depression: "Have you been feeling down, blue, or depressed most of the time over the last few weeks?." A Yes answer would initiate additional follow-up and evaluation focusing on the signs and symptoms above. Suicidal ideation is quite likely to be associated with depression in the terminally ill, even in mild and passive forms.

Delirium and Psychiatric causes. In anxiety, extreme grief, or depression, orientation for person and place is usually preserved, and with encouragement, the patient can concentrate and improve cognitive performance. In patient's clouded consciousness, delirium has a sudden onset (hours or days), a brief and fluctuating course, and rapid improvement when the causative factor is identified and eliminated. Hyperactivity, diminished need for sleep, pressure of speech, delusions, short attention span, and distractibility in acute mania may be confused with the hyper-excitability of delirium.

Delirium Aged. Delirium is one of the most common and important forms of psychopathology in later life. Older people with delirium are susceptible to injuries falls, dehydration, pressure sores, and malnutrition. Almost any complicating illness may bring out a confusional state in an elderly person. A number of factors have been identified that predispose elderly people to delirium, including structural brain disease, reduced capacity for homestatic regulation, impaired vision and hearing, a high prevalence of chronic disease, reduced resistance to acute stress, and age-related changes in the pharmacodynamics of drugs. This is why delirium is a medical emergency.

VIGNETTE

A 60 year old veteran reported to the clinic with confusion that developed suddenly and progressing over a few days. The confusion fluctuated with periods of agitation and restlessness followed by periods of tiredness and indifference. In the interview, the person had difficulty concentrating on familiar tasks and was not able to follow simple commands because he became more and more forgetful. He did not know what day it was, where he was, or even who he was. His speech was jumbled and reflected disorganized thinking. In his diagnosis, of hypoactive delirium, manifested by extreme drowsiness, fatigue, and indifference. As his delirium fluctuated the episodes of lethargy were followed by periods of agitation and hallucinations.

Discussion. The interview itself should focus on establishing a global image of the patient's cognitive functioning. In regarding to Folstein et al (1975) Mini-mental state Examination (MMSE) (see chapter 1) the study reported the mean MMSE score to be 14.3 for delirious patients, versus 29.6 for control subjects. The patient in this vignette is likely to be at his worst when he has been awake for many hours and at the latter part of his day arrives. In this phenomenon, called sundowning, reduced sensory input and fatigue combine to unmask organicity in night time hours. Autonomic manifestations, such as tachycardia, sweating, flushed face, dilated pupils, and elevated blood pressure, are common. The patient with delirium displays reduced ability to extract, process, retain, and retrieve information about his or her environment is impaired, and consequently, he or she is less about to plan, initiate, and sustain goal directed behavior.

The DSM-IV-TR describes by a disturbance of consciousness and a change in cognition that develop rapidly over a short period. (APA,2000) Symptoms of delirium include difficulty sustaining and shifting attention. The person is extremely distractible fan must be repeatedly reminded to focus attention. Disorganized thinking prevails and is reflected by speech that is rambling, irrelevant, pressured, and incoherent, and that unpredictably switches form subject to subject. Reasoning ability and goal-directed behavior are impaired. Disorientation to time and place is common, and impairment of recent memory is invariably evident. Misperception of the environment, including illusions and hallucinations, prevail. The state of awareness may range from that of hypervigilance (heightened awareness to environmental stimuli) to stupor or semi-coma.

Treatment

The first step in the treatment of delirium should be the determination and correction of the underlying causes. While the majority of individuals with delirium have a full recovery with or without treatment, early recognition and intervention usually shortens the duration of the delirium. Additional attention must be given to fluid and electrolyte statues, hypoxia, anoxia, and diabetic problems.

Deborah Y. Liggan, MD

Management of delirium may be non-pharmacological and / or pharmacological. Measures to reduce anxiety and disorientation include keeping lights on low at night, surrounding the patient with quiet familiar objects, family presence, and presence, and keeping a clock and calendar in the visual field. Neuroleptics are used because they help calm the patient and improve mentation. If possible, the neuroleptic should be administered at night so as to facilitate sleep and help restore the disrupted sleep-wake cycle. Haloperidol is most commonly used, but chlorpromazine is often useful particularly in the agitated delirious patient. For severely agitated delirious patients (including those with terminal agitation or terminal restlessness), sedation may be a higher priority than clearing mentation. In this case consider adding meds when the goals of therapy shift to sedation.

Chapter 21: Delirium and Acute Confusional States Examination Review

1. What cardiovascular disorder most often presents with psychiatric?

    A. Elevated dietary sodium levels
    B. Hypertensive encephalopathy
    C. Diastolic blood pressure of less than 60mmHg
    D. A severely elevated serum cholesterol level

2. It is necessary to differentiate a delirium form a dementia by what hallmark differences.

    A. The course of depression fluctuates over a few days
    B. Family history is not contributory in both delirium and depression
    C. Language deficits are dysgraphia in delirium and increased speech latency in depression
    D. Affect is labile in depression

3. What particular kind of memory contents refers to information that relates to the ways in which the memory system functions?

    A. Metamemory
    B. Episodic memory
    C. Generic memory
    D. Semantic memory

4. What disturbance in the sleep wake cycle is often affected in the level of consciousness?

    A. Heightened awareness to environmental stimuli
    B. Fluctuating between hyper-somnolence and insomnia
    C. Vivid dreams and nightmares
    D. All of the above

5. In addition to disturbances in her cognition and orientation, what changes reinforce confusion?

   A. Hearing, speech, and vision
   B. Energy, creativity, and coordination
   C. Personality, speech, and mobility
   D. Appetite, affect, and attitude

6. How do acute and chronic brain dysfunction compare?

   A. The duration of delirium usually lasts 6 months
   B. Thinking is typically disorganized in delirium and impoverished in dementia
   C. Perception is often distorted in dementia
   D. The sleep-wake cycle is often normal for age in delirium

7. Which of the sign and symptoms identified in confused patients correspond with criteria for delirium?

   A. Acute onset (hours to days)
   B. Clouding of consciousness
   C. Perceptual disturbance, disorientation, or memory deficit
   D. All of the above

8. Elderly patients with acute confusional state present with

   A. Reduced cognition
   B. Impaired attention
   C. Disturbance in the sleep wake cycle
   D. All of the above

9. What neurotransmitter is hypothesized to be involved in delirium within the reticular formation?

   A. Serotonin
   B. Acetylcholine
   C. Dopamine
   D. Glutamate

10. What area of the brainstem is the principal site regulating attention and arousal?

    A. The hippocampus
    B. The frontal lobe
    C. The reticular formation
    D. The occipital lobe

Chapter 21: Delirium and Acute Confusional States Examination Answers

1. B
2. C
3. A
4. D
5. C
6. B
7. D
8. D
9. B
10. C

Chapter 22

Dementia

Diagnostic. The term dementia usually denotes a clinical syndrome composed failing memory and impairment of other intellectual functions due to chromic progressive degenerative disease of the brain. Cognitively, a decline in memory functioning is typically the first symptom observed, although language and/or visuospatial problems also can be first symptoms.

Memory. In as much as memory is important for orientation to person, place, and time, orientation can be progressively affected during the course of a dementing illness. For example, patients with dementia may forget how to get back to their rooms after going to the bathroom. But no matter how severe the disorientation seems, patients show no impairment in their level of consciousness. Let us place emphasis on dementia because it is not merely a problem of memory. Affected persons may be disoriented in time (not knowing what day of the week, day of the month, or even what year it is), in place (place not knowing where they are), and inn person (not knowing themselves or others who are around them). It reduces the abilities to learn reason, retain, or recall past experience and there is also loss of patterns of thought, feelings, and activities. Additional mental and behavioral problems often affect people who have dementia. It may influence quality of life, caregivers, and the need for nursing home placement.

Age. Dementia is a serious loss of cognitive ability in a previous unimpaired person, beyond what might be expected from normal aging. Dementia is not part of normal aging any more than gastrointestinal bleeding is a part of growing old. It is the major cause of long term disability in old age. Recent research has advanced our understanding of the boundary between normal aging and dementia. In normal aging the patient may have some loss of cognitive function, but it is nor progressive and does not cause impairments in social and occupational functioning. Dementia breakdown: symptoms of dementia can be classified as either irreversible or reversible, depending upon the causes of the disease. For example, the causes of dementia depend on the age at which symptoms begin. The term mild cognitive impairment has been used to describe the group of older individuals who have greater than expected memory impairment for their age, but do not meet the criteria for dementia. In the elderly population (usually defined in this situation as over 65 years of age) a large majority of cases of dementia takes place.

Cultural differences can complicate the perception, definition, and diagnosis of dementia. For example, in some societies the very concept of dementia does not exist, as changes in cognition with increasing age may be attributed to normal aging.

Dementia syndromes can be divided into major categories based on the location of pathologic changes in the central nervous system.

Cortical dementias are caused by pathologic changes in the cerebral cortex. The most common causes of cortical dementia are Alzheimer's disease and Pick's disease.

Alzheimer's disease. In 1907, the German psychiatrist, Alois Alzheimer first described the condition that later assumed his name. He described a 51year old woman with a 4 year course of progressive dementia. Although Alzheimer disease has been described at every period of adult life, a majority of these patients have been in their late fifties or younger. Alzheimer's type dementia has shown linkage to chromosomes 1, 14, and 21.

Senile plaques, also referred to as amyloid plaques, more strongly indicate Alzheimer's disease, although they are also seen in normal aging. This is the most common and important degenerative disease of the brain. Dementing processes that affect the cortex, primarily dementia, can affect patients' language abilities. The language difficulty may be characterized by a vague, stereotyped, imprecise, or circumstantial locution, and patients may also have difficulty naming objects. The DSM-5 diagnostic criteria for dementia of the Alzheimer's type emphasize the presence of memory impairment and the associated presence of at least one other symptom of cognitive decline (aphasia, apraxia, agnosia, or abnormal executive functioning). The patient's speech is halting because of failure to recall the needed word. The same difficulty interrupts writing. Vocabulary becomes restricted and expressive language stereotyped and inflexible.

Five limited deficits have been observed in Alzheimer disease:

1. **Korsakoff amnesic state.** The early stages of Alzheimer disease may be dominated by a disproportionate failure of retentive memory, with integrity of other cognitive abilities. In such patients, immediate memory, tested buy the capacity to repeat a series of members or words, is essentially intact; it is the longer-term (retentive) memory that fails, such a restricted disabilities constitutes the senile amnesic state.

2. **Dysnomia.** The forgetting of words, especially proper names, may first bring the patient to a physician. Every sentence is broken by a pause and search for the wanted word. A useful test for the failure to find names (dysnomia), which is probably the most common abnormality of language in this disease.

3. **Spatial disorientation.** Parietal lobe function, commonly deranged in in the course of Alzheimer disease, may fail while other functions are relatively preserved Losing one's way in familiar surroundings, inability to interpret a road map, distinguish right

from left, park or garage a car, and difficulty in setting the table or dressing are all manifestations of a special failure to orient the schema of one's body with that of surrounding space.

4. **Paranoia and other personality changes.** Frequently, at some point in the dementing process, the most prominent event in the development of senile dementia is the occurrence of paranoia or bizarre behavior. The patient becomes convinced that relatives are stealing his or her possessions or that an elderly and even infirm husband or wife is guilt y of infidelity.

5. **Gait disorder.** While it is true that most patients with Alzheimer disease walk normally until relatively late in their illness, not infrequently in the older patient, a short-stepped gait and poor balance may call attention to the disease and worsen slowly for several years before other manifestations become evident.

Table 22-1 DSM-IV-TR Diagnostic Criteria for Dementia of the Alzheimer's Type

A. The development of multiple cognitive deficits manifested by both

1. Memory impairment (impaired ability to learn new information or to recall previously learned information)
2. One (or more) of the following cognitive disturbances:

   a. Aphasia (language disturbance)
   b. Apraxia (impaired ability to carry out motor activities despite intact motor function)
   c. Agnosia (failure to recognize or identify objects despite intact sensory function)
   d. Disturbance in executive functioning (i.e. planning, organizing, sequencing, abstracting)

B. The cognitive deficits in Criteria A1 and A2 each cause significant impairment in social or occupational functioning and represent a significant decline from a previous level of functioning.

C. The course is characterized by gradual onset and continuing cognitive decline.

D. The cognitive deficits in Criteria A1 and A2 are not due to any of the following:

  1. Other central nervous system conditions that cause progressive deficits in memory and cognition (e.g. cerebrovascular disease, Parkinson's disease, Huntington's disease, subdural hematoma, normal-pressure hydrocephalus, brain tumor)

  2. Systemic conditions that are known to cause dementia (e.g. hypothyroidism, vitamin B12 or folic acid deficiency, hypercalcemia, neurosyphilis, HIV infection)

  3. Substance-induced conditions

E. The deficits do not occur exclusively during the course of a delirium.

F. The disturbance is not better accounted for by another Axis I disorder (e.g. Major Depressive Disorder, Schizophrenia)

A year old married man with two children has been followed by a multidisciplinary team at Department of Veterans Affairs (VA) geriatric research and clinical center for the past 5 years. The occasion for this evaluation is his wife, who requested residential placement for her husband.

The patient was first evaluated 10 years ago when his wife observed changes in his memory and behavior and suggested that they seek medical advice. At this time, he acknowledged that he had been aware of increasing memory problems for at least the past 5 years. He said that he frequently forgot his keys or would go into the house to get his keys or would go into the house to get something and then forget what he wanted.

His wife noted that he had changed from an outgoing, pleasant person to one who avoided conversation. She said that he also seemed hostile at times for no apparent reason. Instead, he was in good health and was not taking any medications. His alcohol consumption was limited to two to three days a day. He had not significant medical or psychiatric history and no significant family history for either cognitive or psychiatric disorders.

Three years later, his wife contacted the VA center for treatment of her husband's cognitive and behavior symptoms. The neurological examination demonstrated and absence of focal abnormalities and he was hesitant and had difficulty with sustained attention, which made determination of visual fields difficult. There was no evidence of any disturbance of mood. On examination of his sensorium, he was disoriented about place and date; he missed the actual date by 2 years and 1 month. However, he seemed to comprehend most of the questions and was aware that he was experiencing cognitive difficulties.

Discussion. The progressive nature of symptoms associated with dementia has been described according to stages (Stanely, Blair + Beare, 2005; NIA, 2007):

- **Stage 1.** No apparent symptoms. In the first stage of the illness, there is no apparent decline in memory.
- **Stage 2.** Forgetfulness. The individual begins to lose things or forget names of people. Losses in short-term memory are common.
- **Stage 3.** Mild cognitive decline. The individual may get lost when driving his or her car. Concentration may be interrupted. There is difficulty recalling names or words, which becomes noticeable to family and close associates.
- **Stage 4.** Mild to moderate cognitive decline; confusion. At this stage, the individual may forget major events in personal history, such as his or her own child's birthday; experience declining ability to perform tasks, such as shopping and managing personal finances. He or she may deny that a problem exists by covering up memory loss with confabulation (creating imaginary events to fill in memory gaps).
- **Stage 5.** Moderate cognitive decline; early dementia. In the early stages of dementia, some patients present

initially with visuospatial orientation. The individual loses the ability to perform some activities of daily living (ADLs) independently, such as hygiene, dressing, and grooming, and require some assistance to manage these on an ongoing basis. And the razor is no longer correctly applied to the face.

- **Stage 6.** Moderate-to-severe cognitive decline; middle dementia. At this stage; middle dementia. A t this stage, the individual may be unable to recall recent major life events or even the name of his or her spouse. Disorientation to surroundings is common, and the person may be unable to recall the day, season, or year. The person is unable to manage ADLs without assistance. Urinary and fecal incontinence are common. Sleeping becomes a problem. Psychomotor symptoms include wandering, obsessiveness, agitation, and aggression. Symptoms seem to worsen in the late afternoon and evening—a phenomenon termed sundowing. Institutional care is usually required at this stage because depression, agitation, and violent behavior may occur. Delusions are common. For example, the spouse accused of being an imposter or the patient talks to imaginary persons, or to his own reflections in the mirror.

- **Stage 7.** Severe cognitive decline; late dementia. During late-stage dementia, the person becomes more chair bound or bedbound. Muscles are rigid, contractures may develop, and primitive reflexes may be present.

- Appetite decreases and dysphagia is present; aspiration is common. Speech and language are severely impaired, with greatly decreased verbal communication. The person may no longer recognize any family members. They eventually forget their own name and may not recognize their spouse. Bowel and bladder incontinence are present and caregivers are needed to complete most ADLs for the person. The sleep-wake cycle is greatly altered, and the person spends a lot of time dozing and appears socially withdrawn and more unaware of the environment or surroundings.

Dementia due to Pick's Disease

Pick's disease was first described in 1892 by Arnold Pick, a professor of psychiatry at the University of Prague. The clinical picture is strikingly similar to that of Alzheimer's disease. However, the clinical features are those of progressive dementia with severe loss of speech function.

Pick's disease is a progressive degenerative disease beginning in the cerebral cortex of the frontal lobes. Studies also reveal that pathology of Pick's disease results from atrophy in the frontal lobes of the brain, in contrast to Alzheimer's disease, which is more widely distributed. Patients often have frontal release signs, including dramatic behavioral changes of disinhibition and social inappropriateness.

Pick's Disease is an extremely uncommon cause for prercenile dementia, occurring in age groups from 40 to 65 years. One major difference is that the initial symptom in Pick's disease is usually personality change, whereas the initial symptom in Alzheimer's disease is memory impairment. Features of Kluver- Bucy syndrome (such as hyper-sexualtiy, placidity, and hyperoraity) are much more common in Pick's disease than in Alzheimer's disease.

Subcortical Dementias

Subcortical dementias are caused by pathologic changes in the basal ganglia, thalamus, and brain stem. The most common causes of subcortical dementia are vascular disease, Parkinson's disease, Huntington's chorea, and Lewy body dementia.

Vascular dementia is the second most common form of dementia, ranking after Alzheimer's disease. In this disorder, the clinical syndrome of dementia is due to significant cerebrovascular disease. The blood vessels of the brain are affected, and progressive intellectual deterioration occurs. In vascular dementia, clients suffer the equivalent of small strokes that destroy many areas of the brain. Certain focal neurological signs are commonly seen with vascular dementia, including weaknesses of the limbs, small-stepped gait, and difficulty with

Hypertension or other cardiovascular or other cardiovascular risk factors is usual un vascular dementia but rare in Alzheimer's disease. Nocturnal confusion, relative preservation of personality, emotional liability, somatic complaints, and depression are common in vascular dementia. Higher prevalence has been reported in African Americans compared with Caucasians, and in East Asian countries (e.g. Japan, China). Prevalence is also higher n makes than in females.

Vignette: Vascular Disease

A 72 year-old woman with a history of several small strokes experienced moderate forgetfulness and confusion but was generally calm and pleasant. Keeping track of the date with a calendar and making copious notes to herself, she managed to maintain an independent existence at home. At the super-market checkout counter, she could not find her wallet but insisted she had money to pay her for food. The clerk grew impatient, and the patient became increasingly agitated, tearful, and accusatory. When the store manager was called, she picked up grocery items and began throwing them.

Discussion. Prevention and treatment of Vascular dementia are the same as prevention and treatment of hypertension, atherosclerosis, hyperlipidemia and diabetes.

Dementia Due to Parkinson's disease Parkinson's disease was first described in 1817 by James Parkinson, a British paleontologist and surgeon. In this disease, there is a loss of nerve cells located in the sub-stantia nigra, and dopamine activity is diminished, resulting in involuntary muscle movements, slowness, and rigidity. Tremor in the upper extremities is characteristic. Other early subtle symptoms are decreases in the caliber of handwriting and the volume of the voice; both reflect disturbances in extrapyramidal motor function.

The course of progression can be described in terms of sequential stages: staged typically involves unilateral motor signs with akinesia and rigidity; stage 2 manifests with bilateral motor signs and includes tremor and some alteration pf postural reflexes; in stage 3, a marked loss of postural reflexes occurs; and in stage 4, the Parkinson patient is typically able to walk only with the assistance of a walker.

Parkinson's disease is a slowly progressive neurological condition, characterized by tremor, rigidity, bradykinesia, and postural instability. The dementia associated with Parkinson's disease is characterized by cognitive and motoric slowing, executive dysfunction, and impairment in memory retrieval. Declining cognitive performance in individuals with Parkinson's disease is frequently exacerbated by depression. There is compelling evidence that depression in Parkinson's disease is an intrinsic part of the illness and not simply a reaction to disability. Findings on physical examination include the characteristic abnormal motor signs of resting tremor, evidence of slowness and poverty of movement (such as micrographic), associated movements. This disease is characterized by an expressionless face (clinicians sometimes refer to it as "mask-like face"), slowness of movement (bradykinesia or hypokinetic syndrome), rigidity of extremities and neck, and tremors in the hands. Patients with Parkinson's disease have a gait that is characterized by short wide-based steps (sometimes referred to as fenestrating gait), stopped posture, and scarcity of normal limb movements. The patient also displays involuntary movements at rest.

Dementia Due to Huntington's Chorea

Huntington's disease is an inherited degenerative neurologic disorder first described in 1872 by George Huntington, an American general practitioner. Damage is seen in the areas of the basal ganglia and the cerebral cortex. Progressive cognitive impairment is a core feature of Huntington's disease, with early changes in executive function (i.e. processing speed, organization, and planning) rather than learning and memory. Cognitive and associated behavioral changes often precede the emergence of the typical motor abnormalities of bradykinesia (i.e. slowing of voluntary movement) and chorea (i.e. involuntary jerking movements).

Cognitive Disorder with Lewy Bodies.

Core diagnostic features specified in DSM-5 include fluctuating cognition with pronounced variations in attention and alertness. Recurrent visual hallucinations that is well formed and detailed. And spontaneous features of Parkinsonism, with onset subsequent to the development of cognitive, decline. Suggestive diagnostic features are that symptoms meet criteria for rapid eye movement sleep behavior disorder and severe neuroleptic sensitivity. Individuals with Lewy body's dementia frequently experience repeated falls and syncope and transient episodes of unexplained loss of consciousness.

Reversible Causes of Dementia

Once a definitive diagnosis of dementia has been made, a primary consideration in the treatment of the disorder is the etiology. Focus must be directed to the identification ad resolution of potentially reversible processes.

The treatable forms of dementia include normal- pressure hydrocephalus, pellagra, vitamin B12 and thiamine deficiency states, hypothyroidism and other metabolic and endocrine disorders.

Normal Pressure Hydrocephalus

Normal-pressure hydrocephalus with dementia was described in 1965, when Adams and coworkers reported patients with the triad of dementia, disturbance of gait, and urinary incontinence. Dementia is often mild, although it may be a prominent finding. The usual findings are more of slowness of thought, apathy, lethargy, and psychomotor retardation. Memory dysfunction may be severe, and disorientation can occur late in the course of the disease. Gait disturbance is prominent and may be the initial manifestation. There is spasticity with hyperactive deep tendon reflexes and up going toes; slow, shuffling, unsteady gait; problems in initiating movement; and apraxia of gait. In continence is usually urinary and is perhaps more of an indifference to continence.

The term refers to slow ventricular enlargement, without cortical atrophy due to poor cerebrospinal fluid (CSF) reabsorption. The basic term appears to be a clock to CSF flow, usually in the region of the basal cisternae or cerebral subarachnoid space. A vexing question is the selection of patients for shunt therapy who have normal-pressure hydrocephalus.

Pellagra

Poor diet, often compounded by chronic alcoholism, places the patient at risk for niacin deficiency, which cause the disorder today known as pellagra. Classic pellagra is a disease common in parts of the world were people have a lot of corn in parts of the world were people have a lot of corn in their diet. Nevertheless, among the vegetarian, maize eating people of under developed countries and among the black population in South Africa, pellagra is still a common disease. Manifestations of pellagra include the "four D's": dermatitis (scaly skin sores), diarrhea, dementia, and death. The treatment of pellagra is based on the administration of a high-protein diet in conjunction with niacin supplementation. Since 1940 the prevalence of pellagra has diminished because of the enriching bread with niacin.

Vitamin B12 Deficiency

Vitamin B12 is a nutrient that helps keep the body's nerve on blood cells healthy. Patients can get enough vitamin B12 by eating a variety of foods including: beef, fish, poultry, eggs, milk, and other dairy products. Vitamin B12 is also added to most breakfast cereals and other food products. Vitamin deficiencies and chronic infections may occur many symptoms before dementia occurs other than those who have trouble getting enough vitamin B12 include people who eat little or no animal foods including strict vegetarians and vegans.

The patient first notices general weakness and parenthesis consisting as if tingling, "pins and needles" or other vaguely described sensations. Decreased vibratory sense occurs in the lower extremities, motor weakness, and loss of reflexes. Pallor, a yellow, wasted appearance of the skin, rapid pulse, glossitis, and mild splenomegaly are among the other clinical features of patients with B12 deficiency and pernicious anemia.

Thiamin Deficiency

Tachycardia, heart failure, or certain neurologic signs and symptoms (neuropathy, disorientation, and nystagmus) in a patient with a poor diet, especially the alcoholic, suggests vitamin B1 (thiamin) deficiency. Symptoms include palpitations, shortness of breath, weight loss, anorexia, weakness, and paresthesia (especially of the lower extremities). Chronic use of substances of alcohol can predispose cognitive changes suggested of dementia. For example: Thiamin deficiency results in three forms of beriberi and an encephalaopathy termed Wernicke-Korsakoff syndrome.

The value of a nutritionally adequate diet should be stressed to all patients. Thiamin is abundant in wheat germ, rice bran, soybean flour, yeast, and ham. Other good sources are gooseberries, plums, prunes, raisins, asparagus, beans, broccoli, Brussels sprouts, corn, peas, potatoes, oats, brown rice, mushrooms, meat, poultry, eggs, and milk. Some fish, e.g. tuna, contain thiaminase, an enzyme which destroys thiamin.

Hypothyroidism

Hypothyroidism is the most common endocrine condition to present with dementia. In its severest form, classical myxedema is easy to recognize. Common symptomatology includes slow and hoarse speech, lethargy, intolerance to cold, impaired memory, constipation, and slow movements. Symptoms tend to be insidious and often require months to years to evolve into a complete clinical picture. The skin may appear yellow due to carotene accumulation. Often the tongue is enlarged and thing of the lateral eyebrows are common, with loss of expressiveness and lid drooping. Later in hypothyroidism there accumulates in the dermis, associates with complaints of coarse, dry skin and facial puffiness, and brittleness of the nails and hair. Relatives of patients often report slowing of mentation, particularly alterations in recent memory function, cognition, and somnolence.

Examination of the cardiovascular system often reveals cardiac enlargement and diminished heart sounds. This may reflect pericardial effusion or diastolic hypertension. Muscle strength is usually diminished, and joints may show capsular thickening and excessive synovial fluid. The most important neurologic signs is delay in the relaxation phase of deep tendon reflexes, seen best when ankle jerks are elicited with the patient in the kneeling position. Sometimes these symptoms may be fully reversible with treatment with thyroid hormones.

Chapter 22: Dementia Examination Review

1. Describe the presentation in Alzheimer's disease in which the car cannot be parked or the patient turns in the wrong direction on the way home.

    A. Visuospatial orientation
    B. Disorientation to time or place
    C. Abnormal executive functioning
    D. Emotional changes become very pronounced

2. How disoriented affected persons be I their level of consciousness?

    A. In time – not knowing what day of the week, day of the month, or even what year it is
    B. In place- not knowing where they are
    C. In person- not knowing themselves or others around them
    D. All of the above

3. To what chromosomes is Alzheimer's type dementia shown linkage?

    A. Chromosomes 2, 4, and 6
    B. Chromosomes 5,10, and 15
    C. Chromosomes 1,14, and 21
    D. Chromosomes 10,20, and 25

4. Describe the forgetting of words, especially proper names in Alzheimer's dementia.

    A. Korsakoff amnesic state
    B. Dysnomia
    C. Spatial disorientation
    D. Paranoia behavior

5. Which of the following cognitive disturbances is characterized by an impaired ability to carry out motor activities despite intact motor function?

    A. Aphasia
    B. Apraxia
    C. Agnosia
    D. Abnormal executive functioning

6. Which dementia is a progressive degenerative disease beginning in the cerebral cortex of the frontal lobes?

    A. Alzheimer's disease
    B. Vascular disease
    C. Pick's disease
    D. Parkinson's disease

7. In vascular dementia, what symptoms do patients suffer from most of all?

    A. A series of small strokes
    B. Long-standing hypertension
    C. Cerebrovascular disease
    D. All of the above

8. What diagnostic features are specified in dementia by frequently experiencing repeated falls and syncope and transient episodes of unexplained loss of consciousness?

    A. Cognitive disorders with Lewy bodies
    B. Dementia due to Parkinson's Disease
    C. Dementia due to Huntington's Disease
    D. Normal –Pressure Hydrocephalus

9. What are the characteristics of reversible dementia known as pellagra?

    A. A disease common in parts of the world where there is a lot of corn in the diet

B. The disease has diminished because of the enriching bread with niacin

C. Manifestations include the four D's: dermatitis, diarrhea, dementia, and death

D. All of the above

10. What brain disorder is due to thiamin deficiency?

A. Wernicke-Korsakoff syndrome

B. Hypothyroidism

C. Normal- Pressure Hydrocephalus

D. Pernicious anemia

Chapter 22: Dementia Examination Answers

1. A
2. D
3. C
4. B
5. B
6. C
7. D
8. A
9. D
10. A

Chapter 23

Amnestic Disorder

Amnestic disorders are characterized by an inability to learn new information (short-term memory deficit) despite normal attention, and an inability to recall previously learned information (long-term memory deficit). Events from the remote past often are recalled more easily than recently occurring ones. Amnesia can be a sign or a symptom of a variety of disorders, including medical conditions, such as brain tumors and central nervous system infections, substance-related disorders, and so-called functional disorders such as post-traumatic stress disorder and dissociative disorders. The syndrome differs from the dementia in that there is no impairment in abstract thinking or judgment, no other disturbances of higher cortical function, and no personality change.

Amnesia may have a primary or secondary gain. The woman who is amnestic for the birth of a dead baby achieves primary gain by protecting herself form painful emotions. An example of secondary gain is a soldier who develops sudden amnesia and is removed from combat areas as a result.

Profound amnesia may result in disorientation to place and time, but rarely to self. The individual may engage in confabulation-the creation of imaginary events to fill in memory gaps. Loss of memory from psychological causes is dissociative amnesia. Usually there is sudden anterograde loss of emotion-laden information after a severe physical or psychosocial stress. It occurs most frequently in women in their teens or 20's, or in men during the stress of war. The patient often appears confused and puzzled during the attack, but recovery is typically rapid, spontaneous, and complete.

If, usually after an acute stress, the patient suffers a severe memory loss, leaves home, and acts like a different person, he has dissociative fugue. Although he presents himself well to strangers, on questioning he is usually unaware of his previous (real) identity and may seem somewhat perplexed about his current personal identity. Fugue is more common in alcohol abusers. However, occasional patients function for long periods of time in complex roles, undetected. The return of old memories an the old identity usually occurs abruptly within hours or days, but may not happen for months (or longer).

VIGNETTE

A 50 year old male was seen by the psychiatric resident who had abused alcohol since his teenage years. He was seen by the on call for the ER because, according to the ER physician, the patient seems confused and irrational. The ER physician, noting the patient's somewhat ataxia gait, suspected alcohol intoxication. However, a blood alcohol level was read as undetectable, and electrolytes and CBC were within normal limits. On interview, the patient appeared apathetic and somewhat drowsy. His pulse, blood pressure, and temperature, were elevated, and his pupils were dilated and reactive. He was disoriented to day and date and could recall none of three items after 2 minutes. The patient showed mild nystagmus and difficulty with heel-to-toe walking. A diagnosis of Wernicke-Korsakoff syndrome was made, and the patient improved markedly after administration of thiamine hydrochloride intravenously.

In the past 4 to 5 years he has shown signs of alcohol addiction and had suffered three times form withdrawal (delirium tremens). For 2 months while drinking heavily for several weeks, he had undergone a period of confusion, hallucinations, and the inability to walk without holding onto objects.

His symptoms were followed by hospitalization, where he was treated with vitamins, an enriched diet, and medications. When he went home, his wife noted that he did not know his way around the house, did not remember names, and could not recognize some of his friends and relatives. His wife was concerned because he had no memory of the events that led to his hospitalization or of his hospital stay.

Discussion

As our vignette suggests, dissociative amnesia entails the sudden inability to recall important personal information and goes beyond mere forgetfulness. Four types of dissociative amnesia are usually described. In localized dissociative amnesia-the most common type-there is failure to recall all events occurring during a circumscribed period of time, usually just following some traumatic event. In selective dissociative amnesia, the patient fails to recall some, but not all, of the events occurring during some specific time period. Less common is so-called generalized amnesia, in which the amnesia continues in anterograde fashion up to and including the present. His severe alcohol abuse exhibited the syndrome commonly referred to as an alcoholic blackout. He awakes in the morning with a conscious awareness of being unable to remember a period the night before during which he was intoxicated. Sometimes, specific behaviors (hiding money in a secret place and provoking fights) are associated with the blackouts.

The amnesic syndrome is most commonly seen as a portion of the Wernicke-Korsakoff syndrome, which is a disorder seen most often in alcoholic patients. This syndrome was first described by the Russian psychiatrist Sergei Korsakoff in 1887. In 1881, Karl Wernicke described the other features of this disorder. The Wernicke portion is characterized by global confusion, opthalmoplegia, nystagmus, and ataxia. The Korakoff portion of this syndrome is characterized by significant deficits in the learning and normal processing of new information and material. In the Korsakoff amnesic syndrome, newly presented material appears to be temporarily registered but cannot be retained for more than a few minutes (anterograde amnesia or failure of learning). There is always an associated defect in the recall and reproduction of memories that had been formed several days, or weeks, or even years before the onset of the illness (retrograde amnesia).

The statement is often made that the Korakoff patient fills the gaps in his memory with confabulation is generally considered to be a specific feature of Korsakoff psychosis.

Table 23-1 DSM-5. Diagnostic Criteria for Dissociative Amnesia

A. An inability to recall important autobiographical information, usually of a traumatic or stressfull nature, that is inconsistent with ordinary forgetting. NOTE: Dissociative amnesia most often consist of localized or selective amnesia for a specific event or events; or generalized amnesia for identity and life history.

B. The symptoms cause clinically significant distress or impairment in social, occupational, or othr important areas of functioning.

C. The disturbance is not attribute to the physiological effects of a substance (e.g. alcohol or other drug of abuse, a medication) or a neurological or other medical condition (e.g. partial complex seizures, transient global amnesia, sequelae of a closed head injury/traumatic brain injury, other neurological condition).

D. The disturbance is not better explained by dissociative identity disorder, posttraumatic stress disorder, acute stress disorder, somatic symptom disorder, or major or mild neurocognitive disorder.

Specify: with dissociative fugue. Apparently purposeful travel or bewildered wandering that is associated with amnesia for identity or for other important autobiographical information.

Amnesia has a variety of possible causes (Erickson, 1990). Psychiatric conditions include:

Amnesia may often accompany severe depressive or anxiety states. Somnambulism may superficially resemble some fugues but has marked clouding of consciousness. PTSD, somatoform disorders, and other dissociative states often include amnesia.

Some individuals will continue to deny that they have a problem despite evidence to the contrary. Others may acknowledge that a problem exists, but appear unconcerned. The term persisting is used to indicate that the symptoms exist long after the effects of substance intoxication or withdrawal have subsided. Apathy lack of initiative, and emotional blandness are common. The person may appear friendly and agreeable, but the emotionality is superficial. The onset of symptoms may be insidious, depending on the pathological process causing the amnestic disorder. The diagnosis si specified further by indicating whether the symptoms are transient (present for not more than 1 month) or chronic (present for more than 1 month).

Organic processes (usually involving the temporal lobes) account for the majority of cases of significant memory loss in adults. Unilateral damage may sometimes be sufficient to produce memory impairment, particularly in the cases of left-sided temporal lobe and thalamic structures (Benson, 1978).

The processes include intoxication or withdrawal form drugs or alcohol, various dementias, acute ro chronic metabolic conditions (e.g. hypoglycemia), brain trauma (e.g. post-concussive amnesia), brain tumors (particularly in the temporal lobes), cerebrovascular accidents, epilepsy (particularly temporal lobe epilepsy), and various degenerative or infectious CNS diseases.

Transient Global Amnesia

This is the name applied by Fisher and Adams to a particular type of memory disorder that occurs not infrequently in middle-aged and elderly persons and is characterized by an episode of amnesia and bewilderment lasting for several hours. (Fisher and Adams, 1958; Shuping et al, 1980). The patient's symptoms have their basis in a defect in memory for events of the present and the recent past. During the attack there is no impairment in the state of consciousness and no overt sign of seizures activity, and personal identification is intact, as are motor, sensory, and reflex functions. The patient is alert, in contact with his surroundings, and capable of high-level intellectual activity and language function during the attack. These episodes typically last for only a few minutes or hours, or hours, ending with a rapid, spontaneous restoration of intact cognitive function. As soon as the attack has ended, no abnormality of mental function is apparent.

Transient amnestic syndromes can occur from cerebrovascular disease, cardiac arrhythmias, migraine headache, thyroid disorders, and epilepsy (Bourgeois, Seaman, and Servis, 2003). Transietn global amnesia is most often caused by transient ischemic attacks (TIAs) that affect limbic midline brain structures. Transient global amnesia is a sudden, self-limited, massive loss of memory in middle-aged or elderly patients due to a temporary (presumably vascular) cause. This syndrome presents as an acute period of memory loss conisiting of two components: an ongoing anterograde amnesia that persists for several hours, and a retrograde amnesia that lasts a few weeks. The amnesia terminates abruptly and the entire episode usually lasts less than 24 hours.

Treatment Modalities

Amnesitc patients may be confused or frightened; therefore, a calm, reassuring approach is needed. Many cases of dissociative amnesia resolve spontaneously when the individual is removed from the stressful situation. For other, more refractory conditions, intravenous administration of amobarbital is useful in the retrieved of lost memories. Most clinicians recommend supportive psychotherapy also to reinforce adjustment to the psychological impact of the retrieved memories and the emotions associated with them.

In some instances, psychotherapy is used as the primary treatment. Techniques of persuasion and free or directed association are used to help the client remember. In other cases, hypnosis may be required to mobilize the memories. Once the memories are obtained through hypnosis, psychotherapy may be employed to help the client integrate the memories into his or her conscious state.

Treatment for dissociative fugue should focus on helping the patient come to terms with the traumatic event or stressor that caused the disorder. Recovery form dissociative fugue is usually rapid, spontaneous, and complete. In some instances, manipulation of the environment or psychotherapeutic support may help to diminish stress or help the client adapt to stress in the future, When the fugue is prolonged, techniques of gentle encouragement, persuasion, or directed association may be helpful, either alone or in combination with hypnosis or amobarbital interviews.

Various kinds of interactive therapies explore the trauma and work on building the patient's coping mechanisms; prevent further recurrence. Cognitive therapy may be useful in helping the client attempt a change in inappropriate or irrational thinking patterns. Creative therapies (e.g. art therapy, music therapy) are also constructive in allowing clients to express and explore thoughts and emotions in safe ways. Group therapy can be helpful in providing the client with ongoing support form supportive peers. Family therapy sessions may be used to explore the trauma that precipitated the fugue episode and to educate family members about the dissociative disorder.

Chapter 23: Amnesitc Disorder Examination Review

1. What symptoms characterize amnestic disorders by problems with memory function?

   A. Anterograde amnesia
   B. Retrograde amnesia
   C. Confabulation amnesia
   D. All of the above

2. What amnestic disorder is caused by the thiamine deficiency, usually associated with excessive, prolonged ingestion of alcohol?

   A. Korsakoff's Syndrome
   B. Bilateral sixth nerve palsy
   C. Residual amnesic gap
   D. Acute confusional states

3. What medications are the most commonly used prescription drugs associated with amnesia, especially if combined with alcohol?

   A. Antipsychotic Agents
   B. Benzodiazepines
   C. Anti-parkinsonism Agents
   D. Antimanic and mood-stabilizing agents

4. What symptom is characterized by disorientation, apathy, confusion, and inattention?

   A. Nystagmus
   B. Ataxia
   C. Global confusional state
   D. Bilateral sixth nerve palsy

5. In what type of dissociative amnesia is there failure to recall all events occurring during a circumscribed period of time, usually just following some traumatic event?

    A. Localized dissociative amnesia
    B. Selective dissociative amnesia
    C. Generalized dissociative amnesia
    D. Continuous dissociative amnesia

6. What midtemporal lobe structures are involved in amnestic disorder?

    A. Hippocampus
    B. Mamillary bodies
    C. Amygdala
    D. All of the above

7. What form of amnestic disorder is characterized by an abrupt episode of profound antergrade amnesia and a variable inability to recall events that occur during the episode?

    A. Transient global amnesia
    B. Anterograde amnesia
    C. Retrograde amnesia
    D. Clouding of consciousness

8. What organic condition is associated with amnesia in the clinical features of nystagmus, ataxia, and neuropathy?

    A. Transient global amnesia
    B. Hippocampal infarction
    C. Wernicke-Korsakoff Syndrome
    D. Cerebral amoxia

9. What condition is featured by hypervigilance, affective blunting, and flashbacks that may be accompanied by unusual behaviors?

   A. Borderline personality disorder
   B. Posttraumatic disorder
   C. Conversion disorder
   D. Dissociative fugue

10. What alcohol-related neuro-psychiatric syndrome are characterized by thiamine deficiency, ataxia, ophthalmoplegia, and nustagmus?

   A. Delirium tremens
   B. Alcohol hallucinosis
   C. Alcohol idiosyncratic intoxication
   D. Alcohol amnestic disorder

Chapter 23: Amnestic Disorder Examination Answers

1. D
2. A
3. B
4. C
5. A
6. D
7. A
8. C
9. B
10. D

Reference 5

Adams RD, Victor M, Ropper Aly. Principles of Neurology.6th Ed. McGraw-Hill Co,1997.

4 Albert M.L. Clinical Neurology of Aging. Oxford University Press, 1984.

5 Albert M, Butters N, and Brandt J. Patterns of remote memory in amnesic and dementing patients. Archives of Neurology 38: 401-408, 1981.

6 American Psychiatric Association. Diagnostic and Statistical Manual of Mental Disorders, 4th Ed. Text Revision, Washington, DC, 2000.

10 Beck BJ. Neuropsychiatric manifestations of diffuse Lewy body disease. Journal of Geriatric Psychiatry, Neurology 8(3): 189-196, 1995.

11 Benson DF. Amnesia. South Medical Journal 71: 1221-1228, 1978.

12 Bersen EV. Delirium in the Elderly. Journal of Geriatric Psychiatry, Neurology: 1:127, 1988.

13 Blass JP, Gibson GE. Abnormality of a Thiamine Requiring Enzyme in Patients with Wernicke-Korsakoff Syndrome Syndrome. New England Journal of Medicine. 297: 1367.1977.

15 Bondareff W, Mount joy CQ, Wischik CM, et al. Evidence of Subtypes of Alzheimer's disease and implications for etiology. Archives of General Psychiatry.50: 350-356. 1993.

19 Brietbart Ward Strout D. Deliirium in the terminally ill. Clinics in Geriatric Medicine, 16(2): 357-372,2000.

21 Brandt J, Folstein SE, Fosltein MF. Differnential cognitive impairment in Alzheimer's disease and Huntington's disease. Ann Neurol; 23:555. 1988.

22 Butters N, Cerak LS. Alcoholic Korsakoff Syndrome. New York: Academic Press, 1980.

23 Calne DB, Langston JW, Aetiology of Parkinson's Disease. Lancet 2: 1457.1983.

24 Caine ED, Lynes JM. Delirium, Dementia, and amnestic and other cognitive disorders. In: Sadock BJ, Sadock VA, eds. Kaplan + Sadock's Comprehensive Textbook of Psychiatry, 7th Ed. Vol 1. Baltimore: Lippincott Williams +Wilkins, 854. 2000.

25 Caplan L, Chedru F, Lheritte F, et al. Transient Global Amnesia and Migraine. Neurology 31: 1167. 1981.

Coery-Blum J, Galasko D, and Thal LJ. Is it Alzheimer's? A strategy for Diagnosis. IM Intern Medical Specialty 16: 28-37, 1995.

31 Emery VOB and Oxman TE. Dementia: Presentations, Differential Diagnosis, and Nosology. Johns Hopkins University Press, 2nd Ed. 2003.

35 Fisher CM, Transient Global Amnesia: Precipitating Activities and other observations. Archives of Neurology 39: 605.1982.

36 Fisher CM, Adams RD: Transient global Anesia, Acta Neurol Scan 40 (Suppl 9): 1. 1964.

37 Fisher CM, Adams RD. Transient global amnesia. Trans Am Neurol Association; 83: 143-146. 1958.

38 Fisher C. Amnesia States in war neuroses: the psychogenesis of fugues. Psychoanalyst Q. 14: 437-468, 1945.

40 Foslstein MF, Folstein SE, McHugh PR-Mini-Mental State: a practical method for grading the cognitive state of patients for the clinician. JOuranl of Psychiatric Research; 12: 189-198.1975.

41 Forstl H, Sattel H, and Bahro M. Alzheimer's Dissease: Clinical Features. Internal Rev Psych. 5: 327-349, 1993.

44Gray KF. Dementia: Lewy Body Disease. Geriatric Psychiatric New 2(2): 6, 1996.

45 Greer N, Rossom R, and Anderson P, et al. Delirium: Screening, Prevention and Diagnosis: A systematic Review of the Evidence. Washington, DC: Department of Veterans Affairs, US. 2011.

46 Harper PS. The epidemiology of Huntington's disease. Hum Genet 89: 365-376, 1992.

50 Horel JA. The Neuroanatomy of Amnesia. Brain. 101403.1978.

51 Inouye SK. Delirium and other mental status problems in the older patients. In: Goldman L, Ausiello D, eds. Cecil Medicine, 23rd ED. Philadelphia, PA. Sounders Elsevier; chapter 26. 2007

53 Jernigan TL, Arne LO. When Alcoholism Affects Memory Functions. Alcohol Health + Research World 19 No 2: 104-108, Spring 1995.

55 Kendel ER, Schwartz J. H., Jessell TM. Principles of Neural Science. 3rd Ed. Elsevier Science Publishing Co, 1991.

57 Khachaturian ZS. Diagnosis of Alzheimer's disease. Archives of Neurology 42: 1097-1105, 1985.

58 Kishi Y, Iwasaki Y, Takezawa K, et al. Delirium in critical care unit patients admitted through an emergency room. General Hospital Psychiatry 17 (5): 371-379, 1995.

59 Kopelman MD. The Korsakof Syndrome. Britsih Jornal of Psychiatry 166: 154-173. 1995.

60 Koponen H, Stenback U, Mattila E, et al. Delirium aong elderly persons admitted to a psychiatric hospital: Clinical course

during the acute stage and one –year follow-up. Acta Psychiatric Scand; 79: 579-585.1989.

64 Lipowski ZJ. Delirium (acute confusional states). JAMA 258: 1789-1792.1987.

65Lipowski ZJ. Transient cognitive disorders (delirium, acute confusional states) in the elderly. American Journal of Psychiatry 140: 1426-1436.1983.

67 Liptzin B, Levokoff SE. An empiriacal study of delirium subtypes. British Journal of Psychiatry; 161: 843-845.1992.

68 Mayeux R, Stern Y. Subcortical Dementia. Archives of Neurology. 44: 129. 1987.

87 Stern RG, Mohs RC, Davidson M, et al. A longitudinal study of Alzheimer's disease. American Journal of Psychiatry 151: 390-396. 1994.

Shuping JR, Rollinson RD, Toole JF. Transient global amnesia. Ann Neurol; 7: 281-285.1980

83 Sirven JI, Malamut B.L. Clincical Neurology f the Older Adult, Lippincott Willias & Wilkins, 2002.

88 Stern G, Lees A. Parkinson's Disease: the Facts. New York: Oxford University Press, 1982.

90 Terry RD, Katzman R, Bick KL. Alzheimer Disease. New York, Raven Press. 1994.

92 Veterans Administraraton Cooperative Study Group on Antihypertensive Study Gourp on Antihypertensive Agents: Effects of treatment on morbidity in hypertension. Results in patients with diastolic blood pressures averaging 115 through 129 mm Hg. JAMA 202: 1028, 1967.

Section Six

Recovery from Mental Illness

> *Recovery is a process of change through which individuals.*
> *Improve their health and wellness, live a self- directed*
> *Life, and strive to reach their full potential.*
> *SAMHSA*

Substance Abuse and Mental Health Services Administration (SAMHSA) defines recovery as a process of change through which individuals improve their health and wellness, live a self-directed life, and strive to reach their full potential. Lasting recovery is achieved when the patient is willing to make basic and comprehensive changes in habit, attitude, and lifestyle. This section outlines and illustrates a comprehensive approach to recovery that has evolved over the several years during which anxiety problems are treated. These levels are as follows: Strategies for dealing with physical presentation, such as: (1) shallow breathing, (2) muscle tension, (3) bodily effects of cumulative stress, and (4) nutritional and dietary factors (such as excess caffeine or sugar in the diet). With our new knowledge of the brain, medications and treatment, psychotherapy, nutritional therapy, convulsive therapy are expressed for mental illnesses that have changed dramatically.

Chapter 24

Psychiatric Medicines

Pharmacokinetic interactions describe how the body handles a drug; pharmaco -dynamic interactions describe the effects of a drug on the body. In a parallel fashion pharmacokinetic drug interactions refer to plasma concentrations of drugs, and the pharmacodynamic drug interactions refer to receptor activities of drugs. The principle divisions of pharmacokinetics are drug absorption, distribution, metabolism, and excretion.

Absorption. A psycho therapeutic drug must first reach the blood on its way to the brain, unless it is directly administered into the cerebrospinal fluid or the brain. Orally administered drugs must dissolve in the fluid of the gastrointestinal tract, before the body can absorb them.

Distribution. The distribution of a drug to the brain is determined by the blood-brain barrier, the brain's regional blood flow, and the drug's affinity with its receptors in the brain. Both high blood flow and affinity favor the distribution of the drug to the brain. The volume of distribution is a measure of the apparent space in the body available to contain the drug. The volume of distribution can also vary with the patient's age, sex, and disease state.

Metabolism and Excretion. The processes of metabolism and excretion metabolism are often called 'biotransformation'. The four major metabolic routes for drugs are oxidation, reduction, hydrolysis, and conjugation. The liver is the principal site of metabolism and bile, feces, and urine are the major routes of excretion. Psychoactive drugs are also excreted in sweat, saliva, tears, and milk. Therefore, mothers who are taking psychotherapeutic drugs should not breast feed their children.

Medications have at least two names: a generic name that reflects their chemistry followed by a specific brand name, created by the pharmaceutical company that developed the generic drug for commercial use.

Table 24-1: Psychiatric Medicines

Popular Name	Scientific Name	Use
Amidate	Etomidate	Anesthetic
Amytal	Amobarbital	Anesthetic/Sedative
Anapsine	Droperidol	Anesthetic
Anectine	Succinylcholine	Muscle Relaxant
Artane	Trihexyphenidil	Anti-Parkinson
Ativan	Lorazepam	Sedative
Atropine	Atropine	Anti-cholinergic
Benadryl	Diphenhydramine	Sedative
Brevital	Methohexital	Anesthetic
Capoten	Captopril	Anti-hypertensive
Clozaril	Clozapine	Atyp. Anti-psychotic
Cogentin	Benzotropine	Anti-Parkinson
Coumadin	Warfarin	Anticoagulant
Dentrium	Dantrolene	Muscle Relaxant
Depakote	Divalproex	AntiConvulsant
Diprivan	Propofol	Anesthetic
Elavil	Amitriptyline	Antidepressant (TCA)

Popular Name	Scientific Name	Use
Haldol	Haloperidol	Anti-psychotic
Ketalar	Ketamine	Anesthetic
Klonipin	Clonazepam	Sedative
Lanoxin	Digoxin	Cardiac Stimulant
Lithobid	Lithium	Anti-Manic
Metrazol	Pentylenetetrazol	Induces Seizures
Miltown	Meprobamate	Anxiolytic
Moban	Molindone	Anti-psychotic
Nardil	Phenelzine	Antidepressant (MAOI)
Navane	Thiothixene	Anti-psychotic
Norpamin	Desipramine	Antidepressant (TCA)
Pamelor	Nortriptyline	Antidepressant (TCA)
Parlodel	Bromocriptine	Dopamine Agonist
Paxil	Paroxetine	Antidepressant (SSRI)
Pentothal	Thiopental	Anesthetic
Prolixin	Fluphenazine	Anti-psychotic

Popular Name	Scientific Name	Use
Prozac	Fluoxetine	Antidepressant (SSRI)
Risperdal	Risperidone	Atypical Anti-psychotic
Robinul	Glycopyrrolate	Anticholinergic
Romazicon	Flumazenil	Benzodiazepine Antag.
Sinemet	L-dopa	Dopamine Agonist
Sinequan	Doxepin	Antidepressant (TCA)
Tegretol	Carbamazepine	Anticonvulsant
Thorazine	Chlorpromazine	Anti-psychotic
Tofranil	Imipramine	Antidepressant (TCA)
Trilafon	Perphenazine	Anti-psychotic
Valium	Diazepam	Sedative
Versed	Midazolam	Sedative
Xanax	Alprazolam	Anxiolytic
Zoloft	Sertraline	Antidepressant (SSRI)
Zyprexa	Olanzapine	Atypical Anti-psychotic

Mood Stabilizers. The term mood stabilizer is widely used but does not have an official definition. The ideal mood stabilizer is a single agent, that does just that; stabilizes mood, so that manic or depressive symptoms or at least aren't so severe as to disrupt the person's life work and relationships.

The medication that comes closest to this idea is Lithium. Lithium was the first medication proven to stabilize mood in bipolar disorder and also to prevent manic or depressive episodes from returning. So Lithium is still the first choice for bipolar I, depressive, or manic episodes. Lithium has been known to have mood calming properties since at least A.D. 200, when a greek doctor named Galen used it in baths for people with mental illness. Various Lithium bromide compounds were marketed to the public in the 1800's, but were found to be highly toxic. For example, the soft drink 7Up used to have Lithium in it.

John Cade was an Australian physician who theorized that there were toxic compounds in the urine in the patients of what was then called manic depressive illness. He happened upon Lithium by accident. His experiment involved injecting uric acid mixed with Lithium into the blood stream of guinea pigs. Injection with lithium calmed the animals down ad made them less active. Cade then thought to try lithium with a human, which was one of his most severely ill manic patients. The patient responded very well and for the first time was able to function outside a hospital.

Common side effects of Lithium include: thirst, retaining water, frequent urination, fatigue, diarrhea, or a metallic taste in the mouth. Other side effects require more creative solutions: frequent urination, for example, can be reduced by taking Lithium once during the day instead of several times a day; thirst can be controlled by drinking more water, chewing on ice chips, or using sugarless cough drops. More troublesome side effects include weight gain, sluggishness, or problems with memory, shaky hands, development or flare-up of skin conditions (such as acne, or psoriasis), or stomach discomfort or pain. Some people develop hypothyroidism, a condition in which the thyroid gland does not produce enough hormone. Kidney functioning (i.e. the ability of the kidney to concentrate urine) can also be affected if Lithium is taken over a long period of time.

It's not unusual for doctors to recommend thyroid medications because people with bipolar disorder often have hypothyroidism, and certain mood stabilizers such as Lithium, tend to suppress thyroid hormones. This is useful to know if you're feeling fatigued or slowed down on Lithium. A thyroid supplement may help bring the patient back to a normal energy level. Having a normal thyroid level may also increase the chances that the patient will respond to an anti-depressant.

AntiDepressant Drugs. There are five broad categories of antidepressant drugs: the standard tricyclic compounds, the heterocyclic compounds, the selective serotonergic agents, the selective dopamine reuptake blockers, and the Monoamine Oxidase inhibitors (MAOIs). Each of the antidepressants has a different potency in blocking reuptake of one of the major central neurotransmitters: norepinephrine, serotonin, and dopamine. Desipramine (Norpramin) is the most potent norepinephrine reuptake inhibitor; Fluoxetine(Prozac) is the most potent serotonin reuptake inhibitor; and Bupropion (Wellbutrin) is the most potent dopamine reuptake inhibitor.

MAOIs carry an increase risk, however, in that they may trigger a hypertensive crisis or cerebrovascular accident in patients taking them in conjunction with tyramine-containing foods. The patient should be instructed carefully about these dietary instructions. That is patients taking these drugs must not eat pickled herring, sardines, anchovies, chicken livers, canned or processed meats, pods of broad beans, canned figs, yeast extract, or fermented cheeses.

AntiConvulsants. Check the patient's anticonvulsants blood concentration and folic acid concentration because many anticonvulsants produce folic acid deficiency. If the patient's folic acid concentration is low, check the vitamin B-12 concentration, since they tend to fall together. It was discovered by accident that certain anticonvulsant (anti-seizure medications) were helpful in calming agitated behavior. In addition, look for cognitive deficits. Although controlling the seizures can produce a marked improvement in cognitive functioning, anticonvulsants can produce cognitive impairment. The symptoms include: sedation, sluggishness, poor concentration, and memory impairment. And the short term toxic effects include: nystagmus, ataxia, dysarthria, tremor, hyper-reflexia or hypo-reflexia, lethargy, nausea, vomiting, slurred speech, hypotension, and coma.

Carbamazepine, an anticonvulsant appears to be comparable to Lithium in controlling mania and an effective adjunct to lithium in treating rapid cycling (Denicoff et al. 1997). The most common side effects are sedation, nausea, and mild memory impairment (for example, difficulty finding words). These side effects are usually related to the dose taken and often disappear after a few weeks or months of treatment. Some people also experience blurry vision, constipation or loss of muscle coordination. There is less of a problem with weight gain while on Carbamazepene which is why some people prefer it. People taking Carbamazepine can develop a mild elevation in liver enzymes, which can be identified through regular liver function tests. The doctor prescribing this drug will probably discontinue it if the patient develops signs of hepatitis, such as feeling sluggish or experiencing stomach pain or other gastrointestinal problems. The most serious side effect of carbamazepine – although quite rare – is a bone marrow reaction called agranulocytosis, which involves a dramatic drop in white blood cells. Fever, infection, sore throat, sores in the mouth and easy bruising or bleeding are all symptoms (Ketter et al. 1998).

Lamotrigine, another anticonvulsant used the treatment on epilepsy, is being used more and more for people with bipolar depression. It has become fairly popular in the last ten years because of its side effect profile (Geddes et al.2009). Lamotrigine is easier to take than Lithium or Valproate because it is less likely to cause serious weight gain, tremors, or other unpleasant side effects. Typically, the side effects are temporary and include problems with physical coordination, dizziness, vision, nausea, vomiting, and headaches (Malhi et al. 2009). There are some concerns about this drug because 5% to 10% of people who use it, develop a benign skin rash within 2 to 8 weeks of beginning treatment. This typically mild rash can, in rare instances (1 in 1,000) lead to serious skin conditions, such as Stevens-Johnson Syndrome, a potentially life threatening condition involving a blistering or a burning of the skin tissue or lining of the mucous membrane often accompanied by fever.

Divalproex sodium, which is also called valproate or valproic acid, is an anticonvulsant that has been used for decades to treat epilepsy and other seizure disorders. Many anticonvulsant drugs have mood stabilizing properties. It probably works in several ways; including reducing activity of the protein kinase C pathway and enhancing the action of the inhibitory neurotransmitter GABA (Manji et al.2003). It has replaced Lithium as a first choice therapy in the United States, probably due more to drug company marketing than research evidence (Thase, 2006).

There are at least three reasons why a physician might prescribe Divalproex rather than Lithium(Bowden,2009). First, if the patient has mixed episodes it may be more effective. Second, it seems to work a bit more quickly, even within as few as 3- 5 days after the onset after a major manic episode. In contrast to lithium, the dosage can usually be raised rapidly without severe side effects. Third, there is evidence that people have less severe side effects with Divalproex than with

Lithium. Because Divalproex is broken down by the liver, and can also affect the production of blood platelets. For this reason, the doctor should conduct liver enzyme tests and blood platelet counts at regular interavals. Some people also develop hair loss or hair thinning. More worrisome is significant weight gain, which can contribute to other medical problems (for example, high blood pressure, heart disease, or diabetes).

AntiPsychotics. This group of drugs represents the major treatment for some of the most disturbed patients seen by psychiatrists. That is why, dramatic progress has been made in the treatment of schizophrenia in the last decade. Although there is still no cure, new medication help reduce symptoms and offer hope for a longer, happier life (Jenike 1985; Spar and LaRue 1990).

Traditional antipsychotic medications for schizophrenia, prescribed since the early 1950's, are called neuroleptics. They have been effective in suppressing the hallucinations, delusions, and disorganized thinking of schizophrenia (the positive symptoms). Thorazine is one of the best known of these neuroleptics because it works on the dopamine system, decreasing the amount and overactivity of dopamine in the brain- the presumed cause of the positive symptoms. Unfortunately, the neuroleptics are not effective in relieving the negative symptoms of schizophrenia: lack of interest in activities and people, decreased motivation and self-care, reduce ability for communication and emotional expression. These symptoms can be extremely disabling since they tend to result in withdrawal and social isolation.

Moreover, many patients do not respond to the neuroleptic medications, or if they do, they usually suffer disturbing side effects such as: muscle spasms, Parkinson's- like tremors, stiff gait, slowed speech, and sexual dysfunction. The most serious side effect is tardive dyskinesia, a dreadful condition, sometimes irreversible in which a person experiences repetitive involuntary movements such as lip smacking, facial grimacing, and abnormal gestures.

Anxiolytics. Benzodiazepines are usually the anxiolytic drugs of choice; however, evaluate the anxiety and the associated symptoms thoroughly before prescribing a benzodiazepine, such as Alprazolam (Xanax), Clonazepam (Klonopin), and Lorazepam (Ativan) are effective in stopping panic attacks. Start with a low dosage and increase the dosage as needed unitl it is clearly effective. Many patients carry a Benzodiazepine tablet with them and derive considerable relief from simply knowing that it is there, even if they never take it. Judicious use of benzodiazepines may actually allow psychotherapy, behavioral therapy, or psychoanalytic work to proceed more efficiently and productively with the ultimate goal of further reduction in anxiety without drugs. Clomipramine (Anafranil), Fluvoxamine (Luvox), and Fluoxetine (Prozac) are potent inhibitors of serotonin reuptake and are drugs of first choice in treating Obsessive Compulsive Disorder.

Drug Use and Mental Health. In the best-case scenario, a medication regimen should accomplish three things:

1. Control and help resolve an episode that has already developed
2. Delay future episodes and minimize the severity of those that do occur.
3. Reduce the severity of the symptoms experienced between episodes.

There are simple systems for ensuring that your patient takes prescribed medications. These can include some of the following strategies: Create text messages to be sent to his or her self periodically as a reminder. Some cellular phones and personal digital assistants (PDA's) can be programmed to send text messages at set times. Your client can also use one of several software programs, such as email program (Microsoft Office Outlook or Gmail by Google, for example) as a reminder either by email or phone. Some reminder tools are also available for free on www.moodtracker.com. You can set your watch or cellular phone alarm as a reminder to take medications.

Some people put a note on the bathroom mirror to remind them to take their medications, especially if they have to take them at morning and night, which are the two times they are most likely to be in their bathrooms. Or the patient may put a note on his or her front door that says, "Did you take your meds today?." Note the times for the medication dosage as an appointment in the daily calendar or PDA.

Purchase a pill dispenser that helps remind oneself of the medication needed to take each day. A pill dispenser also facilitates taking medication in ones purse or briefcase so that if you don't go home on a given night or some emergency separates medications, there will always be a supply of medication. For people who travel frequently, when crossing borders, it's best to keep medications in their prescription bottles so that if you're traveling with controlled substances such as Klonopin (Clonazepam), you won't risk being arrested for importation of a controlled substance. The prescribed information will be on the containers.

Finally, keep a medication log which can help motivate you to take medications regularly while keeping track of side effects and intake of other substances that may interact with prescribed medications.

Medication Record Sheet

Name: Family Physician:

EXAMPLE

Generic Name	Instructions	Reason for Therapy	Duration	Side Effects
What is the name of your medication? What is the pill dosage?	When and how do you take this medication? With meals? With water? How many times a day?	Why are you taking the medication?	How long have you been taking this medication?	What are the side effects you experience when taking this medication?
Example: Ranitidine. 150 mg	Example: 1 tablet, twice a day, with meals	Example: Acid Reflux Disease Heartburn	Example: 6 months	Example: Headache, cramps, bloating, etc.

Generic Name	Instructions	Reason For Therapy	Duration	Side Effects

Chapter 24: Psychiatric Medicines Examination Review

1. Medications used to treat anxiety in low doses in the elderly include

    a. Benzodiazepines
    b. Tricyclics
    c. MAOI's
    d. SSRI's

2. Which one of the general treatment principles augments medicine therapy?

    a. Do not touch the patient
    b. Discourage self-esteem
    c. Promote the quality of the patient's current environment
    d. Do not be reachable by telephone

3. What determine the distribution of a drug to the brain?

    a. Biotransformation
    b. Oxidation
    c. Hydrolysis
    d. Patient's age, sex, and disease state.

4. What was the first medication proven to stabilize mood in bipolar disorder?

    a. Haloperidol
    b. Amitriptyline
    c. Lithium
    d. Divalproex

5. What should be monitored if the patient's folic acid concentration is low?

    a. Vitamin B-12 concentration
    b. Cognitive activity
    c. Rapid speech
    d. Frequency of seizures

6. Which medicines inhibits serotonin reuptake by presynaptic neurons?

    a. Risperidone
    b. Fluoxetine
    c. Diazepam
    d. Phenelzine
    e.

7. What is medication-induced postural tremor usually notable?

    a. By taking the total daily dosage at one time
    b. In outstretched hands, especially in the fingers
    c. During times of lowest drug levels
    d. All of the above

8. What drugs should be avoided during MAOI treatment?

    a. Anesthetics
    b. Tricyclic antidepressants
    c. Dopamine antagonist
    d. Anto-psychotics

9. What symptoms result in drug-induced parkinsonism?

    a. Bradykinesia
    b. Cogwheeling
    c. Stooped posture
    d. All of the above

10. What categories make up anti-depressant drug?

    a. Anti-seizure medications
    b. Neuroleptics
    c. Heterocyclic compounds
    d. Anxiolytics

Chapter 24: Psychiatric Medicines Examination Answers

1. A
2. C
3. D
4. C
5. A
6. B
7. B
8. A
9. D
10. C

Chapter 25

Pain Management

History of Pain Medicine

The early concept of pain as a form of punishment for sinful activity is as old as humankind. Christians believed that pain during childbirth, for example. Was a consequence of Eve's sin and was transferred to them directly by God. It was not until 1847, when Queen Victoria was administered chloroform by James Simpson for the delivery of her eighth child, Prince Leopold, that Christians accepted the idea that it was not heresy to promote painless childbirth. To fully appreciate the historical significance of pain, it is important to reflect on the origins of the "pain patient." The word pain comes from the Latin word "poena," which means "punishment." Then the word patient is derived from the Latin word "patior," meaning "to endure suffering or pain." Thus, it is not too outrageous to appreciate that, in ancient days, persons who experienced pain were interpreted to have received punishment in the form of the gods or offered up to appease the goads for transgressions. Today, the task of medicine is to preserve and restore health and to relieve suffering. Understanding pain management is essential to these goals.

Even the deeply religious find it hard to make sense of chronic pain- Why is God doing this to me? And their bewilderment often leads to despair. Anxiety and depression are planets in orbit about the dark sun of pain. Claiming that proper pain treatment requires special knowledge, so we emphasize that our medical system needs to give control of relief to the doctor, not the patient.

Living with Pain. If the study of pain is to have a scientific foundation it is essential to measure it. Diaries are a specific type of numerical rating scale in which repeated ratings are taken. Consider how bad pain is at its worst, how bad pain is most of the time, and how bad pain is at its least. And how pain changes with treatment.

Order of Questions in the Pain History:

1. Allowing patients to tell their own history in relatively unhurried fashion exemplifies the old clinical maximum "healing begins with the history."
2. Sometimes patients relate the onset of pain to the occurrence of some meaningful event in their lives even though the pain is not related. One may also gather a tentative summary of physicians who have previously treated the patient under these circumstances.
3. This temporal benchmark includes the differentiation between acute pain, which is usually of recent, well-defined onset and expected to end in days or weeks; and chronic pain, which is remote, of ill-defined onset, and with unpredictable duration.
4. Although there is tremendous variation in how patients describe pain, the following terms are useful:
   - Hyperpathia- an unpleasant dysesthesia or abnormal sensation characterized by an exaggerated pain response to either noxious or non-noxious stimulation.
   - Allodynia-a situation in which a non-noxious stimulus is perceived as painful.
   - Hyperalgesia-an increased pain response to a noxious stimulus.
   - Nociceptive pains may be sharp if musculoskeletal, gnawing or aching if muscular, and crampy if originating from an internal viscus.

- Neuropathic pains are more difficult to describe and may be more difficult to describe and may be more diffuse; they may be burning, lancinating, sharp, or tearing.

5. Individuals vary widely in their stoicism and their description of pain intensity. A visual Analogue scale score ranges from 1 to 10 is often useful in helping one interpret the patient's description of pain.

6. The physician next attempts to understand the location of the pain and any radiation of pain. In the assessment, pain may be focal (experienced at one site), multifocal, or generalized.

7. Medical conditions that include a remote history of cancer, or a present history of diabetes mellitus or collagen vascular disease should be tight.

8. This question sets the stage for assessing whether earlier diagnoses have been correct and which future treatments might be useful.

9. All medication should e confirmed as to dose and duration of use. Since this is an opportunity to discover injudicious drug use, possible interactions, and past successes and failures, the question represents an important moment in the patient history and one that often calls for certification from sources other than the patient.

10. Certain conditions are clearly associated with inciting factors. These include lifting of Valsalva maneuvers for producing abdominal hernia pain, herniated disk pain, and pain associated with spinal conditions. In other instances, vascular headaches may be worsened by vaso-active substances (e.g. nitrites, chocolate, tyramine containing compounds, and alcohol).

11. When a pain is very obscure and its treatment has been in effective to date, it is time to inquire of the exact circumstances- social, martial, and economic- under which the pain arose. This inquiry includes job and marital satisfaction, sexual activity, length of a work lost, avocations

abandoned, and social and religious activities before and after onset of the pain.

12. A history of psychiatric illness or addictive behavior in a recovering person does not preclude a legitimate current pain syndrome.

Mankind has undoughtably experienced pain since the beginning of time. Early man attributed pain to demons, evil humors, and dead spirits. Much later, pain was felt to be a punishment form the God's. Today, the task of medicine is to preserve and restore health and to relieve suffering. Understanding pain is essential to these goals.

It is a great help to managing pain by keeping a pain diary with a record of daily activity and pain scores during a typical day, In this way you can determine how the pain effects your life and factors may influence the pain.

A tool that measures pain intensity: may help you to communicate your level of pain.

0-----1-----2-----3-----4-----5-----6-----7-----8-----9-----10
No Pain Mild Moderate Severe Very Severe Worst Possible Pain

How do we apply the pain diary and intensity scale to our pain?

Every evaluation of a client with pain should begin with a comprehensive pain history. It is important to have a standardized format to decrease chances of missing important to have a standardized format to decrease chances of missing important information and to minimize having the client lead the interview. You can manage headaches by answering the following questions in the pain diary:

- Where is the headache located on one side of the head or over the whole scalp?
- Does t he pain radiate into the neck or eyes?
- Is the pain made worse by light, noise, or position?
- What time of day do headaches occur?

Abdominal Pain. Irritable bowel syndrome is very common disorder associated with abdominal pain and alternating constipation and diarrhea, with no recognized organic cause. In the abdomen pain may be called pressure, cramping, bloating, tearing, exploding and the like. It is common for the pain to be meal related and have disturbed bowel habits-either constipation or diarrhea or both. This syndrome usually occurs in people with chronic emotional distress, who have been under psychic or physical stress. Many of these patients suffer from depression, neurosis, and alcoholism; either can occur with near obstruction. You can manage abdominal pain by answering the following questions in the pain diary:

> ➤ Are you aggravated or relived by factors such as eating or drinking, less than 45 minutes implies gastric origin more than an hour or more implies pancreas biliary track or small intestine.
> ➤ Consider activity or inactivity: are there certain movements that aggravate, so bumps in the road increase the pain, does sneezing or coughing affect it?
> ➤ Have you lost weight due to malignancy or decreased caloric intake secondary to pain>
> ➤ Do symptoms such as diarrhea and constipation, mostly relate to small intestine and colon?

Arthritis. The skeletal system goes through a variety of changes throughout life. Any involvement in pain management demands an appreciation of the cast difference between the acute and chronic pain. The former is self-limiting in the majority of cases. The later is not. Many of the disappointments are due to failure in understanding the difference. Tendons, ligaments, and joint capsules loose elasticity with age. The term arthritis refers to inflammation within a joint. Pain is the most common initial symptom. Blumer (1987) compared patients with dysthymic pain disorders and those with documented rheumatoid arthritis. The results are summarized in Table 25-1`. How applicable these differences are to pain disorders is not clear, but we might expect many similarities. The pain is described as dull and aching and is made worse by movement. Pain is made worse when the joint and slow move is referred to as stiffness. Joint stiffness typically with rest and improves with rest. Stiffness typically upon rising in the morning and after activities is usually mild and usually last less than fifteen to thirty minutes. Loss of function resulting from pain, may involve activities such as: bathing, dressing, feeding, grooming, and toileting. Because the condition is essentially irreversible the goals of management are provide relief from pain, minimize further damage to the involved joints, and keep you functioning independently. You manage arthritis pain, stiffness, and loss of function, by answering the following questions in the pain diary:

> For example, gout usually commonly attacks the great toe, foot, or knee. And pseudogout typically strike the knee, wrist, or shoulder.
> What aggravates it? Do symptoms frequently occur with motion or activity and is relived by rest?
> Is the pattern of joint involvement often provides additional clues about the correct diagnosis?
> What functional losses have you occurred?

Low Back Pain is one oftthe most common human affliction, let us examine low back pain, which is one of the over 70% of people in developed counties that will experience low back pain at sometime in thier lives. Low back pain is most common between the ages of 35 and 65. The diagnosis of low back pain is made heavy physical work, frequent bending, twisting, lifting, pulling, and pushing, and repetitive work. Examples include pain referred to the opposite kidney; pain referred from the diaphragm to the tip of the shoulder, and the pain of myocholdria escema being felt in the chest wall, or running into the kneck. It is relieved by rest or by activities that are opposite that aggravate the pain. For example, if extension of the spine aggravates the pain, often gentle flexion will ease it. Although, acute symptoms will subside with rest proper back care should become a way of life for you. That means you should be instructed to sleep on your side, or back, legs, and hips in a position of flexion. And you should be cautioned against the prone position which increases in size of the lumber spine. Most important, symptomatic measures consist of local heat or warm baths.

Low back pain is managed by answering the following the questions in the pain diary:

> ➤ When and under what circumstances did the pain begin, and was it clearly associated with an injury?
> ➤ Can you determine what factors aggravate it and which relieve it?
> ➤ Do you suffer from insidious (working or spreading harmfully in a stealthy manner) onset morning stiffness, and improvement with exercise?
> ➤ What is its relationship to such stereotypical movements such as forward bending, coughing, sneeze, and strain?

Coping with pain. Prayer is the most frequently reported way individuals use religion to cope with pain. It is reasonable to expect that when you are experiencing pain your utilization of coping mechanisms include prayer will increase. It is essential to emphasize that the church plays a cental role in the community by providing social support, a context for coping, and a frame work for engaging in trial issues.

Table 25-1. Rheumatoid arthritis and dysthymic pain disorder: a comparison

RHEUMATOID ARTHRITIS	DYSTHYMIC PAIN DISORDER
Onset of pain mostly gradual	Onset usually sudden
Pain variable in intensity	Pain usually continuous
Depressive traits not common	Depressive traits common
Rare history of past physical abuse	Physical abuse history more common
Normal work history	Excessive work history

Questions in the pain diary:

- When is the patient's attention asked to focus on a topic other than pain?
- Is the pain constant or periodic?

Does it travel or radiate?

Have there been any recent changes in the pattern?

- Has the pain resulted in any functional limitations?
- Has it caused any changes in the client's ability to participate in life, including employment and recreational activities?

Family. The question now arises of how the family should be involved in rehabilitation efforts.

- ➤ The family must undergo its own rehabilitation regardless of the special needs of the patient.
- ➤ The extent to which the family should be involved directly in the rehabilitation process for the patient, however, depends on the following factors:

1. Comprehensive analysis of the patient's linguistic abilities and communicative competence.
2. Psychological analysis of the patient and family.
3. Communication environment analysis.
4. Developing a rehabilitation plan.

Acute/ Chronic Pain. Any involvement in pain management demands an appreciation of the vast difference between acute and chronic pain. The former is self-limiting in the majority of cases: the latter is not. Many of the disappointments in managing chronic pain are due to failure in understanding this difference.

Table 25-2 Essential differences between acute and chronic pain

CHRONIC PAIN	ACUTE PAIN
Vague or remote trigger	Recent, obvious trigger
No apparent biological function	Serves a protective function
Depression and irritability common	Anxiety is common
Unpredictable duration	Lasts hours to days
May not have obvious association	Associated injury or illness

Acute: Duration of less than 6 months

Chronic: Duration of 6 months or longer

Note: The following is not considered to be a mental disorder and is included here to facilitate differential diagnosis.

Pain Disorder Associated with a General Medical Condition:

A general medical condition has a major role in the onset severity, exacerbation, or maintenance of the pain. It is a great help to manage of the pain by keeping a pain diary with a record of daily activity and pain scores during a typical day. In this way it can be determined how the pain effects life and factors that may influence the pain.

A tool that quantifies pain intensity may help communicate level of pain. [**Pain Intensity Scale**]

Pain Intensity Scale (enter this number in the column "Pain scale rating.")

0	1	2	3	4	5	6	7	8	9	10
No Pain										Worst Pain

Date	Time	Pain Scale Rating	Medicine and Dose	Other Pain relief methods	Side Effects form Pain Medicine

Today, we will describe the validity and reliability of popular pain scales in the elderly. You can use a rating scale to describe:

- How bad your pain is at its worst.
- How bad your pain is most of the time.
- How bad your pain is at its least.
- How your pain changes with treatment.

It is not unusual for patients with endogenous depression to have pain as the predominant symptom. And most patients with chronic pain of all types are depressed. Wells and colleagues (1989) have convincingly corroborated this clinical impression. They surveyed a large number of depressed and chronic pain patients and found that those with chronic pain were often depressed and those who were depressed often had pain as a prominent symptom. Fields (1991) has elaborated a theoretical explanation of the overlap of pain and depression. In such cases one is faced with an extremely difficult clinical problem-that of determining whether a depressive state is primary or secondary. Empirical treatment with antidepressant medication or electroconvulsive therapy is one way out of the dilemma.

If the pain disappears or recedes to a minor arthritic ache or some similar trivial disorder, one can conclude that depression was the primary problem. If the depression lifts as the pain is brought under medical control, one may assume that it was secondary.

Pain is defined by the International Association for the study of Pain as "an unpleasant sensory and emotional experience associated with actual or potential tissue damage or described in terms of such damage." One aspect of pain is nociception, a complex series of electrochemical events that occur between a site of active tissue damage and the perception of pain.

Nocicpetion is made up of four processes:

1. Transduction- Noxious stimuli are translated into electric activity at the sensory endings of nerves.
2. Transmission: Impulses are propagated throughout the sensory nervous system.
3. Modulation: Nociceptive transmissions are modified by a number of neural influences.
4. Perception: Transduction, transmission, and modulation are developed into the subjective, sensory, and emotional experience of pain.

Table 25-3. DSM-5. Diagnostic Criteria for Pain Disorder

A. Pain in one or more anatomical sites is the predominant focus of the clinical presentation and is of sufficient severity to warrant clinical attention.

B. The pain causes clinically significant distress or impairment in social, occupational, or other important areas in functioning.

C. Psychological factors are judged to have an important role in the onset, severity, exacerbation, or maintenance of the pain.

D. The symptom Pain Intensity Scale or deficit is not intentionally produced or feigned (as in Factitious Disorder or Malingering).

E. The pain is not better accounted for by a Mood, Anxiety, or Psychotic Disorder and does not meet criteria for Dyspareunia.

Code as follows:

Pain Disorder Associated With Psychological Factors: psychological factors are judged to have the major role in the onset, severity, exacerbation, or maintenance of the pain. (If a general medical condition is present, it does not have a major role in the onset, severity, exacerbation, or maintenance of the pain.) This type of Pain Disorder is not diagnosed if criteria are also met for Somatization Disorder. *Specify if:*

Acute: duration is less than 6 months

Chronic: duration of 6 months or longer

Pain Disorder Associated With Both Psychological Factors and a General Medical Condition: both psychological factors and a general medical condition are judged to have important roles in the onset, severity, exacerbation, or maintenance of the pain. The associated general medical condition or anatomical site of the pain is coded on Axis III.

Specify if:

Acute: duration is less than 6 months

Chronic: duration of 6 months or longer

Note: the following is not considered to be a mental disorder and is not included her to facilitate differential diagnosis. **Pain Disorder Associated With a General Medical Condition:** a general medical condition has a major tole in the onset, severity, exacerbation, or maintenance of the pain. (If psychological factors are present, they are not judged to have a major role in the onset, severity, exacerbation, or maintenance of the pain.) The diagnostic code for the pain is selected based on t he associated general medical condition if one has been established or on the anatomical location of the pain if the underlying general medical condition is not et clearly established-for example, low back, sciatic, pelvic, headache, facial, chest, jont, bone, abdominal, breast, renal ear, eye, throat, tooth, and urinary.

VIGNETTE

A 40 year old veteran man with a long history of Parkinson's Disease presented to the clinic complaining of constitutional symptoms including fever and a 30 pound weight loss. He experienced pain at night or with lying down; increasingly in his left buttock and left thigh pain with dysesthesias and a constant burning sensation. He had a marked increase in back pain a night secondary to a benign neoplasm affecting tissues in or near the spinal column. His morning stiffness lasted for hours as a hallmark symptoms of an inflammatory of the spine. His history of trauma characterized acute, localized bone pain because he sustained an acute fracture of a vertebrae. His visceral pain occurs in conjunction with back pain as symptoms of dysfunction in another organ symptom.

How has the pain intensity changed since the onset? These symptoms of dyspepsia, abdominal pain, or a change in bowel habits. In addition, his visceral pain had colicky, severe tearing, or episodic low back pain. The patient's nervous system accurately express it self to the therapist, especially when the patient's attention was asked to focus on a topic other than pain and the patient was not aware that movement is being observed.

Discussion. Special Surgery in New York, 200 patient's with osteoarthritis who participated in a weekly exercise program reported a significant drop in pain and an improvement in quality of life. The program included tai chi, yoga, dance and other forms of exercise, tailored to people with osteoarthritis. Other studies show that exercise eases chronic back pain. When scientists at Tel Aviv University compared six-week programs of brisk walking versus strength training work ours in patients with chronic low-back pain, both improved functioning and reduced pain (Jaret, 2013). Treating the psychological consequences of chronic pain is equally important. Acute pain is typically a symptom of injury or disease. The goal of the treatment of acute low back pain is to eliminate it and return the patient to the previous functional level. But when pain persists, it becomes a disorder in its own right, with its own set of symptoms. These often included depression and ager. Psychiatric medications bot only improve mood, both also take the edge off pain.

Pain. The connection between stress and pain leads us to move to the main concepts behind this treatment approach:

1. Pain is real, and pain is stress-related
2. Pain triggers stress
3. Stress makes pain worse
4. Stress can be made better or worse by how one thinks about pain.
5. Learning about stress ad how to manage stress, can reduce one's pain.

Because stress makes pain worse, we must ask: What is stress?

Stress often is defined as a biological, emotional, and cognitive (that is, mental) reaction to an event that the subject might not be able to cope with. Let's look at the three parts of a stress reaction:

1. Biological. Stress reactions are biological. Therefore, the biological response to stress includes an increase in blood

pressure, heart rate, and respiration and a decrease in digestive processes.

2. Emotional. One part of the signal travels to the amygdala, where it initiates your emotional response to pain. In addition to biological responses, stress also sets off emotional reactions. Many patients with pain relate that they react to the stress of chronic pain with nervousness, sadness, depression, anger, embarrassment, and shame ot name some of the more common emotions.

3. Cognitive. Stress also sets off cognitive, or mental, reactions. Cognitions are thoughts, images, or beliefs. For example, cognitions include what we tell ourselves about the stress, what we tell ourselves about our ability to cope, and what we think about ourselves. These thoughts, by themselves, can be negative, overwhelming, and stressful. In effect, the way we think –our cognitions- can trigger stress reactions by themselves.

Cancer pain. One important role behavior therapy in the treatment of patient with cancer is the reduction of anxiety and nausea associated with cancer chemotherapy, an example of classical conditioning. Relaxation training can be used for patients who do not respond to modern antiemetic agents. Controlled studies demonstrate that such treatment is effective in reducing anxiety, nausea, and vomiting.

A second role of behavior therapy is to enhance coping with cancer. Fawzy et al. (1993) used a structured 6 week group intervention with components including health education, stress management, coping skills, and supportive group psychotherapy.

Cancer pain exists in two categories: nociceptive and neuropathic pain.

Questions in the pain diary:

*   Once the diagnosis of cancer has been established, how does therapy include some type of pain control?

- As patients live longer, how does the need for effective pain control increase for improving the quality of life?
- Is spinal analgesia an important technique in the management of intractable cancer pain?
- How does the incidence of pain varies depend on the type of neoplasm, stage, and extent fo spread?

Patients with advanced or terminal cancer are more likely than those in the early stages to have pain as their chief complaint. In recent years, advances in cancer treatment have improved survival among cancer patients. As patients live longer, the need for effective pain control has gained increased importance for improving quality of life.

Chapter 25: Pain Management Examination Review

1. Research suggests that the major psychological dimensions of pain include all except:

    A. Sensory-discriminative
    B. Motivational-affective
    C. Activity-interaction
    D. Cognitive-evaluative

2. The most frequently reported psychiatric diagnosis among acute pain patients is

    A. Depression
    B. Sleep Disorders
    C. Eating Disorders
    D. Anxiety

3. The most common nociceptors re

    A. Mechanosensory nociceptors
    B. Mechanothermal nociceptors
    C. Polymodal C fiber nociceptors
    D. Thermoreceptive nociceptors

4. Anti-dromic impulses in primary nociceptor afferents result in an increase in

    A. Substance P
    B. Potassium
    C. Prostaglandins
    D. SRS-A

5. What medications have promising treatments for chronic pain?

    A. Benzodiazepines
    B. Antianxiety agents
    C. Tricyclic
    D. Analgesics

6. What are the symptoms of dysthymic pain disorder?

    A. Rare history of past physical abuse
    B. Onset of pain is mostly gradual
    C. Current symptoms of physical abuse
    D. Onset of pain is mostly gradual

7. What are the most important risk factors for low back pain?

    A. Female ender
    B. Symptoms during adolescence
    C. Morning stiffness lasting for hours
    D. All of the above

8. Cancer pain can be conceptualized in two categories:

    A. Nociceptive and neuropathic
    B. Embolism and thrombosis
    C. Visceral and peptic pain
    D. Hydronephrosis and micturition

9. What type of pain disorder is thought to show alexithymia, i.e. the inability to appreciate and verbalize feelings?

    A. Peptic pain
    B. Dysthymic pain
    C. Visceral pain
    D. Psychogenic pain

10. What is an important technique in the management of intractable cancer pain?

    A. Weekly exercise programs
    B. Spinal analgesia
    C. Ideomotor apraxia
    D. Chemotherapy

Chapter 25: Pain Management Examination Answer

1. C
2. D
3. C
4. A
5. C
6. B
7. C
8. A
9. B
10. B

Chapter 26

Psychotherapy as a Treatment Procedure

Psychotherapy is a generic term that covers a wide variety of theories and techniques, all of which have articulate spokespersons and supporters, and make claims of success. This chapter is concerned with how you as a therapist can make your groups most effective.

Freud believed that the sense of sudden alienation and unreality associated with depersonalization arises form a twofold defensive process: first, repression is activated in order to fend off unacceptable impulses, but fails to do so; next, the unacceptable feelings are masked as unreal. Freud believed that in melancholia, hostile feelings that were once directed at the self, which- through introjection- has subsumed the lost object. The history of phobias disorders is intimately bound up with Freud's theories concerning, "the transformation of undischarged sexual energy," repression, and symbolization. We have already alluded to the psychoanalytic formulation of phobic disorders.

Despite much controversy over Freud's views, our modern understanding of social and simple phobia is influenced by psychoanalytic theory. In Freud's later formulation of phobias, anxiety was not the result of repression but the cause of repression; that is, anxiety prompts the ego to employ repression as a defense against an unacceptable impulse, one that is generally sexual in nature. This is the concept of "signal anxiety": anxiety signals the ego to employ repression as a defense. Freud made important contributions to our psychodynamic concept of manic- depressive illness. Freud made important contributions to our psychodynamic concept of manic-depressive illness. Freud suggested that I melancholia the ambivalently regarded lost object is incorporated into the ego (introjection).

Although Sigmund Freud (1856-1939) is best known for his work on the "neuroses," he contributed some fundamental ideas in the area of paranoid psychoses and schizophrenia. Essentially, Freud regarded schizophrenia as a regression to a primitive narcissistic state- one in which libido is withdrawn from objects (i.e. other people) and directed into the self. Clinically, Freud's hypothesis seems to fit the very regressed, uncommunicative schizophrenic patient, who spends all day rocking, muttering, and responding to internal stimuli. Freud also delineated the role of projection states, although his focus on homosexual urges has not been borne out in all cases. If Freud had done nothing else but separate "anxiety neurosis" from the hodgepodge of symptoms known as "neurasthenia," he would have made a significant contribution to psychiatry. But Freud did a great deal more. First, he recognized that anxiety could be distinguished from depression on the basis of the "motor manifestations" of anxiety (e.g. dyspnea and palpitations). Second, Freud appreciated that anxiety could be manifested either as a chronic state or as discrete attacks, although he used the term "anxiety neuroses" to encompass both forms of the disorder. Of course, Freud's preeminent contribution to the theory of anxiety involved the idea that anxiety is a signal to the ego that some unacceptable able drive is pressing for awareness and discharge.

The hostility once present I the actual relationship is then directed against the incorporated love object. This is experienced as self-hatred and the usual signs and symptoms of major depression. Freud eventually explained mania as a fusion of the ego and superego, freeing up the energy previously used in the conflict between these two parts of the psyche. Freud postulated two broad resonses to trauma: 1) attempts to remember or repeat the trauma and 2) attempts to avoid or fend off such memories and repetitions. Both mechanisms may be involved in the development of PTSD. In essence, the psychoanalytic view holds that a particular trauma in the here and now may reactivate an unresolved childhood conflict. The ego is overwhelmed, and the aggressive drives the id gain the upper hand.

Jung —Interest in the analytic psychology of Carl Jung remains strong in certain religious circles and shows signs of increasing. It is a mixture of a formal, or Catholic, psychoanalytic psychology (with its appealing intellectualism) and a less formal, or Protestant, counseling psychology approach (with its appealing freedom of choice). Indeed, two of the foremost interpreters of Jungian thought for the ecumenical religious audience, Morton Kelsey and John Sanford, are Episcopalians who share a deep and abiding interest in aesthetics, ritual, symbolism and the depth of dimensions of religious experience.

Ludwig Binswagner (1881-) a disciple of Eugen Bleuler, and one of the early followers of Freud, succeeded his father as medical director of the Sanatorium Bellevue in Kreuzlingen, Switzerland. Existential analysis does not have in mind the solidity of the structure of the inner life- history, but rather the solidity of the transcendental structure preceding a prior, and all psychic structures as the very condition of this possibility. Binswanger regards mental illness as twisted, distorted modes of experience in their own right. Above all, he demands that man should not be viewed as an object of the analyst's detached scientific inquiry.

Carl Rogers is an advocate of limited intense relationships in the encounter movement. What really goes on in an encounter group? It is is a question often asked by persons who are contemplating joining one, or who are puzzled by the statements of people who have had the experience. That is why encounter groups focus on problem solving techniques, self-improvement, and increased goals awareness.

Plan of Action for Therapy Sessions

Depression- Karasu (1990) explores the current status of psychotherapy for depression, describing and contrasting the three predominant psychotherapeutic approaches- psychodynamic, cognitive, and interpersonal. They are conceptually different but complementary with regard to theory, major strategies, goals, mechanisms of change, and advantages and limitations. Karasu presents advantages and disadvantages of each of the three psychotherapeutic approaches. Problems of a psychodynamic approach are: overuse of catharsis, pitfalls of a regressive transference, negative response to therapist silence, and undue priority given to individual dynamics and the dyadic relationship. A major advantage of cognitive therapy is that the therapist intervenes directly. It is used to interrupt thought patterns and actively help patients learn and practice logical alternatives. Finally, fundamental asset of interpersonal therapy is that it addresses the broader social context of depressive risk and engages the family in treatment. A plan of actions for therapy sessions defines specific interventions targeted at resolving the identified problem. Sadock and Sadock (2003) state:

Each session begins with the question, "How have things been since we last met?" to focus on current mood states and their association with recent interactions. The basic techniques for handling each problem area are clarifying positive and negative feelings states, identifying past models for relationships, guiding, and encouraging the patient in examining and choosing alternative courses of action.

VIGNETTE

A 50 year old woman reported to the our patient clinic to bear on the chief people in her life, by receiving guidance, explanation, suggestions, or direct request, so that she can help her approach the many aspects of treatments. In adult psychiatry when a negligent husband of a depressed woman may be counciled to be more attentive to his wife. Certain obvious errors need to be avoided which a doctor which can often be seem to make. Authoritative statements must not be made about maters which are in fact thoughtful e.g. what the course of an anxiety neurosis will be, how long it will take the patient to recover etc. The clinician should also avoid statement which will increase the patient level of anxiety and result in dis-organization at a time in the discussion when composure is needed, e.g. when the interview is ending and the patient has to be in a condition to cope with ordinary responsibilities.

Psychotherapy for Mood.

The cognitive- behavioral approach to depression has a good deal of empirical support (Rush et al,1977). It emphasizes the irrational and self-defeating cognitions that often underline severe depression. Interpersonal psychotherapy (IPT) for depression is a brief weekly treatment (12 to 16 sessions) for ambulatory, non-bipolar, nonpsychotic depressed persons. It is based on the premise that understanding and renegotiating the interpersonal context of a depressive episode will facilitate recovery and prevent relapse. In IPT, depression is viewed from three perspectives:

1. Symptom formation, including depressive affect and vegetative signs;
2. Social and interpersonal relations, based on current interaction and emphasizing the four common problems-grief, role disputes, role-transitions, and interpersonal deficits; and
3. Personality, in the form of enduring traits, such as inhibitions of expressing anger and other emotions and tendencies toward perfectionism and self-criticism.

Psychotherapy for Anxiety Disorders

Horowitz (1986, 1989) notes that psychotherapy of PTSD begins with the establishment of a safe relationship and with the patient's telling the story of the traumatic events. Because patients usually seek treatment during the intrusive phase of PTSD, therapeutic efforts are aimed at helping the patient modulate the often overwhelming flood of memories, feelings, and ideas surrounding the trauma. This may involve the use of behavioral approaches, such as relaxation techniques or systematic desensitization. Much of supporting evidence in the area of psychosocial approaches to treatment of panic disorders is anecdotal and it still is not clear what form of psychotherapy is best for this disorder. Cognitive-behavioral approaches benefit many panic disorder-agoraphobia patients. In fact, the basic Reality Therapy was developed in the mid 1960's by the American psychiatrist William Glassner. (1995)

The therapy is based n control theory and suggests that all individuals are responsible for what they choose to do. It includes the principle that human beings are born with the following five basic needs:

- Power (includes achievement, competence, and accomplishment)
- Belonging (includes social groups, as well as families and loved ones)
- Freedom (includes independence and personal autonomy)
- Fun (includes enjoyment and pleasure)
- Survival (includes physiological needs, such as food, shelter, sexual expression)

Personality development is viewed as an attempt to fulfill these five basic needs. In reality therapy, emphasis is on the present the "here and now." Pat behavior is addressed only as it impacts present choices or future behavior. A primary function of the therapist is to assist the client in dealing with getting needs met in the present. The therapist helps the client identify needs that are not being met, correlate the unmet needs to current ineffective behaviors, and make conscious choices to change to more effective patterns of behavior in an effort to satisfy basic needs.

In Reality Therapy, psychopathology is viewed in terms of ineffective behaviors. The concept of responsibility is emphasized.

- Accepting responsibility for one's own behavior is equated with mental health.
- An individual who behaves responsibly is able to fulfill his or her basic needs without interfering with others' attempts at need fulfillment
- An important part of the therapist's role is serving as a positive role model for responsible behavior

Individual Psychotherapy for Schizophrenia

Establishing a relationship is often particularly difficult because the individual with schizophrenia is desperately lonely yet defends against closeness and trust. He or she is likely to respond to attempts at closeness with suspiciousness, anxiety, aggression, or regression. Successful intervention may be achieved with honesty, simple directness, and a manner that respects the client's privacy and human dignity. Exaggerated warmth and professions of friendship are likely to be met with confusion and suspicion.

Individual Psychotherapy for Anxiety Disorders

Most clients experience a marked lessening of anxiety when given the opportunity to discuss their difficulties with a concerned and sympathetic therapist. Sadock and Sadock (2003) state that focuses on helping patients understand the hypothesized unconscious meaning of the anxiety, the symbolism of the avoided situation, the need to repress impulses, and the secondary gains of the symptoms. The psychotherapist also can use logical and rational explanations to increase the client's understanding about various situations that create anxiety in his or her life.

Individual Psychotherapy for Chronic Pain

Debates about the objectives and the process of psychotherapy are also to be found in the literature. Karasu (1980) lists the objectives of psychotherapy as consisting of any or all of the following:

1. Achieving relief when in crisis
2. Obtaining the reduction or elimination of symptoms
3. Moving toward the strengthening of defenses and intergrative capacities
4. Reaching a resolution or rearrangement of conflicts and
5. Achieving personality changes leading to more adaptive functioning.

Bellak(1977) emphasizes the learning process. He sees the need for learning to be linked to

1. A Sound Theory of Personailty
2. Hypotheses directed at the development of psychopathology
3. Interrelated propositions developed from 1 and 2, which direct the patient to restructure maladaptive patterns into adaptive ones.

Cognitive Therapy for Depression and Mania

In cognitive therapy, the individual is taught to control thought distortions that are considered to be a factor in the development and maintenance of mood disorders. (Miklowitz and Scott,2009). In the cognitive model, depression is characterized by a triad of negative distortions related to expectations of the environment, self, and future. The environment and activities within it are viewed as unsatisfying, the self is unrealistically devalued, and the future is perceived as hopeless.

In the same model, mania is characterized by exaggeratedly positive cognitions and perceptions. The individual perceives the self as highly valued and powerful. The general goals in cognitive therapy are to obtain symptom relief as quickly as possible, to assist the client in identifying dysfunctional patterns of thinking and behaving, and to guide the client to evidence and logic that effectively tests the validity of the dysfunctional thinking.

Examples of automatic thoughts in depression include:

- Personalizing (I'm the only one who failed)
- All or nothing (I'm a complete failure)
- Mind Reading (He thinks I'm foolish)
- Discounting Positives (the other questions were so easy. Any dummy could have gotten them right)

Examples of automatic thought in main include:

- Personalizing (she's this happy only when she's with me)
- All or nothing (Everything I do is great)
- Mind Reading (she thinks I'm wonderful)
- Discounting negatives (none of those mistakes are really important)

The Cognitive Therapy for Anxiety Disorder

The cognitive model relates how individuals respond in stressful situations to their subjective cognitive appraisal of the event. Anxiety is experienced when the cognitive appraisal is one of danger with which the individual perceives that he or she is unable to cope:

Impaired cognition can contribute to anxiety disorders when the individual's appraisal are chronically negative. Automatic negative appraisals provoke self-doubts, negative evaluations, and negative predictions. Anxiety is maintained by this dysfunctional appraisal of a situation. Cognitive therapy strives the assist the individual to reduce anxiety responses by altering cognitive distortions. Anxiety is described as being the result of exaggerated, automatic thinking. Cognitive therapy for anxiety is brief and time limited, usually lasting from 5 to 20 sessions. Brief therapy discourages the client's dependency on the therapist, which is prevalent in Anxiety Disorders, and encourages the client's self-sufficiency. A sound therapeutic relationship is a necessary condition for effective cognitive therapy. The client mist be able to talk openly about fears and feelings for the therapeutic process to occur. A major part of treatment consists of encouraging the client to face frightening situations to be able to view them realistically, and talking about them is one way of achieving this. Rather than offering suggestions and explanations, the therapist uses questions to encourage the client to correct his or her anxiety-producing thoughts. The client is encouraged to become aware of the thoughts, examine them for cognitive distortions, substitute more balanced thoughts, and patterns of thinking. Cognitive therapy is very structured and orderly, which is important for the anxious client who is often confused and lacks self-assurance. The premise is that one develops anxiety because he or she has learned inappropriate ways of handling life experiences.

Family Therapy for Depression and Mania

The ultimate objectives in working with families of clients with mood disorders are to resolve the symptoms and initiate or restore adaptive family functioning. Some studies with bipolar disorders have shown that behavioral family treatment combined with medication substantially reduces relapse.

Sadock and Sadock (2003) stated that family therapy is indicated if the disorder jeopardizes the a patient's marriage or family functioning or if the mood disorders is promoted or maintained by the family situation. Family therapy examines the role of the mood disordered member in the overall psychological wellbeing of the whole family; it also examines the role of the entire family in the maintenance of the patient's symptoms.

Group Psychotherapy is a form of treatment in which beneficial changes in emotionally disturbed patients occur as a result of their interactions with other patients and a t least one trained professional therapist in a group setting. Therapeutic results include both relief of symptoms and resolution of intra-psychic and interpersonal problems. The therapist's tools are clinical experience and applied theories of individual psychodynamics and interpersonal systems.

History of group Psychotherapy

- The first psychotherapy group ws described in 1907 by Joseph Pratt, a Boston internist, who developed a group method of education and improving the morale of patient's with tuberculosis.

- Around 1910, Jacob Moreno in Europe began using theatrical techniques to have patients act out problem situations in a groups setting; this later became known a psychodrama.
- In the late 1920s and early 1930s, a number of psychiatrists began applying psychoanalytic theory to groups, emphasizing issues of transference, free association, and recapitulation of family problems
- During the late 1930's and early 1940's, Kurt Lewin began emphasizing the importance of group member interactions and introduced the notion of group dynamics, a phenomenon describing actions in group as being more than the sum of individual interactions.
- The need to train more therapists in the theory of group dynamics became obvious after World War II, when large numbers of veterans requiring psychiatric assistance began to overburden the personnel resources of the mental health system.

Evidence from controlled studies attest to the usefulness of a group psychotherapy.

- A number of reviews have concluded that group psychotherapy is effective for patients with personality and anxiety disorders; substance-related disorder; schizophrenia; depressive and stable bipolar disorders; and medical illnesses, including asthma, myocardial infarction, obesity, chronic pain, and ulcers.

Contraindications to Groups Psychotherapy

- Group psychotherapy is not for everyone. Over-stimulation in the group environment causes patients with acute manic episodes to become more hyperactive and pressured, although recent evidence suggests that patients with stable bipolar disorders do well in homogeneous groups.

- Patients with severe antisocial personality disorders who are more interested in manipulating others than in improving their interpersonal relationships usually hinder group progress.

Four main phases of group development

Group dynamics--- Each individual in the groups is affected by his or her perceptions of what other members think and feel about various issues. These are called a group norm. Most conceptual models portray four main phases of group development.

1. The first phase is characterized by hesitant participation and the establishment of initial group norms. During this phase, the members should be able to perceive some common purpose in being there and declare their individual goals, while the therapist works in a quiet way to encourage the establishment of bonds between.

2. The second phase is characterized by conflict, dominance, and the establishment of a hierarchy (pecking order) among the patterns. The therapist is often seen as an appropriate figure to be rebelled against, and fantasies may be entertained of excluding the therapist from the group. Several patients may band together to attack verbally or exclude a particular patient form their discussions, thereby identifying that patient as the group scapegoat.

3. In the third phase, true group cohesiveness is established along with a sense of intimacy and mutual affection and need for each other. Overdependence on a rebellion against the therapist has been worked through, and the therapist is reintegrated with the group. A great deal of productive group work can be accomplished in the third phase

4. The fourth phase occurs when the group terminates. It may last for several sessions as the members say good bye, review their progress, and prepare for life without the group.

Compare outpatients vs. inpatient groups.

Psychiatric outpatients tend to value their group experience for (1)giving them feedback on interpersonal behavior, (2) allowing then an opportunity to vent repressed feeling, (3) giving them a sense of acceptance by other people, and (4) helping them discover unconscious motivations for what they do.

In contrast, psychiatric patients tend to value their group experience for (1) giving them feelings of optimism through watching other patients improve and leave the hospital, (2) giving them a sense of acceptance by other people, (3) improving self-esteem through their ability to help others, and (4) allowing them to feel less isolated.

Group therapy for people with schizophrenia generally focuses on real-life plans, problems, and relationships. Some investigators doubt that dynamic interpretation and insight therapy are valuable for typical patients with schizophrenia. But group therapy is effective in reducing social isolation, increasing the sense of cohesiveness, and improving reality testing for patients with schizophrenia.

Group Therapy for schizophrenia has been most useful over the long-term course of the illness. The social interaction, sense of cohesiveness, identification, and reality testing achieved within the group setting have proven to be highly therapeutic process for these clients.

Psychotherapy for Schizophrenia and Related Disorders

McGlashan (1986) has admirably reviewed the psychosocial treatment of schizophrenia. This is an issue that tends to polarize psychotherapists, because it touches on two fundamental clinical questions: Does psychotherapy really work in schizophrenia, and what are its potential risks?

A number of controlled outcome studies suggest that individual psychotherapy of the traditional exploratory type is not effective in schizophrenia (May and Simpson, 1980).Two caveats are in order. First, almost all the studies in this area have significant methodological flaws (e.g. the use of inexperienced therapists, poor definition of technique). Second, the available literature does not test or call into question the importance of the individual relationship between doctor and patient. The individual clinician remains central to any treatment effort, if only to coordinate other treatment modalities and provide ongoing evaluation (Cancro, 1983). The best general approach to psychotherapy with schizophrenic patients is a friendly, matter-of-fact, reality oriented one that minimizes exploration of unconscious material. On the other hand, dealing with here-and –now feelings of anger, demoralization, or anxiety is very important in maintaining the therapeutic alliance. In addition, a good deal of evidence has pointed toward the usefulness of what might be termed "family education therapy" in the treatment of schizophrenia. Treatment may be directed not at showing families how they caused their loved one's schizophrenia, but at informing them about schizophrenia its nature, likely course, and exacerbating factors. In particular, families are taught the prodromal signs of relapse and the ways in which inappropriate emotional expression may promote relapse (McGlashan, 1986). This approach will also help to decrease the patient's level of stress and reduce risk of relapse. It should be noted that group therapy is not recommended because patients with delusional disorder tend to be suspicious and hyper-vigulant and are prone to misinterpret situations that may arise in the curse of the therapy.

Functions of a Group

Sampson and Marthas (1990) have outlined eight functions that groups serve for their members.

1. **Socialization**. The cultural group into which we are born begins the process of teaching social norms.
2. **Support.** Individuals derive a feeling of security from group involvement.
3. **Task Completion**. Group members provide assistance in endeavors that are beyond the capacity of one individual

alone or when results can be achieved more effectively as a team.

4. **Camaraderie**. Members of a group provide the joy and pleasure that individuals seek form interactions with significant others.

5. **Informational.** Learning takes place within groups.

6. **Normative.** This function relates to the ways in which groups enforce the established norms.

7. **Empowerment**. Groups help to bring about conditions by providing support to individual members who seek to bring about change.

8. **Governance.** An example of the governing function is that of rules being made by committees within a larger organization.

Suggested Guidelines for a twelve Step Support Group for Families of Veterans (Mason,1990)

WELCOME

My name is _____. I am a family members of a veteran. We want to welcome you to the _____ night meeting of the families of veteran support group. Would you join me I a moment of silence to compose ourselves

Let us join hands while I read this statement of purpose:

Look around you and you will see people who have experienced many of the same things you may have experienced. Veterans of war develop certain characteristics. One may be re-experiencing the trauma through obsessive thoughts nightmares, flashbacks, sudden reemergence of survival behaviors, and emotional overloads, rages, or deep depressions. Another characteristic emotional numbing, may include a sense of not really being a person, feelings of not fitting in. Feeling that one has no emotions, and not being able to feel emotions in situations calling intimacy, tenderness, sexuality, of grief. Hyper-vigilance includes being unable to relax. Having frequent startle responses, continual of anxiety, and attacks of panic. Survivor guilt includes self-destructive behaviors, depresson, and a feeling of guilt at surviving when others did not. Each of these normal reactions to traumatic experiences can have a profound and painful effect on the family. Especially if family members do not understand that they are normal.

If these issues have caused us time and again to put aside our own needs and concerns to try to help our veterans, we may have developed patterns for coping which are not working in the way we hoped they would.

At this time I have asked _____ to read the preamble.

PREAMBLE

We are a fellowship of people who share experience, strength and hope with each other in order to deal with the effects of war on our lives. The only requirement for membership is the sincere desire to make life better for ourselves and our family. We do not wish to make life better for ourselves and our families. We do not wish to blame but rather to understand the effects of war on people and how those effects can affect the family members. Thereby becoming free to grow and accept responsibility for our own lives. We are a self-supporting group through our won contributions. We are not allied with any sect., denomination, politics, organization, or institution. We do not wish to engage in any controversy or endorse or oppose any cause.

The primary purpose of our group is to learn to deal with the effects on our lives of our veteran's experiences and survivor skills, and to develop healthy patterns to cope with these.

I have asked _____ to read the twelve steps.

Here are the steps we took which are suggested as a program of recovery:

1. We admitted we were powerless over the effects of war on ourselves and our families. That our lives had become unmanageable.
2. Came to believe that a power greater than ourselves could restore ourselves to sanity
3. Made a decision to turn our will and our lives over to the care of our Higher Power as we understood our Higher Power.
4. Made a searching and fearless moral inventory of ourselves.
5. Admitted to our Higher Power ourselves, and to another human being the exact nature of our wrongs.
6. Were entirely ready to have our Higher Power removed our shortcomings
7. Humbly asked our Higher Power to remove our shortcomings
8. Made a list of all people we have harmed and became willing to make a mends to them all.
9. Made direct amends to such people where ever possible, except when to do so would injure them or others.
10. Continued to take personal inventory when we were wrong, promptly admitted it.
11. Sought through prayer and meditation to improve our conscious with our Higher Power as we understood our Higher Power, praying only for knowledge of our Higher Power's will for us and for the power to carry that out.
12. Having had a spiritual awakening as the result of these steps, we tried to carry this message to others, and to practice these principles in all our affairs.

Embry (1990) outlined seven major parameters for effective psychotherapy in war veterans with chronic PTSD: 1) Initial rapport building, 2) limit setting and supportive confrontation, 3) affective modeling, 4) defocusing on stress and focusing on current life events, 5) sensitivity to transference-countertransference issues, 6) understanding of secondary gain, and 7) therapist's maintenance for a positive treatment attitude.

Chapter 26: Psychotherapy Examination Review

1. What thoughts make up the cognitive model of depression?

    a. A negative view of the self
    b. A negative interpretation of present and past experience
    c. A negative expectation of the future
    d. All of the above

2. What is the most suitable approach to individual psychotherapy for schizophrenia?

    a. Reality-oriented individual therapy
    b. Group therapy
    c. Family therapy
    d. Miliey therapy

3. In the cognitive model, depression is characterized by distortions related to what expectations?

    a. Of the environment
    b. Of the self
    c. Of the future
    d. All of the above

4. What therapeutic processes determine which the client must imagine situations that are extremely frightening for a prolonged period of time?

    a. Flooding
    b. Automatic thinking
    c. Relaxation training
    d. All of the above

5. What psychotherapies are based on the Freudian theory of a dynamic unconscious, psychic determination, and unconscious conflict?

    a. Individual analysis
    b. Existential analysis

    c.   Psychoanalysis

    d.   Aversive therapy

6.   Patients with poor frustration tolerance and poor reality testing are best treated with

    a.   Supportive psychotherapy

    b.   Insight-oriented psychotherapy

    c.   Expressive therapy

    d.   Intensive psychoanalytic psychotherapy

7.   What make up the cognitive therapy approach?

    a.   Eliciting automatic thoughts

    b.   Identifying maladaptive underlying assumptions

    c.   Testing the validity of maladaptive assumptions

    d.   All of the above

8.   What is broadly defined as the experience f feelings toward a person that in fact belongs to another form the past?

    a.   Countertransference

    b.   Transference

    c.   Resistance

    d.   Free association

9.   Which of the following statements are true regarding psychotherapy of addicted individuals?

    a.   Services for legal aid, job counseling, and medical attention are provided

    b.   Symptoms such as shame, guilt, and isolation may be treated by psychotherapy

    c.   Psychotherapy is not efficacious for the treatment of depression

    d.   All of the above

10. Insight –oriented psychotherapy arose in the 1930's from psychoanalytic theory. Which statement is true regarding the suitability of patients with schizophrenia for this type fo psychotherapy?

    a. No patient with schizophrenia should be treated with insight-oriented psychotherapy
    b. Patients who have failed to respond to long-term hospitalization may benefit from intensive outpatient therapy
    c. Outpatients who have had good premorbid functioning, have had minimal residual deficits, and have retained the capacity for self-observation and humor would benefit
    d. Patients who experienced onset of the illness in adolescence would benefit

Chapter 26: Psychotherapy Examination Answers

1. D
2. A
3. D
4. A
5. C
6. A
7. D
8. B
9. B
10. C

Chapter 27

Nutritional Therapy

The broad outlines of good nutrition are well known: eat more foods rich in vitamins, minerals, fiber, and phytochemicals (fruits, vegetables, whole grains, and low-fat animal products), and fewer foods rich in saturated and trans fats, cholesterol, refined sugars, and salt (meat, cheese hydrogenated shortening, egg yolks, soft drinks, sweet baked goods and salty processed foods).

This is a good time to put a question in your introspection list. How about "have I noticed how my mood changes when I eat spicy food"? Richard Wurtman, M.D. and Judith Wurtman, PHD, scientists at the Massachusetts Institute of Technology (MIT), first linked food with mood when they found that the sugar and starch in carbohydrates foods boosted a powerful brain chemical called "serotonin." Soon they linked serotonin and other neuro-transmitters to every mood, emotion or craving. For instance, they noted that eating carbohydrate-rich foods (breads, cereals, pasta, fruits and starchy vegetables such as potatoes, winter squash or corn) elevated serotonin levels, helps the patient feel more relaxed and calm; high protein foods (nonfat dairy products such as cottage cheese, yogurt or milk; or beans, peas, nuts and also soy products, such as tofu or soy milk) has the opposite effect. They release other substances that stimulate thoughts and reactions more quickly, or feel more alert and energetic.

Box 27.1 Dietary Guidelines

- **Reduce fat intake to less than or equal to 30% of calories.**
- **Increase fiber intake to 20-30 g/d with an upper limit of 35g.**
- **Include a variety of vegetables and fruits in the daily diet.**
- **Avoid obesity**
- **Consume alcoholic beverages in moderation, if at all.**
- **Minimize consumption of salt-cured, salt-pickled, or smoked foods.**

The goals and methods of nutritional therapy vary according to the patient's clinical situation. It is essential that veterans agree on the appropriate methods and interpretation of data so that a consensus on key issues can be achieved and evidence-based policy recommendations provided to government agencies and consumers.

Vitamins, Minerals, and the Brain. Folate insufficiency has long been recognized as a potential cause of accelerated loss of mental abilities in older adults. Clearly, folate and folic acid are staunched supporters of brain health, especially, healthy brain aging.

Choline is a B-vitamin- like nutrient that is required for the synthesis of essential components of nerve and brain cell membranes. The rate of synthesis of these components is governed by the availability of choline in the brain, which itself is determined by dietary choline intake. In contrast, dietary supplementation with choline prevents such avoidable loss of brain cell integrity.

Because Vitamin E is a strong antioxidant, especially in tissues with large ratios of cell membranes to total cell volume (such as the brain), it has long been thought that this vitamin must play an important health – sustaining role in protecting brain membrane lipids from oxidation. These findings confirm that vitamin E is a strong antioxidant protector within the human brain and promotes a healthy brain.

The usefulness of any nutrient to the brain depends on the ability of that nutrient to reach and enter the brain. Several systems, together called the blood –brain barrier, work to regulate the nature and amount of both desirable and undesirable compounds and nutrients that can gain access to the human brain. For example, selenium is a very beneficial antioxidant for the central nervous system, once it passes through the blood-brain barrier.

Vitamins, Minerals, and the Cardiovascular System. Vitamin C and vitamin E inhibit the oxidation of cholesterol in the blood and stimulates the immune system to remove from the circulation any cholesterol-containing particles that have become oxidized. These actions both protect the cardiovascular system from damage that can be caused by oxidized cholesterol and decrease the overall level of blood vessel- damaging inflammation in the body.

Maintaining the proper degree of sensitivity to stimuli that allows blood vessels to swell or constrict according to the body's needs is an unappreciated function of the calcium that is circulating in the blood-stream. If there is not enough calcium available, blood vessels become stiff and tend to lose their ability to relax – a situation that causes the blood pressure to remain elevated even when the body does not need the extra pressure to distribute blood where it is needed.

The heart muscle is sensitive to all aspects of it's environment, including the amount of magnesium available to it. In recent research, magnesium reduces the toxicity of the oxidative substances that are produced during normal cardiac contractions. Magnesium also acts to stabilize the electrical excitability of the heart muscle, promotes normal cardiac rhythmicity, and increases the efficiency of energy used by the myocardium. In addition to actions within the heart itself, magnesium also helps maintain the patency of blood vessels, with positive effects on the maintenance of healthy blood pressure regulation. Daily magnesium intakes of 300 mg also relaxes skeletal muscles and fosters restful sleep in individuals prone to leg cramps at night.

Vitamins, Minerals, and Blood Glucose Regulation. Chromium is a vital cofactor that allows insulin to effectively stimulate the transfer of glucose from the blood into cells. The functions of chromium are so important that daily dietary supplementation with chromium can improve insulin sensitivity, restore, and maintain healthy blood glucose regulation, and reduce the risk of developing adult onset (Type II) diabetes.

In addition to chromium, adequate magnesium intake is required for maintenance of stable insulin sensitivity. As dietary magnesium intake goes up, insulin is able to act more efficiently and less insulin is needed to help muscle cells obtain glucose from the blood.

In addition to chromium and magnesium, the trace mineral, vanadium also plays important roles in healthy blood sugar control. Dietary supplementation with vanadium increases the ability to move glucose from the blood into muscle cells – promoting normalization of blood glucose regulation.

Vitamins, Minerals, and the Immune System. –The many roles for Vitamin D that have been discovered in the last decade include contributions to the strength and robustness of the immune system. Vitamin D appears to interact in a coordinated manner with cells near a new wound, increasing the ability of the body to maintain a barrier against bacteria while a wound heals.

One of the major functions of vitamin C is to work with the cells in the immune system, to kill foreign invaders such as bacteria and viruses. This group concluded that vitamin C strengthened the human immune system and increased the ability to defend against pathogenic organisms.

The intriguing role of zinc as an essential trace element for immune function is well established. If zinc is not available in sufficient amounts, immune cell functions are compromised; for example, some types of lymphocytes confuse some normal cells for invaders that must be destroyed. In addition, the lethality of the white blood cells called "natural killer cells "against invading organisms is dependent on zinc supplies.

Selenium is a facilitator of immune system function. In addition to its antioxidant roles, which support many immune activities indirectly through tissue and cellular protection, selenium increases the efficiency of the cellular immune response to pathogenic invasion.

Stimulants: Caffeine. Of all the dietary factors that can aggravate anxiety and trigger panic attacks, caffeine is the most notorious. In particular, the effects of caffeine on a simulated task was examined. The results show beneficial effects of caffeine and confirm findings by using laboratory tasks. Studies conducted by the military have also shown that caffeine can improve a critical military task, mainly, sentry duty. Caffeine has a directly stimulating effect on several different bodily systems. It increases the level of the neurotransmitter norepinepherine in the brain, causing clients to feel alert and awake. It also produces the same physiological arousal response that is triggered when subjected to stress – increased sympathetic nervous system activity and a release of adrenaline. It is contained not only in coffee but in many types of tea, cola beverages, chocolate candy, coco, and over-the-counter drugs. It is contained not only in coffee but in many types of tea, cola beverages, chocolate candy, cocoa, and over- the- drugs. In short, too much caffeine can keep you in a chronically tense, aroused condition, leaving you more vulnerable to more generalized anxiety as well as panic attacks.

As with any addictive drug, chronic caffeine consumption leads to increased tolerance and a potential for withdrawal symptoms. If the client has been drinking five cups of coffee a day and abruptly cuts down to one a day, withdrawal reactions may include fatigue, depression, and headaches. Therefore, it is better to taper off gradually over a period of a few months.

Stimulants: Nicotine. Because it is as strong a stimulant as caffeine, nicotine causes increased physiological arousal, vasoconstriction, and makes the user's heart to work harder. Smokers often object to this notion and claim that having a cigarrete tends to calm their nerves. Research has proven, however, that smokers tend to be more anxious than nonsmokers and tend to sleep less well than non-smokers.

Stimulants: Salt. Excessive salt stresses the body in two ways: (1) it can deplete the body of potassium, a mineral that's important to the proper functioning of the nervous system; and (2) it raises blood pressure, putting extra strain on the heart and arteries and hastening arteriosclerosis. You can reduce the amount of salt consumed by avoiding the use of table salt, using a natural salt substitute (such as tamari) both in cooking and on the table, and limiting salty meats, salty snack foods, and other processed foods containing salt. As a rule of thumb, it's good to limit salt intake to one gram or teaspoon per day. And if you must buy processed foods, choose those that are labeled low sodium or salt-free.

Hormones in Meat. Red meat, pork, and most commercially available forms of chicken are derived from animals that have been fed hormones to promote fast weight gain and growth. One particular hormone, diethylstilbestrol (DES), has come to the public's attention because implicated in the development of breast cancer and fibroid tumors.

Try to reduce consumption of red meat, pork, and commercially available poultry, replacing it with organically raised beef, poultry, and fish such as cod, halibut, salmon, snapper, sole, trout, or turbot.

Food Allergies. How can you find out whether food allergies are aggravating problems with anxiety? For some people, food allergies can definitely be a contributing factor to excessive anxiety and mood swings. If you suspect this to be a problem, try experimenting with elimination methods.

Blood Sugar/ Diabetes. Disregulation of excess sugar metabolism can lead to high levels of blood sugar diabetes. For an even larger number of individuals, the problem is just the opposite-periodic drops in blood sugar level below normal, a condition that is popularly termed hypoglycemia. Typically, this occurs about two to three hours after eating a meal. It can also occur simply in response to stress, since the patient's body burns up sugar very rapidly under stress. What causes blood sugar to hall below normal is an excessive release of insulin by the pancreas. Insulin is a hormone that causes sugar in the blood stream to be taken up by the cells. The most common subjective symptoms of hypoglycemia are light-headedness, anxiety, trembling, feelings of unsteadiness or weakness, irritability, and palpitations. A non-clinical way to diagnose hypoglycemia is to determine whether the patient has any of these symptoms three or four hours after a meal and whether they go away as soon as the patient has something to eat.

Glucagon affects many of the same metabolic pathways as insulin, but its influence is opposite. Glucagon affects may of the same metabolic pathways as insulin, but its influence is opposite. A blood glucose levels fall, the release of glucagon from the pancreas is stimulated. The principal target of the glucagon is the liver, where it stimulates the conversion of glycogen to glucose. High levels of amino acids stimulate and fatty acids inhibit the release of glucagon. The conversion of non-glucose substrates such as amino acids into glucose levels are raised. Glucagon affects lipid metabolism, encouraging the production of ketone bodies, which are used as a source of energy my muscle, sparing glucose for the brain. Because of the opposing actions of insulin and glucagon, it has been suggested that the ratio between these hormones is important. After a high- carbohydrate meal, the molar ratio of insulin to glucagon can be as high as 30. Before breakfast the ratio is about 2 and after a fast of 1 or 2 days, the ratio may be less than 0.5. From the perspective of ensuring a supply of energy to the brain, a series of stages, from eating to prolonged starvation, can be distinguished:

1. In the post absorptive stage that follows a meal, glucose is released into the bloodstream following digestion. Glucose stimulates the release of insulin form the pancreas, which stimulates the liver to synthesize glycogen.
2. A major function of the liver is to take up glucose, after a meal when it is plentiful and to release it later as required. Glycogen in muscle can be used locally but is not released as glucose into the blood stream.
3. When fasting exceeds some eight hours, the process supplying glucose to the blood and hence the brain and other glucose-consuming tissues such as erythrocytes.
4. The production of glucose depends to a large extent on the breakdown of muscle protein. Because 1.75g of muscle is required to produce 1g of glucose, about 150g of protein a day will be used to

Amino Acids. In the past few years, amino acids, which are the natural contituents of protein, have come into use in the treatment of both anxiety disorders and depression. (Larson,2001; Ross,2003). The amino acid tryptophan is a natural precursor to the neurotransmitter serotonin. It is significant that serotonin is involved in regulating many body functions, including mood, sleep, appetite, and pain threshold. It also produces a feeling of calmness and well-being and deficiencies have been linked to anxiety. As an alternative to tryptophan, consider trying gamma-aminobutyric acid (GABA, for short). GABA has a mildly tranquilizing effect, although it is not as potent as prescription drugs, it does have the advantage of having few side effects and being non-addictive. It is a good idea to take GABA either on an empty stomach or with a carbohydrate snack (such as a piece of toast, crackers, cereal, or rice cakes). Carbohydrate foods actually enhance the calming or sedative effect. Avoid taking GABA with protein in doing so, but the protein (which is made up of many different amino acids) will tend to complete with absorption of GABA.

Since depression frequently accompanies anxiety, it's important to consider two amino acids that have been used effectively to treat these disorders. Both Phenylalanine and tyrosine increase the amount of a neurotransmitter substance in the brain known as norepinephrine, a substance whose deficiency has been implicated as a contributing cause of anxiety and depression.

Omega-3 Fatty Acids are important for brain and neurological health. Without sufficient levels of omega-3 fatty acids, nerve cell membranes are less fluid and may cause nerve cells to react slowly and misfire. Recent studies have found omega-3 supplementation to be helpful in diminishing symptoms of depression and mood instability. The best source of omega-3 fatty acids is wild fish (especially salmon and sardines), meat, and fowl.

Supplements for Anxiety. B Vitamins and Vitamin C. It is widely known that during times of stress your body tends to rapidly deplete stores of B vitamins and Vitamin C. Many people find that monitoring these vitamin levels makes a noticeable difference in their energy level and resiliency to stress.

The B vitamins are necessary to help maintain the proper functioning of the nervous system deficiencies, especially of vitamin B1, B2, B6 and B12 can lead to anxiety, irritability, restlessness, fatigue, and even emotional instability. Vitamin C is well known for enhancing the immune system and promoting healing from infection, disease, and injury. Less well known is the fact that vitamin C helps to support the adrenal glands, whose proper functioning is necessary to your ability to cope with stress.

Cultural Themes of Nutrition

The Diagnostic and Statistical Manual of Mental Disorders, 4th Edition, Text Revision (DSM-IV-TR) American Psychiatric Association (APA, 2000), recognizes various symptoms that are associated with specific cultures and that may be expressed differently from those of the dominant American culture. Society and culture have a great deal of influence on eating behaviors. In this text, we focus on eating as social activity on which seldom does and event of any social significance occur without the presence of food.

Diet/Arabian Americans. Arabian Cooking shares may general characteristics. Spices and herbs include cinnamon, allspice, cloves, ginger cumin, mint, parsley, bay leaves, garlic, and onions. Bread accompanies every meal and is viewed as a gift from God. Lamb and chicken are the most popular meats. Muslims are prohibited from eating pork and pork products. Food is eaten with the right had because it is regarded as clean. Eating properly, consuming nutritious foods, and fasting are believed to cure disease. Gastrointestinal complaints are the most frequent reason for seeking health care. Lactose intolerance is common.

Diet/Jewish Americans. For Jewish people who follow the dietary laws, a tremendous amount of attention is given to the slaughter, preparation, and consumption of food. There are religious laws that dictate which foods are permissible. The term Kosher means "fit to eat," and following these guidelines is thought to be a commandment of God. Meat may be eaten only if the permitted animal has been slaughtered, cooked, or served following Kosher guidelines. Pigs are considered unclean, and pork and pork products are forbidden. Dairy products and meat may not be mixed together in cooking, serving, or eating.

Diet/ Northern European Americans. Northern European Americans, particularly those who achieve middle-class socioeconomic status, value preventive medicine and primary health care. Beef and certain sea foods, such as lobster, are regarded as high-status foods among many people in this culture (Giger and Daidhizar, 2004). However, changing food habits may bring both good and bad news. The good news is that people are learning to eat healthier by decreasing the amount of fat and increasing the nutrients in their diets. The bad news is that Americans still enjoy fast food, and it conforms to their fast-paced lifestyles.

Diet/ African Americans. The diet of most African American differs little from that of the mainstream culture. However, some African American follow their heritage and still enjoy what has come to be known as "soul" food. Some of these foods include collard greens, beans, corn, friend chicken, black-eyed peas, grits, okra, and cornbread. These foods are now considered typical Southern favorites and are regularly consumed and enjoyed by most individuals who inhabit the Southern region of the United States.

Diet/Native Americans. Nutritional deficiencies are not uncommon among tribal Native Americans. Fruits and green vegetables are often scarce in many of the federally defined Indian geographical regions. Meat and corn products are identified as preferred foods. Fiber intake is often of the saturated variety. A large b=number of Native American living on or neat reservations recognized by the federal or state government receive commodility foods supplied by the U.S. Department of Agriculutre's food distribution program (U.S. Department of Agriculture, 2004).

Diet/Asian Americans. Restoring the balance of Yin and Yang is the fundamental concept of Asian health practices (Spector,2004). Yin and Yang represent opposite forces of energy, such as negative/ positive, dark/light, cold/hot, hard/soft, and feminine/masculine. When there is a disruption in the balance of these forces of energy, illness can occur. Rice, vegetables, and fish are the main staple foods of Asian Americans. Milk is seldom consumed because a large majority of Asian Ameicans experience lactose intolerance. With Western acculturation, their diet is changing, and unfortunately, with more meat being consumed, the percentage of fat in the diet is increasing. Foods, medicines, and herbs are classified according to their hot and cold properties and are used to restore balance between Yin and Yang, (hot and cold) thereby restoring health.

Diet/Hispanic Americans. The three major subgroups that make up the Hispanic population are Mexican Americans, Puerto Ricans, and Cubans. Hispanics tend to eat more rice, but less pasta and ready-to-eat cereals than their non-Hispanic white counterparts. With the exception of tomatoes, Hispanics are also less likely to consume vegetables, although they have a slightly higher consumption of fruits. They are also more likely to eat beef, but less likely to eat processed eats such as hotdogs, sausage, and luncheon meats. Analysis of the macronutrient content of the diet reveals that Hispanics, especially Mexican Americans, have a lower intake of total fat and higher intake of dietary fiber compared to non-Hispanic white populations, with much of the dietary fiber coming from legumes. Approaches for improving the health of Hispanics need to be broad-based and consider the complexities of a variety of lifestyle factors. Nutrition education programs aimed at improving the quality of the Hispanic diet- including a reliance on beans, rice, and tortillas- and a change on others- such as reduced consumption of high-fat dairy products and less use of fat in cooking. In addition, they tend to have higher intakes of proteins, vitamins A and C, folic acid, and calcium than other cultural groups.

VIGNETTE

A 40-year-old male veteran with a strong alcoholic history entered the VA hospital for severe epigastric pain and vomiting. Physical examination, initial X-rays and serum amylase level was consisted with acute pancreatitis. The patient was treated with nasogastric suction and intravenous fluids. It was anticipated that a nothing-by-mouth, nasogastric suction regimen was required for less than a week, after which time he should be able to be started on feeding and nutritional rehabilitation.

On nutrition assessment after rehydration, he was found to have body weight that was 80% of ideal and 80% of his usual weight. Skinfold and muscle area measurements were consistent with moderate protein malnutrition. He experienced imbalanced nutrition, less than body requirements related to depressed mood, loss of appetite or lack of interest in food, evidenced by weight loss, poor muscle tone, pale conjunctiva and mucous membranes, poor skin turgor, and weakness. He complained of insomnia, weight loss, decreased libido and suicidal ideation over the past 2 months, which he attributed to the recent breakup of his marriage. A careful history revealed that over the past 6 weeks, the patient had been drinking a half a bottle of whiskey per day, and at times substantially more than this.

Recovery began within hours after the administration of thiamine. Under the influence of thiamine or an adequate diet, the patient rapidly became more alert and attentive and more capable of taking part in mental testing. However, he did not recover completely from ataxia. He was left with a slow shuffling, wide based gait and inability to wale tandem. It was so severe that he could not stand or walk without support. It was important that he showed signs of alcohol withdrawal, i.e. hallucinations and other disorders of perception, confusion, agitation, tremor, and overactivity of autonomic nervous system function. Spontaneous speech was minimal and many questions were unanswered, and the patient suspended conversation in the middle of a sentence and drifted off to sleep.

Discussion. What is the current protein-calorie nutritional status of the patient? This a key question in formulating a nutrition support plans. While taking the patient's history and performing the physical examination, the physician must be aware of the manifestations of the various nutritional disorders for which the patient with disease is at desk. Korsakoff psychosis refers to a unique mental disorder in which retentive memory is impaired out of all proportion to other cognitive functions in an otherwise alert and responsive patient. This disorder, like Wernicke disease, is often associated with alcoholism and malnutrition. However, it may be a symptom of various other disorders that have their basis in lesions of the diencephalon or the temporal lobes.

Alcoholism is an important factor in the causation of nutritional diseases of the nervous system. This is true because alcohol acts mainly by displacing food in the diet but also by adding carbohydrate calories (alcohol is burned almost entirely as carbohydrate), thus increasing the need for thiamine. For nutria tonal therapy to be effective, reasonable goals must be established. There is some evidence as well that alcohol impairs the absorption of thiamine and other B-vitamins form the gastrointestinal tract. That is why thiamine should be given prior to the patient's first meal in order to avoid depleting body stores of thiamine used for carbohydrates metabolism. Consultation with clinical dietitians and physicians who maintain an updated interest in clinical nutrition will result in the most effective use of nutritional therapy.

Nutritional Therapy

Green Tea for Relaxation. The amino acid, L-theanine, is unique to tea leaves and is primarily obtained in the diet by drinking green tea. Studies demonstrated that the consumption of L-theanine increases the release of dopamine and serotonin in the brain and increases brain alpha- wave activity, a sign of relaxation and increasing calmness. This research suggests that the consumption of 200mg of L-theanine about one hour before bedtime can help a difficult sleeper relax while trying to fall asleep. Tea, especially green tea, is great for the heart. It helps keep arteries clear, the heart pumping strong and cholesterol at bay Green tea catechins also prevent heart attacks. There is some scientific evidence that drinking tea helps to maintain healthy aortic function and the delivery of oxygenated blood to the heart muscle while reducing the risk of aortic occlusion and ischemic heart disease. In other words, the vessels expand to allow more blood to pass when more oxygenated blood is needed, especially to the heart muscle. Green tea contributes to the maintenance of healthy body weight in several ways.

In men and women, the degree of body fatness, whether expressed as percent body fat or the ratio of waist circumference to hip circumference, decreases as green tea intake increases. (Wu, Lu, Chang et al. 2003).

Herbal Remedies. Herbs have been used for hundreds of years to promote camlness and relaxation. (Tierra, 1998). Herbs that have been most helpful for monitoring states of anxiety include Ginko biloba, Kava, Valerian, Saint-John's Wort. And Passionflower. Early in the process of evaluating the performance- enhancing attributes of a feed or ingredient it becomes essential to identify the active compound in the food. This is important for a number of reasons, including having the ability to titrate dose against response and to allow comparison of efficacy of different preparations of same food.

For example, Ginkgo biloba is an herb reported to improve peripheral and brain blood flow, to improve learning and memory, and slow the rate of the mental degeneration in Alzheimer's patients.

Kava is a natural tranquilizer that has become a popular relaxer in the United States in recent years. Small doses produce a sense of well-being, while large doses can produce lethargy, incur drowsiness, and reduce muscle tension. In European countries, such as Germany and Switzerland, Kava has been approved for treatment of insomnia and anxiety. It appears that Kava may tone down the activity of the limbic system, particularly the amygdala, which is a brain center associated with anxiety.

Valerian is a herbal tranquilizer and sedative that is widely used in alleviating mild to moderate anxiety and insomnia, yet it has fewer side effects and is non-addictive. Valerian is also not as likely as prescription tranquilizers to impair memory and concentration or cause lethargy and drowsiness, and will not cause a hangover the next day if used for sleep. Long experience indicates valerian as an especially safe herb. However, long-term use at high doses has been associated with side effects such as headache, excitability, restlessness, agitation, and palpitations.

Saint John's Wort, also known as hypericum, has a long history of use. It was recommended by Hippocrates for anxiety more than two thousand years ago. Currently, it is being used to treat symptoms of mild to moderate depression, as well as anxiety. It's important to keep in mind that hypericum takes four to six weeks to reach therapeutic effectiveness. If the patient does not see any benefit in the first two to three weeks, don't get discouraged and stop. It is necessary to stick with the plan for at least one month.

Passion flower is a good natural tranquilizer considered by many to be as effective as valerian. In higher doses, it is often used to treat insomnia, as it both relieves nervous tension and relaxes muscles.

Flu-fighting foods. When the flu season was about to begin to get a flu shot and do what is required so that health prepares disease prevention. To help cut down on illness, it's important that family members and those who work around people 65 and older get vaccinated. And don't forget to boost the body's immune system with these natural flu-fighting foods.

- Black-eye Peas. The nutritious legumes are rich in Zinc, a trace mineral that keeps the immune system in working order. Pinto beans, peanuts, roasted pumpkin seeds and wheat germ are other good choices.
- Carrots. They're rich in beta-carotene, which your body uses to ward off respiratory infections. Other good sources are dark green vegetables, sweet potatoes, pumpkin and winter squash.
- Tea. Green, black and oolong tea all contain naturally occurring compounds that reduce the risk of flu, including quercetin, a powerful anti-oxidant, and L-theanine, and amino acid found naturally only in tea. Decaffeinated teas also contain amino acid, but herbal teas do not.
- Yogurt Probiotics, the beneficial bacteria found in yogurt and other fermented foods, strengthen the immune system. Not a fan of yogurt? Try cottage cheese, kimchi (a fermented Korean dish made of seasoned vegetables) or sauerkraut instead.
- Tomatoes. Vitamin C- rich tomatoes help fight colds and flu by boosting the body's natural defense system in the same way their citrusy relatives do. One medium tomato provides 40% of the daily vitamin C, so have a glass of tomato juice at lunch and treat yourself to pasta with tomato sauce.
- Mushrooms. These nutritional powerhouses heighten the body's resistance to viral infections by increasing the activity of natural killer cells, a vital part of the immune system. They are also rich in selenium; Low levels of this element have been linked with an increased risk of developing more severe flu.

- Almonds. These popular nuts are a rich source of the antioxidant Vitamin E, which helps your body Ward off viral infections. To maximize vitamin E absorption, opt for chopped almonds, almond butter or almond oil.

Nutrition and Cancer. Nutrition and the cancer patient- The relationship between diet and cancer has been of interest for many years. Research has shown a correlation between dietary fats and several cancers. (Colon, breast, prostate) The key issue is whether there is correlation between the risk of complications and the degree of nutrition. Why is dietary fiber important in cancer prevention? For example, In colon cancer high-fiber diets are associated with lessoned risk, perhaps because they speed travel time of food within the bowels. This is best accomplished by eating fiber rich foods at each meal, such as whole grain cereals, breads, pastas, beans, leafy vegetables, fruits, nuts, and seeds. Dietary fiber is the part of foods or plant origin. It doesn't come from any foods the come from animals, because fiber provides bulk to our diets and helps to maintain a healthy colon.

Dietary fiber is important in cancer prevention. Cancer of the breast is one of the oldest and best known types of cancer. A number of observations suggest that breast cancer risk is influenced by diet. Particularly, consumption of fats. Metastasis or advanced breast cancer is the presents of disease at distant sites such as the bone, lung or liver. Therefore, symptoms may include pain from n=bone metastasis, breathlessness id spreads to the lung, or abdominal discomfort from liver involvement. Some researchers have suggested a possible relationship between prostate cancer and low-fat intake. Prostate cancer is now the most common male caner in the United Sates. Risk factors include age, family history or prostate cancer, black race, and possible higher dietary fat intake. Prostate cancer metastasizes predominantly to bone. This results in pain weakness, paralysis, and even death.

Can eating fish be protective against cancer? Oily fish such as salmon, herring, mackerel, halibut, and tuna contain oils rich in Omega-3 fatty acids. It is recommended to eat foods rich in omega-3 several times each week. Fish is a good source but berries, mushrooms, and Brussels sprouts are also dietary sources of omega-3 fatty acids. Liquid dietary supplements in the form of milk shakes and commercial preparations are excellent if tolerated.

Dietary Toxins. Many health problems can be expected to require diet modification, of which a few examples follow. Once you master the intricate interaction between what you eat and its effect on your body and mind, you inlock powerful and scientifically proven tool to use in the quest for maintaining or improving your personal health.

Chinese Restaurant Syndrome. Monosodium Glutamate (MSG) is used as a flavor enhancer in many foods. The syndrome of neurotoxicity typically occurs when foods containing MSG are consumed on an empty stomach. Rapid absorption of this chemical results in headache, flushing, bronchospasm, burning, and facial pressure. The syndrome usually resolves within one hour. During this time, most patients reports a sense of fear and distress. The burning symptoms are intense and frequently spread to the neck, torso, and abdomen.

Seafood toxins. Ciguatera poisoning is the most common type of seafood poisoning in the world. The ciguatoxin is heat stable, odorless, and tasteless and is most commonly found in red snapper, grouper, sea bass, and amberjack. Most episodes of toxicity occur 2 to 6 hours following ingestion. The characteristic manifestation of ciguatera poisoning include headaches, the sensation of loose painful teeth, a strange metallic taste, circumoral numbness, that may progress to involve the tongue and throat. It is then that the patient experiences onset of gastrointestinal problems in abdominal pain, nausea, vomiting, and profuse watery diarrhea for 24 to 48 hours.

Botulism Toxin. Food- borne botulism has traditionally been associated with home processed foods. The toxin is inactivated by heat, so transmission occurs from unheated or inadequately prepared foods. The toxin is carried via the bloodstream to the neuromuscular junction, where it binds irreversibly leading to paralysis. This is significant because food-borne botulism may be proceeded by gastrointestinal symptoms such as cramps, nausea, vomiting, and diarrhea. The incubation period of food-borne botulism is usually between 12 and 36 hours. It is important to note that a clear sensorium is usually present because the toxin does not penetrate the brain parenchyma. Although mortality has improved with the advances in critical care and application of equine botulism antitoxin. The recovery period may be protracted, as it requires the re-innervation of paralyzed muscle fibers.

We know that everything the patients eats and drinks has an effect on both mind and body. By eating right, increasing physical activity, and reducing the risk through wise choices, you can stay healthy throughout your life. In summary, studying dietary toxins leads to making smart eating choices is essential to living a healthy, happy, and successful life.

Chapter 27: Nutritional Therapy Examination Review

1. Which vitamin inhibits the oxidation of cholesterol in the blood and stimulates the immune system to remove from the circulation any cholesterol-containing particles that have become oxidized?

    A. Vitamin A
    B. Vitamin B
    C. Vitamin D
    D. Vitamin E

2. What cofactors allow insulin to effectively stimulate the transfer of glucose from the blood into cells?

    A. Chromium
    B. Choline
    C. Folate
    D. Zinc

3. What are the reasons for an inadequate nutritional intake in the elderly?

    A. Lack of pleasure in this activity
    B. Many forget to eat due to dementia.
    C. Tremors that interfere with the ability to feed oneself
    D. Cultural habits promoting management of foods by families

4. Of all the dietary factors that can aggravate anxiety and trigger panic attacks, which is the most notorious?

    A. Sodium
    B. Caffeine
    C. Calcium
    D. Magnesium

5. What dietary guideline are promoted in elderly patients?

    A. Increase fat intake to 40% of calories

    B. Decrease fiber intake to 10-15g/d

    C. Frequent alcoholic beverages

    D. Minimize consumption of salt-cured, salt-pickled, or smoked foods

6. What is the principal target of glucagon?

    A. The Liver

    B. The Heart

    C. The Brain

    D. The Kidneys

7. Why is dietary fiber important in cancer prevention?

    A. Diets high in calcium slows epithelial cell proliferation in colon cancer.

    B. Relationship between prostate cancer and high-fat intake.

    C. Avoid daily eating foods rich in omega-3 fatty acids.

    D. Encourage taking GABA with protein.

8. Boost the body's immune system with all of the natural flu-fighting foods, except:

    A. Black-Eyed Peas

    B. Potatoes

    C. Carrots

    D. Tomatoes

9. Low levels of this element have been linked with an increased risk of developing more severe flu:

    A. Melatonim

    B. St. John's Wort

    C. Ginkgo Biloba

    D. Selenium

10. Some foods affect mood. What are they?

    A. Sugar and starch in carbohydrate foods boost serotonin in the brain.

    B. High protein foods release substances that stimulate feeling more alert and energetic.

    C. Starchy vegetables such as potatoes, winter quash, or corn helps feeling more relaxed and calm.

    D. All of the above.

Chapter 27: Nutritional Therapy Examination

1. D
2. A
3. C
4. B
5. D
6. A
7. A
8. B
9. D
10. D

Chapter 28

Relaxation Techniques

This chapter on relaxation would not be complete without discussion of the concepts of down time and time management. Down time is exactly what it sounds like-time out from work or other responsibilities to give yourself an opportunity to rest and replenish your energy. There are three kinds of down time, each of which has an important place in developing a more relaxed lifestyle: 1) rest time, 2) recreation time, and 3) relationship time. A common problem in time management is understanding the amount of time required to complete a task. The result is that you end up rushing to try to get something done, or else run into overtime and encroach on time that was needed for the next activity in your schedule. Deep relaxation refers to a distinct physiological state that is the exact opposite of the way each person's body reacts under stress. This state was originally described by Herbert Benson in 1975 as the relaxation response. It involves a series of physiological changes including (Bourne, 1995).

- Decrease in heart rate
- Decrease in respiration rate
- Decrease in blood pressure
- Decrease in skeletal muscle tension
- Decrease in metabolic rate and oxygen consumption
- Decrease in analytical thinking

- Increase in skin resistance
- Increase in skin resistance
- Increase in alpha wave activity in the brain

Abdominal Breathing. Breathing directly reflects the level of tension carried in the body. Under tension, breathing usually becomes shallow and rapid, and occurs high in the chest. When relaxed, the patient breathes more fully, more deeply, and from the abdomen at the same time.

Some of the benefits of abdominal breathing include:

- Increased oxygen supply to the brain and musculature.
- Stimulation of the para-sympathetic nervous system. This branch of applied autonomic nervous system promotes a state of calmness and quiescence.
- Greater feelings of connectedness between mind and body. More efficient excretion of bodily toxins. Many toxic substances in the body are excreted through the lungs.
- Improved concentration, in the mind that is racing, it's difficult to focus attention therefore abdominal breathing will help to quiet mental activity.
- Abdominal breathing by itself can trigger a relaxation response.
- The result is a cluster of symptoms, including rapid heartbeat, dizziness, and tingly sensations that are so similar to the symptoms of panic that they can be indistinguishable. Some of the physiological changes brought on by hyperventilation include:
- Increased alkalinity of nerve cells, which causes them to be more excitable. The result is that each person feels nervous and jittery.
- Decreased carbon dioxide in the blood, which can cause feelings of the heart to pump harder and faster as well as making lights seem brighter and sounds louder.
- Increased construction of blood vessels in the brain, which can cause feelings of dizziness, disorientation, and even a sense of unreality or separateness from the body.

Abdominal Breathing Exercise. Practice the Abdominal Breathing Exercise for five minutes every day for at least two weeks. If possible, find a regular time each day to do this so that your breathing exercise becomes a habit. Once you feel you've gained technique, apply it when you feel stressed or anxious, or when you experience the onset of panic symptoms. By extending your practice of this exercise to a month or longer, you will begin to retrain yourself to breathe from your abdomen. Then the more you can shift the center of your breathing from your chest to your abdomen, the more consistently you will feel relaxed on an ongoing basis.

Abdominal Breathing Exercise Box 28-1

1. Note the level of tension you're feeling. Then place one hand on your abdomen right beneath your rib cage.
2. Inhale slowly and deeply through your nose into the bottom of your lungs, sending the air as low down as you can. In abdominal breathing, the diaphragm- the muscle that separates the lung cavity from the abdominal cavity- moves downward.
3. When you've taken in a full breath, pause for a moment and then exhale slowly through your nose or mouth, depending on your preference.
4. Do ten slow, full abdominal breaths. Try to keep your breathing smooth and regular, without gulping in a big breath or letting you breathe out all at once. Count from ten down to one counting backwards one number with each exhalation. The process should go like this; Slow inhale … Pause … Slow exhale (count ten). Slow inhale … Pause … Slow exhale (count nine). Slow inhale … Pause … Slow exhale (count eight).
5. Extend the exercise by doing two or three sets of abdominal breaths, remember to count backwards from ten to one for each set (each exhalation counts as one number).

Progressive Muscle Relaxation is a systematic technique for achieving a deep state of relaxation. It was developed by Dr. Edmund Jacobson more than fifty years ago. Dr. Jacobson discovered that a muscle could be relaxed by first tensing it for a few seconds and then releasing it. Tensing and releasing various muscle groups throughout the body produces a deep state of relaxation, which Dr. Jacobson found capable of relieving a variety of condition, from high blood pressure to ulcerative colitis. Dr. Jacobson himself once said, "An anxious mind cannot exist in a relaxed body."

Other symptoms that respond well to progressive muscle relaxation include tension headaches, backaches, tightness around the eyes, muscle spasms, and insomnia. That is why in his original book, Progressive Relaxation, Dr. Jacobson developed a series of two hundred different muscle relaxation exercises and a training program that took months to complete.

Passive Muscle Relaxation. A modified version of this technique (called passive progressive relaxation) involves relaxation of the muscles by concentrating on the feeling of relaxation within the muscles, rather than the actual tensing and relaxing of the muscle.

Box 28-2. Progressive Deep Muscle Relaxation Exercises

Forehead. Wrinkle up your forehead by arching your eyebrows and creasing your forehead, hold the tension, and then slowly let go of the tension.	**Right Arm.** Tense your right arm and hand by stretching it out in from of you and clenching your fist tightly, hold it the tension, and then slowly let go of the tension.
Eyes. Squeeze your eyes together tightly, hold the tension, and then slowly let go of the tension.	**Left Arm.** Tense your left arm and hand by stretching it out in front of you, and then slowly let go of the tension.
Nose. Wrinkle up your nose and spread your nostrils, hold the tension, and then slowly let go of the tension.	**Right Leg.** Extend your right leg in front of you (at the height of the chair seat), tense your thigh and leg by pointing your toes inward toward your face, hold the tension, and then slowly let go of the tension.

Tongue. Push your tongue hard against the roof of your mouth, hold the tension, and then slowly let go of the tension.	**Left Leg.** Extend your left leg in front of you, tense your thigh and leg by pointing your toes inward toward your face, hold the tension, and then slowly let go of the tension.
Face. Put a forced smile on your face and spread your face, hold the tension, and then slowly let go of the tension.	**Upper Back.** Tense your back muscles by sitting slightly forward in the chair, bending your elbows and trying to get them to tough each other behind your back, hold the tension, and then slowly let go of the tension.
Jaws. Clench your jaws together tightly, hold the tension, and then slowly let go of the tension.	**Chest.** Tense your chest muscles by pulling your stomach in and thrusting your chest upward and outward, hold the tension, and then slowly let go of the tension.
Lips. Pucker up your lips and spread them, hold the tension, and then slowly let go of the tension.	**Stomach.** Tense your stomach muscles, making them hard by pushing your stomach out, hold the tension, and then slowly let go of the tension.
Neck. Tighten the muscles of your neck by pulling your chin in and shrugging up your shoulders, hold the tension, and then slowly let go of the tension.	**Buttocks and Thighs.** Tense your buttocks and thighs by placing your feet squarely on the floor, hold the tension, and then slowly let go of the tension.

Practice should be engaged in twice daily for a period of 12-15 minutes. Mastery of the technique is after 2-4 weeks of twice daily practice.

Passive Box 28-3: Passive Muscle Relaxation Exercise

Begin by taking two or three deep, abdominal breaths and let yourself settle back into the chair, bed, or wherever you are fully comfortable. Put aside any worries, any uncomfortable, unpleasant thoughts right now. Let yourself be totally in the present moment as you let yourself relax more and more (Pause)

Let each part of your body begin to relax, starting with your feet. Just imagine your feet letting go and relaxing right now. Let go of any excess tension in our feet. Just imagine the tension draining away. As your feet are relaxing, imagine relaxation moving up into your calves unwind and loosen up and let go. (Pause)

Now as your calves are relaxing, allow relaxation to move up into your thighs. Let the muscles in your thighs unwind and smooth out and relax completely. You might begin to feel your legs from your waist down to your feet becoming more and more relaxed. Continue and let relaxation move into your hips.
(Pause)

Soon you might allow relaxation to move into your stomach area. Just let go of any stress in your stomach area- let it all go right now, imagining deep sensations of relaxation spreading all around your abdomen. As your stomach is relaxing, continue to allow relaxation to move up into your chest. All the muscles in your chest can unwind and loosen up and let go. Each time you exhale, imagine breathing away any remaining tension in your chest until your chest feels completely relaxed.
(Pause)

Soon you might allow relaxation to move into your shoulders by just letting deep sensations of calmness and relaxation to spread although the muscles of your shoulders. Then allow the relaxation in your shoulders to move down into your arms, spreading into your upper arms, down into your elbows and forearms, and finally all the way down to your wrists and hands. You can feel relaxation moving into your neck now. All the muscles in your neck just unwind, smooth out, and relax completely.
(Pause)

Then soon, the relaxation can move into your chin and jaws. As they are relaxing, imagine relaxation moving into the area around your eyes. Now let your forehead relax, too. Let the muscles in your forehead smooth out and relax completely, noticing the weight of your head against whatever it's resting on as you allow your entire head to relax completely.
(Pause)

Visualizing a Peaceful Scene

After completing progressive muscle relaxation, it's helpful to experience self-visualizing in the midst of a peaceful scene. Progressive muscle relaxation addresses particular groups of muscles; imagining yourself setting can manifest a global sense of relaxation that is freed from anxious thoughts. The peaceful scene can be a quiet beach, a stream in the mountains, or a calm lake. Don't restrict yourself to reality: you can imagine, if you want to, floating on a cloud or flying on a magic carpet.

This exercise is to design your own peaceful scene. Be sure to describe it in vivid detail, appealing to as many of your senses as possible. It may help to answer the following questions:

Box 28-4 Visualizing a Peaceful Scene Exercise

- What does the scene look like?
- What colors are prominent?
- What sounds are present?
- What time of day is it?
- What is the temperature?
- What are you touching or in physical contact with in the scene?
- What does the air smell like?
- Are you alone or with somebody else?

A relaxing visualization constitutes a light form of self-hypnosis. The whole point of imagining a peaceful scene is to transport yourself from your normal state of restless thinking into an altered state of deep relaxation. Once you have imagined your own ideal peaceful scene, practice returning to it every time you do progressive muscle relaxation, deep breathing, or any other relaxation technique. This will help to reinforce the scene on your mind.

Meditation

There are many ways to meditate. Here's one simple way: just sit comfortably, close your eyes, relax your shoulders, breathe slowly and deeply, and say to yourself over and over, a mantra or "I love you God."

When we meditate (Taub, 2009):

- The body's internal pharmacy and internal healing force are stimulated.
- The brain's electrical activity is calmed though an increase in brain waves associated with deep relaxation.
- The body's metabolic rate slows down, leading to more efficient oxygen consumption.
- Blood pressure and pulse rate both decrease, lessening the work load on the heart.

Meditation really amounts to deep, relaxed breathing, which allows you to calm down your brain waves, refocus and rebalance your energy, and take a brief, mental vacation form the stresses and strains of everyday life. Some people recommend meditating 20 to 30 minutes a day. Others say that meditations a lot like exercise- if you aren't familiar or comfortable with it, just do it for a few minutes each day. Practically anyone can find 5 minutes for this life-enhancing process.

Box 28-5: Guidelines for Practicing Meditation

1. Find a quiet environment. Do what you can to reduce external noise. If this is nor completely possible, paly a record or tape of soft, instrumental sounds, or sounds from nature such as the sound of ocean waves that makes a good background.
2. Reduce muscle tension. If you're feeling tense, spend some time, no more than 10 minutes, relaxing your muscles.
3. Sit properly. Eastern Style. Sit cross-legged on the floor with a cushion or pillow supporting your buttocks. Rest your hands on your thighs. Lean slightly forward so that some of your weight is supported by your thighs as well as your buttocks.

   Western Style (preferred by most Americans). Sit in a comfortable, straight-backed chair, with your feet on the floor and legs uncrossed, hands on your thighs.

4. Set aside 20-30 minutes for meditation. You may wish to set a timer or run a background tape that is 20-30 minutes for long so that you'll know when your done.
5. Make it a regular practice to meditate every day.
6. Meditating is easier if you don't do it on a full stomach or when you are tired.
7. Select a focus for your attention. The most common devices are your own breathing cycle or a mantra.
8. Assume a non-judgmental, passive attitude.
    - Concentrate on whatever you've chosen as an object of meditation but don't force or strain yourself to do so.
    - Every time your concentration wanders from your object of focus, gently bring it back again.
    - The more you let go and refrain from trying to do anything other than gently guiding your attention back to your object of focus.

Relaxation Techniques. In the 1970's Herbert Benson did research on Transcendental Meditation, which he published in his well-known book, <u>The Relaxation Response.</u> The practice of transcendental meditation (TM) evolved within the spiritual disciplines of India. In recent years it has spread to other countries where it is employed, not necessarily for spiritual insight, but in the hope of gaining a tranquil outlook on life. This state of merging is called Nirvana by the Buddhists, Ecstasy by the Christians, Samadhi by the Hindus, Illumination by the Jews, and Tabattal by the Muslims.

Variations of technique are found, though in general TM involves the following procedures:

1. The silent repetition of a word or sound known as a mantra
2. Concentration on the mantra to the exclusion of distracting thoughts
3. Muscular relaxation, adopted by sitting in a relaxed position.

In the 1980's and 1990's, Jon Kabat-Zinn did extensive research on meditation as a method of stress management. Utilizing an approach to meditation, he referred to as mindfulness, his program for stress management is known as mindfulness-based stress reduction.

What if mindfulness practice does not seem to help you quiet down? What if you continue to feel highly agitated and distracted after ten or more minutes of meditation? If this happens, your body maybe too charged up to sit still. The best thing to do is to get physical. Try doing some form of aerobic exercise or take twenty minutes to do a sequence of yoga postures. After you've discharged the energy from your body, try sitting in meditation again (Goldstein, 1993).

Biofeedback. The most dramatic example of behavioral medicine techniques in the treatment of somatic complaints is biofeedback. Neal Miller demonstrated the medical potential of biofeedback by showing that the normally involuntary autonomic nervous system can be operantly conditioned by use of appropriate feedback. In recent years behavioral researchers have been exploring the clinical uses of biofeedback as a means of improving somatic functioning. Biofeedback is often used together with other relaxation techniques such as deep breathing, progressive relaxation, and metal imagery. Biofeedback provides people with prompt and exact information, otherwise unavailable, on heart rate, blood pressure, brain waves, skin temperature, and other autonomic bodily functions.

The particular internal physiological process is detected and amplified by a sensitive electronic recording device. The most common form of biofeedback used in stress management is electromyographic (EMG) feedback. EMG feedback operates by detecting biological signals and providing visual or auditory signals and providing visual or auditory signals linked to this biological system via amplification of the psychophysiological measures (Stoyva and Budzynski, 1993). The person knows instantaneously, through an auditory or visual signal, the rate of the process whether it is too high or too low or just right.

The individual utilizes this continuous feedback to modify the response incrementally in the desired direction through a series of increasingly stringent criterion levels.

Migraine headaches are estimated to afflict up to 10 percent of the general population. Some people have these attacks as often as every few days, others only a few times in their lives.

The headache pain itself is usually on one side, almost as though the head were divided in two by an impermeable wall. A distinction is usually made between classic migraine and common migraine. In classic migraine the person has prodromal symptoms, symptoms experienced before the onset of the headache itself. They take the form of tension, wakefulness, declining energy and drive, and sometimes visual disturbances which are seen first as a shimmering haze, then as zigzag lines.

In both types of migraine it is known that the headache itself is caused by sustained dilation, or increase in size, of the extra-cranial vasculature, principally of the temporal artery which trifurcates to supply the side of the head. Therefore, the headache is initially a pulsing pain on one side of the head, coinciding with each heartbeat as the blood is pumped through the expanded extra-cranial arteries.

Through biofeedback the individual is trained to reduce the amplitude of pulsations in the superficial temporal arteries, in other words to constrict the arteries at the site of the actual migraine headache.

That is why biofeedback has many potential applications. For example in fecal incontinence, through training of the anal sphincter; in hypertension, through displaying blood pressure values and allowing patients to discover methods to control their blood pressure; and in Raynaud's disease, through enhancing temperature control.

Yoga. By definition, yoga is involved with promoting unity of mind, body, and spirit.

It was originally laid out by the philosopher Pantanjali in the second century BC. The series of stretch exercises actually embraces a broad philosophy of life and an elaborate system for personal transformation. Yoga postures, by themselves, provide a very effective means to increase fitness, flexibility, and relaxation. This process of lengthening and energizing on each inhale and relaxing and deepening on each exhale should continue throughout the entire practice session. They can be practiced alone or with a group, as long as it simultaneously increases energy and vitality while calming the mind. Yoga may be compared to progressive muscle relaxation, in that it also involves holding the body in certain flexed positions for a few moments and then relaxing.

Yoga. Always start the warm-up process with attention to your breath, noticing your posture from your comfortable seated position and the effect of the breath on your body and perspective. Balance postures in yoga practice allow you to mimic the realignment of the heart's center with the centering of the mind and body. The two most important elements of balance postures are starting with a deep, flowing breath and finding a fixed point on which to focus your gaze. As you notice how your body is feeling, there may be a couple of finishing postures you will need to perform to make you more comfortable. It is my recommendation that you perform the postures above at the end of every practice.

Standing Postures are best included after a warm-up period and balance postures. With your muscles warm and your body aligned properly, you are ready to challenge your body with heat-building postures that develop strength and stamina. Again, make sure you are practicing at the level that is appropriate for you and how you are feeling today.

Floor Postures. God desires to draw near to each individual. He promises in scripture that if we draw near to Him, Hew will draw near to us (James 4:8). How do you draw near to God? You remove the barriers that create separation.

The most familiar type of yoga practiced in Western countries is hatha yoga. Hatha yoga uses body postures, along with the meditation and breathing exercises, to achieve a balanced, disciplined workout that releases muscle tension; tones the internal rgans; and energizes the mind, body, and spirit, to allow natural healing to occur. The complete routine of poses is designed to work all parts of the body- stretching and toning muscles and keeping joints flexible. Studies have shown that yoga has provided beneficial effects to some individuals with back pain, stress, migraine, insomnia, high blood pressure, rapid heart rates, and limited mobility (Sadock and Sadock, 2003; Steinberg, 2002; Trivieri and Anderson, 2002).

Calming Breath Exercise. This exercise was adapted forom the ancient discipline of yoga. It is a very efficient technique for achieving a deep state of relaxation quickly.

1. Breath from the abdomen, then inhale through your nose slowly to a count of five.
2. Pause and hold your breath to a count of five.
3. Exhale slowly, through your nose or mouth, to a count of five.
4. When you've exhaled completely, take two breaths in your normal rhythm, then repeat steps 1 through 3 in the cycle above.
5. Keep up the exercise for at least three to five minutes. If possible, find a regular time each day to do this so that your breathing exercise becomes a habit.

With proper preparation, yoga can be a safe, effective, and rewarding practice that is suitable for students of all ages and levels of ability (Bordenkircher, 2006).

Recommend that patients practice at least three times per week to see progressive developments in muscle strength, flexibility, balance, and focus. Attempt to perform these postures at about the same time each day. It is best to practice postures with bare feet so that your toes will help in balance ad create better foot health. This will help ensure steady progress and will help ensure steady progress and will help develop a regular routine.

Relax. Remember that yoga is a very individualized practice. You are encouraged to work at your own intention for each class. Therefore you need to set your intention for the class early, and let your postures and attitude reflect that purpose. With deliberate intention, each person can go from stressed to calm in the matter of a few deep breaths. Learning proper breathing techniques that will not only make for a successful yoga practice but will also enhance health, vitality, and emotional well-being off the mat.

Pregnancy. Yoga is generally safe for normal pregnancies with the following exceptions: in the third trimester, students are encouraged to avoid twists, inversions, ab isolation poses, and postures that involve lying on the belly. Always check with your doctor to determine if the practice will be suitable.

VIGNETTE

A middle-aged white woman was referred for intractable headaches following a thorough neurological work-up. She reported a 4 month history of tension-type headaches unaccompanied by migrainous phenomena. Although she had experienced headaches three or four times a year before this periods, the frequency now approximated three times a week, with each episode lasting several hours and occasionally becoming severe enough to interfere with routine domestic duties. Initial use of several over –the-counter analgesics according to her physician's recommendation resulted in some relief, but soon became ineffective. Her primary care physician believed that an evaluation for stress counselling was in order.

On initial examination the patient's cognitive status was unremarkable, and no clear evidence of psychotic, anxiety, substance abuse, or depressive disorders was obvious, although she described increasingly disturbed sleep during the same 4 month period. Her caffeine use was normal (two to three cups of coffee a day). Premarin was her only prescription medication. She consumed alcohol socially and averaged about 2-3 ounces a week. During her psychosocial history she became defensive and annoyed, protesting its irrelevance. At various time, she worried that she was getting old and unattractive or that her husband had a new lover.

Relaxation therapy was effective in relieving her headaches. The headaches is usually throbbing, though it may begin as a dull sensation and take a while to reach maximum intensity. It usually ends within 24 hours, but occasionally persists for 1 to 2 days. Her headaches often begin with various prodromal sensations, such as nauseas, loss of vision in part fo the field of vision, or visual aura. Ordinarily, the prodromal symptoms begin half an hour to an hour prior to the beginning of the headache itself.

Discussion

Headache. Relaxation training is a relatively simple therapeutic technique that is useful in a variety of conditions. For example, a patient who has tension headaches would be told that muscles tense up as a result of anxiety and this can lead to pain, If the patient were to learn to relax his or her muscles, such pain could be lessened. Patients are then seated comfortably in a chair and are taught to tense and then relax each muscle group systematically. Soon they are able to induce relaxation fairly quickly simply by relaxing all their muscles. Patients are encouraged at the same time to visualize a pleasant, relaxing scene or to use a simple mantra to control distracting thoughts. Patients are given a tape recording of relaxation instructions and are encouraged to use the tape for some 20 minutes each day at home.

In migraine headaches, pain usually affects one side of the head. Pain most commonly originates in the muscles of the face, neck, and head; the blood vessels' and the dura mater. The blood vessels dilate and become congested with blood. Pain results from the exertion of pressure on nerves that lie in or around these congested blood vessels. Migraines headaches can occur at any age, but commonly begin in persons between 16 and 30 years of age. They are more common in women than in men and often are associated with various phases of the menstrual cycle (Stewart et.al., 1992). Most throbbing, recurrent headaches are of vascular origin; migraine accounts for the vast majority. Relaxation techniques may significantly decrease the frequency and severity of headaches. These activities help reduce the impact of stress. Patient suffering from migraine headaches, caused by expansion of the blood vessels around the brain, have obtained relief by learning to raise the temperature of their hands. This restores balance to the circulatory system by increasing the flow of blood to the hands and decreasing the amount of blood in the vessels that supply to the brain.

Chapter 28: Relaxation Examination Review

1. What are the more common methods by which you can achieve a state of deep relaxation?

    A. Abdominal Breathing
    B. Progressive Muscle Relaxation
    C. Biofeedback
    D. All of the above

2. The relaxation response involves a series of physiological changes including

    A. Increase in heart rate
    B. Increase in blood pressure
    C. Increase in alpha wave activity in the brain
    D. Increase in metabolic rate and oxygen consumption

3. Herbert benson described the relaxation response in 1975 to involve a series of physiological changes including

    A. Increase in heart
    B. Increase in respiration rate
    C. Decrease in metabolic rate and oxygen consumption
    D. Decrease in alpha wave activity in the brain

4. The practice of transcendental meditation involves which procedures

    A. The silent repletion of a word or a sound known as a mantra
    B. Concentration on the mantra to the exclusion of distracting thoughts
    C. Muscular relaxation, adopted by sitting in a relaxed postion
    D. All of the above

5. Applying which relaxation training to patients with PTSD can lead to control over the physiological and motor components of the disorder?

   A. Progressive muscle relaxation
   B. Hypnosis
   C. Biofeedback
   D. All of the above

6. In what way will a patient experience a relaxation response?

   A. Heart rate will increase
   B. Breathing becomes slower and deeper
   C. Blood pressure increases
   D. All of the above

7. What relaxation technique is derived from self-suggestion and suggestions about the reaxing feeling a heaviness of the neuromuscular system, warmth in the abdominal area, a steady strong heart rate, and effortless respiration?

   A. Autogenics
   B. Guided Imagery
   C. Sensory deprivation
   D. Self-hypnosis

8. The practice of transcendental meditation involves which of the following procedures:

   A. The silent repetition of a word or sound known as a mantra
   B. Concentration on the mantra to the exclusion of distracting thoughts
   C. Muscular relaxation, adopted by sitting in a relaxation, adopted by sitting in a relaxed position.
   D. All of the above.

9. Who is responsible for the development of progressive muscle relaxation?

    A. Dr. Edmund Jacobson discovered that a muscle could be relaxed by first tensing it for a few seconds and then releasing it

    B. Jon Kabat-Zinn originally described the relaxation response

    C. Herbert Benson did extensive research on meditation as a method of stress management

    D. Matt Redman documented that with deliberate intention each person can go from stressed to calm in the matter of a few deep breaths

10. What are the most important elements of balance postures?

    A. Starting with a deep, flowing breath

    B. Finding a fixed point on which to focus your gaze

    C. Mimic the realignment of the heart's center with the centering of the mind and body

    D. All of the above

Chapter 28: Relaxation Examination Answers

1. D
2. C
3. C
4. D
5. D
6. B
7. A
8. D
9. A
10. D

Chapter 29

Electroconvulsive Therapy (ECT)

Electroconvulsive therapy is not a trifling or inconsequently procedure to be delegated to a junior resident or casually administered, unassisted, in the office. It is unique among psychiatric treatments: a significant medical intervention requiring general anesthesia and entailing risks, however small, of morbidity and mortality. The psychiatrist administering ECT adopts a role most like that of his medical and surgical colleagues. To perform it well requires an intimate knowledge of the physiology and biochemistry of induced seizures, an understanding of the pharmacology of anesthetic agents, familiarity with the physical properties of the electrical stimulus used, and the confidence and skill to lead a treatment team in the event of a medical emergency.

Dr. Max Fink discusses the development of ECT from its discovery in 1934, its acceptance and widespread use for two decades until it was largely replaced by the introduction of psychotropic drugs in the 1950's, and its revival in the past twenty years as a viable treatment now that undesirable side effects have been largely removed. When ECT was revived in the late 1970's, the principal concern was its effects on cognition and memory.

The electrical stimulus produces a grandma seizure consisting of a brief tonic phase followed by a more prolonged chronic phase. This treatment relieves symptoms more quickly and lastingly than the use of psychotropic drugs. The seizure of ECT is initiated when the quantity (charge) of electrons id driven through the brain with sufficient voltage to generate the energy required to depolarize cell membranes. The seizure threshold is crossed when sufficient neurons have been depolarized to initiate cortical propagation (spatial summation) of an excitatory process that ultimately reaches the brainstem, presumably activating a pacemaker to begin firing rhythmically and repeatedly, and through its projections, ultimately causing the rest of the brain to discharge in unison.

- In clinical trials, safely use caffeine
- For anesthesia, usually use barbiturates
- A tourniquet applied to an extremity

How is the patient prepared for treatment?

- Treatments are usually given in the morning. In the first decades of ECT use, treatment was given in the evening, allowing patients to return home after being sedated by the treatment. In the present practice, personal considerations mandate morning treatments.
- Because some people become nauseated by anesthetic, the patient consumes neither food, nor liquid after midnight, which prevents vomited food from entering the lungs.
- Consent: The essential element of informed consent always includes:

  1. A full explanation of the procedures in laymen's terms;
  2. A presentations of the risk and potential benefits of the treatment offered;
  3. Statements that the patient may withdraw his/her consent at any time and for any reason.

What does the patient experiences in the procedure from preparation to recovery?

Anesthesia and muscle relaxation are usually administered to ensure patient comfort during ECT. These techniques are administered to ensure patient comfort during ECT. It is used primarily for psychiatric inpatients, and it is common for an anesthetist or anesthesiologist in administering the treatment. The APA Task Force on Electroconvulsive Therapy (American Psychiatric Association, 2001) recommended pretreatment with an anticholinergic drug such as atropine to decrease the morbidity of cardiac Brady-arrhythmias and aspiration.

General anesthesia is induced only to the degree that a light comma is produced, using a fast-acting anesthetic such as methohexital, which has fewer cardiac side effects than slower-acting barbiturates such as thiopental. Once the patient is anesthetized, intravenous succinylcholine is used for muscular relaxation. Once the succinylcholine is administered, the patient is administered, the patients is ventilation with 100% oxygen until muscle fasciculation's occur and motoric relaxation of the patient is accomplished. Modern ECT devices allow for simultaneous monitoring of the EEG and ECG before, during, and after the ECT procedures. Patients neither remember nor feel the treatment. In addition, there should be frequent monitoring of blood pressure, pulse rate, and blood oxygen saturation with pulse ox meter.

In the Seizure EEG, we look for four distinct phases: a rapid build-up of spike activity, a prolonged period of spike and slow waves, a period of high-voltage slow waves, and an exact end point at which the electrical energy is momentarily silenced. For anesthesia, usually use barbiturates, and dosage should be adjusted to minimum effective amount because higher dosages will increase the seizure threshold and prolong the apneic period. In clinical trials, safely 6 use caffeine augmented bi-lateral ECT. They found that per-administration of caffeine was associated with a significant increase in seizure duration, but not with any decrease in seizure threshold. A tourniquet applied to an extremity can be used to prevent distribution of muscle relaxant and may allow the seizure to be observed in that extremity. Routine technical information dictate that three electrodes are put in place for the EEG; two stimulating electrodes for the electrical stimulus; four for the ECG and heart rate; and two to measure motor movements during treatment.

In the Recovery Area, the staff documents stabilization of vital signs within margin of pre-ECT parameters and verifies a return of alertness and orientation. After the treatment, the patient may be in a dreamy state, perhaps concerned about not knowing where he is or what is expected of him/her. Occasionally, a patient will vomit when the anesthetic wars off. If a patient has the kind of muscular soreness and stiffness that follows intensive exercise, he may get relief from an analgesic. A backache is a sign that the dose of muscle relaxant was not adequate; it can be adjusted in subsequent treatments.

Post-ictal Care: The goal of the post-ictal phase is primarily that of maintaining an adequate airway until the return of spontaneous respiration and, eventually, alertness. The anesthetic specialist continues forced ventilation until the patient is breathing on his own, at which time he is transferred to a recovery area under the observation of trained staff until awakening. Headache occurs in about one third of all patient after ECT and usually responds to aspirin and if severe, to ibuprofen. Cognitive deficits after ECT include disturbances of orientation, memory, and general cognition. Patients often become confused and may not know where they are when they awaken. This may be frightening, but the confusion disappears within a few hours. Memory for recent events, mainly for the period of illness and the treatments, may be disturbed. Dates, names of friends, public events, telephone numbers, and addresses may be difficult to re-call. In most patients, the memory difficulty is gone within four weeks after the last treatment.

VIGNETTE

A 65 year-old African American woman with a history of recurrent psychotic depression was referred to our service because of poor medication response, serious medication side effects, or very severe symptoms. During her illness, she has cycles of bipolar depression consisting of periods of depressed mood, crying spells, loss of interest in usual activities, insomnia, loss of appetite and weight, difficulty with concentration, feelings of helplessness, and thoughts of suicide. During these episodes, she also has psychotic symptoms such as multiple voices commanding her to take a drug overdose, slit her wrists, and hang herself in the shower. The presence of the psychotic subtype in this patient is a good prognostic indicator for a response to ECT, as is her age. She has had infrequent relapses, which respond well to a brief course (3-4 treatments), and often does not require inpatient hospitalization. ECT is an appropriate strategy given her lack of response to or intolerance of adequate trials of antidepressant medications and neuroleptic agents. In addition, the presence of suicidal ideation with a plan for constitutes first-line treatment for psychotic depression. She received a total of 145 treatments over 7 years. Given the severity of her depression and her history of multiple episodes, her treatment team also recommended combining ECT with an antidepressant medication to prevent a relapse, tapering the ECT rather than abruptly discontinuing it on remission, and adding a mood stabilizer to the antidepressant to prevent a relapse. Maintenance ECT is also reasonable strategy because it is considered to be an effective way of preventing relapses and recurrence in patients with major psychiatric disorders who have shownan initial response to ECT.

Discussion. It is important to remember that ECT for the treatment of an acute depressive episode is usually reserved for those patients who have failed pharmaco-therapy, cannot tolerate medications because of side effects or other comorbid medical problems, and /or who pose immediate danger to self or others and cannot wait for medications to take effect. Maintenance ECT follows and index course of ECT and seeks to prevent relapse of depression. It is especially often featuring depression with psychotic features. All the rapid cyclers (100%) and most patient with delusional depression (80%) attained full or partial remission with maintenance ECT.

We recommend ECT for the patient in the vignette for several reasons. Give the severity of her depression and her history of multiple episodes, we recommend combining ECT with an anti-depressant medication to prevent a relapse, tapering the ECT rather than abruptly discontinuing it on remission, and adding a mood stabilizer to the antidepressant to prevent relapse. Maintenance ECT would be appropriate given her lack of a response to or intolerance of adequate trials of antidepressant medications and neuroleptic agents. In addition the presence of suicidal ideation with a plan for suicide underscores the need for a rapidly acting and definitive treatment. The presence of the psychotic subtype in this patient is a good prognostic indicator for a response to maintenance ECT, as is her age.

Bipolar depression is a complex and heterogeneous disorder that compromises three broad domains of clinical manifestations: (1) disorders of mood: (2) cognitive function; and (3) neurovegetative functions.

Disorders of Mood: Depression may be defined as a syndrome characterized by a dysfunction of affect or behavior involving multiple signs and symptoms. By far the most common symptom of dysphoric mood is a complaint of feeling sad, "blue," or "down in the dumps." They may also express a sense of "not caring anymore," or feeling guilty for mental recollections. Other features are recurrent thoughts of death, suicidal ideation, wishes to be dead, or planned suicide attempts. When delusions occur, they are almost always mood-congruent and reflect the hopelessness of the patient.

Cognitive function: Bipolar depression is often a recurrent illness; therefore, measures must be taken to sustain remission after a successful index course of electroconvulsive therapy. Shortly after index ECT, depressed patients may improve in performing tests of attention, immediate learning, and intelligence. Simultaneously, retention of newly learned information (anterograde amnesia) can be impaired. During ECT cognitive function is thought to be due to electrochemical effects on the medial temporal lobe. These cognitive side effects are seen as a major disadvantage of maintenance ECT. Cognitive function assessed by an analyzing Mini-Mental State Exam (MMSE) scores, a common measure of cognitive function, before and after at least a year of maintenance ECT. One drawback to use of the MMSE as our cognitive assessment tool is that it does not monitor retrograde amnesia, which is the type of memory impairment most troublesome to patients. It typically occurs shortly after ECT and is manifested as gaps in the memory of events that occurred before the treatment, retrograde amnesia may extend back several months or years.

Neurovegetative functions: Treatments effects and side effects of ECT depend on the level of applied energy in relation to the individual patient's seizure threshold. One approach to the ECT dose, called seizure-threshold titration, involves giving progressively higher doses during the initial ECT session until the seizures threshold is reached, and then selecting a dose at various percentages above the seizures threshold during subsequent treatment sessions. The dosage of ECT according to the patient's individual seizures threshold is the "gold standard" in ECT therapy. The threshold is known to increase during a course of frequently repeated ECT treatments and to return to baseline 6 months after cessation of treatment. Wild et. al. found significant changes in seizures duration, as measured by EEG and the cuff technique, when treatments were separated by duration exceeding 60 days. This is compatible with a decrease in seizure threshold or a loss of anticonvulsant action after 2 months and indicates the necessity to retitrate seizures threshold after this time. Ethnicity and seizures threshold is an important variable detailed by Dawkins et.al. In this study the data suggest that Black patient s may have higher seizure threshold than white patients at the time of initial ECT treatments. The clinical implications of these findings are that they were more likely to receive concomitant medication that lower seizure threshold.

These ethnic differences, however, may be confound by cultural and socioeconomic factors, as well as the effects of deviation from standard titration.

FREQUENTLY ASKED QUESTIONS?

Who should get ECT?

- Psychiatric diagnosis for many disorders such as depression, mania, catatonia, and schizophrenia, respond well to ECT. Contradictory there are psychiatric diagnosis for which ECT is considered ineffective: dementia and amnesic disorders, substance-related disorders, anxiety and somatoform disorders, factitious disorders, dissociative disorders, sexual dysfunctions, sleep disorders, impulse disorders, and personality disorders.

- Neurologic illnesses that respond well for ECT: Parkinson's disease, epilepsy, delirium, catatonia, Neuroleptic Malignant Syndrome, depression associated with dementia, and depression associated with stroke.

- Systemic diseases that preclude the use of ECT: the safe treatment of a patient with recent myocardial infarction, cerebrovascular injury, or cerebral vascular malformation requires special attention to the control of blood pressure, heart rate, and oxygenation during ECT.

- Pregnancy: ECT has been used safely in all stages of pregnancy; it does not precipitate miscarriage, nor does it affect the development of the fetus. However, it is required that OB/GYN care be readily available.

- Age: The treatment is safe for patients of all ages, from children to elderly. However, adults older than 60 years make up the age group that may have the best response to ECT. Because the seizure threshold increases and drug metabolism increases with age, high stimulus intensities and low anesthetic dosages are often used in the elderly.

- Gender. Sex is a strong predictor of seizure threshold. In study's using constant-current, brief pulse stimulation, male subjects had a much higher seizure threshold than female subjects, requiring an electrical dose that was approximately 70% higher (as measured in charge) to elicit seizures (Sackeim et al. 1987).

How frequent are treatments given?

- It is difficult to predict the number of treatments required after the initial course of ECT, but it is rarely fewer than six. To be of benefit, seizures must be repeated two or three times a week for many weeks. There is no lifetime maximum number of treatments A typical schedule for maintenance ECT provides a treatment 1 week after the initial course is successfully completed, a second in 2 weeks, a third in 3 weeks, and a fourth and subsequent treatments at monthly intervals for up to 6 months. Some patients may not remain well on monthly interval maintenance ECT and will require treatments a t 3 week intervals Usually, the depressed need between three and nine treatments after the successful initial course. Some patients may need years of weekly treatments.

Why is treatment stimulated by induction of a seizure?

- The purpose of the electrical stimulus is to induce a brain seizure. The generalized brain seizure is the central therapeutic event.
- In ECT, the currents from the stimulating electrodes on each temple pass maximally through the central parts of the brain.
- Similar systemic and mental effects have been associated with deficiencies or excesses of the hormones produced by the pituitary, hypo-thalamus, adrenal, parathyroid, testes, and ovary glands.
- For example, each seizure stimulates the hypothalamus to discharge its hormones. Then those in turn stimulate

the pituitary gland to discharge its products which then inhibit the discharge of cortical from the adrenal gland.

- When it was introduced, electro-shock was given without anesthetic, and patients approached each treatment with anxiety, dread, and panic. Some patients sustain fractures; and some died.
- Today, anesthesia, muscle relaxation, and hyper-oxygenation are answers to these problems.

For which behaviors is ECT ineffective:

- Severe character pathology
- Substance abuse and dependence (including alcoholism)
- Sexual identification disorders
- Psychoneuroses (hysterical disorders, Briquet's syndrome, hypochondriasis, panic or anxiety disorders, pain syndromes, obsessive-compulsive disorders)
- Chronicity of illness without flagrant psychopathology
- Recent myocardial infarction (heart attack), cerebrovascular malformation

Chapter 29: Electroconvulsive Therapy
Examination Review

1. What agent is recommended for pretreatment to decrease the morbidity of cardiac brady arrhythmias and aspiration?

    A. Atropine
    B. Methohexital
    C. Thiopental
    D. Succinylcholine

2. What does a backache signal during recovery after ECT treatment?

    A. A light coma is produced during the treatment.
    B. The patient should be ventilated with 50% oxygen
    C. The dose of muscle relaxant was not adequate
    D. The patient was too old to express the stress of induced convulsions

3. When ECT was revived in the late 1970's, what was its principal concern?

    A. Muscular soreness and stiffness
    B. Effects on cognition and memory
    C. A dreamy state about not knowing where he/she is
    D. Profuse vomiting when the anesthetic wears off

4. What makes sex a strong predictor of seizure threshold?

    A. Male subjects had a much higher seizure threshold than female subjects
    B. Male subjects required an electrical dose that was approximately 20% lower to elicit seizures
    C. Use of caffeine in women to increase seizure threshold and shorten the apneic period
    D. As women patient's age, the seizure threshold decreases in a roughly linear correlation.

5. What disorders respond well to ECT?

   A. Dementia
   B. Substance-related Disorders
   C. Personality Disorders
   D. Schizophrenia

6. How does age older than 60 years affect ECT response?

   A. Seizure threshold decreases with age
   B. Drug metabolism decreases with age
   C. Higher stimulus intensities are required with age
   D. Higher anesthetic dosages are required with age

7. What clinical variants of melancholia are exquisitely responsive to ECT?

   A. Catatonic stupor
   B. Mood disorders (only in late stages of pregnancy)
   C. Mental Retardation in an adolescent
   D. Situational maladjustment

8. Before administering anesthesia for ECT, what pretreatment examinations should be performed?

   A. Patients are encouraged to eat a hearty breakfast before ECT.
   B. A dental examination in the elderly
   C. Avoid extra weakness or dizziness, insulin administration should be increased before the treatment.
   D. Spine and Chest X-Rays are routinely done before each treatment

9. How do we judge whether a particular treatment will have the desired effect?

   A. Continuation in the symptoms of mood states
   B. Changes in the EEG recorded during the treatment
   C. A decrease in the serum level of prolactin during the seizure
   D. Continuation in suicidal or homicidal preoccupations

10. How does monitoring a seizure cause profound changes in mental physiology?

    A. Treatments applied to repetitive magnetic pulses to the head without inducing a seizure are equal to ECT

    B. Longer seizure duration (over the 20-second minimum) indicates greater therapeutic impact

    C. Currents from the stimulating electrodes on each temple pass through the central parts of the brain, stimulating the hypothalamus to discharge hormones that elicit a grand-mal seizure

    D. Low-energy electric currents delivered from a battery with electrodes on the scalp were of equal benefit

Chapter 29: Electroconvulsive Therapy
Examination Answers

1. A
2. C
3. B
4. A
5. D
6. C
7. A
8. B
9. B
10. C

Reference Section 6

Abrams R. Electroconvulsive Therapy, 4th Edition. Oxford University Press, 2002.

Abrams R. Electroconvulsive Therapy, 2nd Edition. New York: Oxford University Press, 1992.

Abrams RC. Electroconvulsive Therapy. New York, Oxford University Press, 1988.

Agronin, ME, and Maletta, GJ. Principles and Practice of Geriatric Psychiatry, Lippincott: Williams + Wilkins, 2006.

Aldrich L and Variyam, JN. Acculturation Erodes the Diet Quality of U.S. Hispanics. Food Review. 23: 51- 55, 2000.

American Psychiatriv Association: The Practice of Elecctronconvulsive Therapy: Recommendations for Treatment, Training, and Privileging. A Task Force Report of the American Psychiatric Association, 2nd Edition. Edited by Weiner RD. Washington, DC. American Psychiatric Association, 2001.

American Psychiatric Association. Diagnostic and Statistical Manual of Mental Disrders. 4th Edition, text revised. Washington, DC: American Psychiatric Association, 2000.

Andreasen, NC and Black, DW. Introductory Textbook of Psychiatry. American Psychiatric Publishing, Inc., 2006.

Ashburn MA, Rice L J. The Management of PAIN. Churchill Livingstone, 1998.

Avery D, Lubrano A. Depressions treated with imipramine and ECT: the DeCarolis Study Reconsidered. American Journal of Psychiatry. 136: 559-569,1979.

Barlow D. Clinical Handbook of Psychological Disorders. New York: The Guilford Press, 1993.

Basch MF. Doing Psychotherapy. Basic Books, Inc. 1980.

Beck AT. and Emery G. Anxiety Disorders and Phobias: A Cognitive Perspective. Basic Books: A member of the Perseus Books Group, 1985.

Beck JS. Cognitive Therapy: Basics and Beyond. The Guilford Press: NY, 1995.

Bellak L. Brief Psychoanalytic Psychotherapy of nonpsychotic depression. American Journal of Psychotherapy. 35: 160-172. 1981.

Bellak L. Once Over: What is Psychotherapy? Journal of Nervous Mental Disorders: 165. 1977.

Benson, H. Beyond the Relaxation Response. New York: Berkley Books, 1985

Benson, H. The Relaxation Response. New York: Morrow, 1975.

Benton D and Parker PY. Breakfast blood glucose and cognition. American Journal of Clinical Nutrition,. 67: 7725-7785. 1998.

Bernard HS. MacKenzie KR. Basics of Group Psychotherapy. The Guilford Press: New York, 1994.

Bernstein, JG. Handbook of Drug Therapy in Psychiatry. Mosby Year Book, 1995.

Blackwell B, Merskey H, Kellner R. Treatments of Psychiatric Disorders, Vol. 3. Washington, DC. American Psychiatric Association, 1989.

Blumer D and Heilbronn D. Chronic pain as a variant of depressive disease. The pain –prone disorder. Journal of Nervous and Mental Disease: 170, 381-406. 1982.

Blanchard EB, Andrasik F, Ahles TA, et al. Migraine and Tension Headache: A meta-analytic review. Behavior Therapy, 11: 613-631. 1980.

Bickel H. Digestion and Absorption of Nutrients. Ft Lee: New Jersey. J.K. Burgess, 1983.

Binswanger L. Sigmund Freud: Reminiscenes of a Friendship. New York: Grune and Stratton, 1957.

Birch BB. Power Yoga: the total strength and flexibility workout. A Fireside Book: Simon & Schuster, 1995.

Bonica JJ, ed: Definitions in Taxonomy of Pain. In The Management of Pain. Philadelphia; Lea and Febiger, 1990.

Bordenkircher S. Yoga for Christians: A Christ- Centered Approach to Physical and Spiritual Helath. W Publishing Group, 2006.

Bourne EJ. The Anxiety and Phobia Workbook. 5th Edition. New Harbinger Publication, Inc. 2010.

Bowden CL. Anticonvulsants in bipolar disorder: Current research and practice and future directions. Bipolar Disorders, 11 (Suppl.2), 20-33, 2009.

Cancro R. Individual Psychotherapy in the Treatment of Chronic Schizophrenic Patients. American Journal of Psychotherapy. 37: 493-501. 1983.

Carrington, P. Freedom in Meditation. New York: Anchor Press/Doubleday, 1977.

Coffey CE. The Clinical Science of Electroconvulsive Therapy. Progress in Psychiatry, Number 38, 1993.

Committee on Military Nutrition Research, Food and Nutrition Board, Institute of Medicine. Caffeine for the Sustainment of Mental Task Performance: Formulations for Military Operations. Washington, DC. National Academics Press, 2001.

Copeland ME. Wellness Recovery Action Plan (WRAP). Peach Press, 2001.

Coery G. Theory and Practice of Counseling and Psychotherapy 4th Edition. Monterey: CA. Brooks Cole, 1990.

Crow TJ, Johnstone EC. Controlled trials of Electroconvulsive Therapy. Annual New York Acadamey of Science. 462: 12-29,1986.

Dawkins K, Ekstrom RD, Hill MA, et al. Ethnicity and Seizure Threshold, Programs. Neuro-Psychopharmacology and Biology of Psychiatry, 24: 1289-1298, 2000.

Denicoff KD, Smith-Jackson EE, Disney ER, et al. Comparative prophylactic efficacy of lithium, carbamazepine, and the combination in bipolar disorder. Journal of Clinical Psychiatry. 58, 470-478. 1997.

Dubovsky SL. Using Electroconvulsive Therapy, in Comprehensive Textbook of Psychiatry/ VI, 6th Edition, Vol.2 Wiliams+Wilkins, 1995.

Dubovsky SL. Electrconvulsive therapy for patients with neurological disease. Hospital Community Psychiatry. 37: 819-825, 1986.

Dudek S. Nutrition Handbook for Nursing Practice. Lippincott-Raven Publishers, 1997.

Durkin HE. The Group in Depth. New York: International Univerisities Press, 1964.

Edwards T. Living in the Presence. San Francisco: Harper, 1987.

Ehrenwald J. The History of Psychotherapy: from Healing Magic to Encounter. Jason Aronson, Inc., 1976.

Embry CK. Psychothrapeutic Interventions in Chronic Post-Traumatic Stress Disorder, in Post-Traumatic stress: Etiology, Phenomenology, and Treatment. American Psychiatric Press, Washington, DC, 1990.

Endler NS. The Origins of Electroconvulsive Therapy (ECT). Convulsive Therapy. 4: 5-23. 1988.

Ends E. J. and Page C.W. A Study of Three Types of Group Psychotherapy with Hospitalized male Inebriates. Q. J. Study of Alcohol 18, 1957.

Escott-Stump S., Nutrition and Diagnosis- Related Care. Lippincott. Williams+ Wilkins, 2002.

Ferrel BA, Stein WM, Beck JC. The Geriactric Pain Measure: validity, reliability and factor analysis. Journal American Geriatric Society; 48: 1669- 1673. 2000.

Fields HL. Depression and Pain: A Neurobiological-model. Neuropsychiatric, Neuropsychology, Behavior Neurology. 4: 83, 1991.

Fields HL, ed: Pain Syndromes in Neurology. London: Butterworth, 1990.

Fink M. Electroconvulsive Therapy: A Guide for Professional and Their Patients. Oxford University Press, 2009.

Fink M. ECT for Parkinson's Disease? (editorial). Convulsive Therapy. 189-191. 1988.

Fink M. Electroshock: Restoring the Mind. Oxford University Press, 1999.

Foster R. Meditative Prayer. Madison: Wisconsin. Inter Varsity, 1983.

Foulkes S.H. Group-analytic dynamics with specific reference to psycho-analytic concepts. International Journal of Group Psychotherapy. 7: 40-53, 1975.

Foulkes S.H. Introduction to Group analytic psychotherapy. London: Heineman, 1948.

Frances A, Clarkin J, Perry S. Diffential Therapeutics in Psychiatry: The Art and Science of Treatment Selection. New York. Brunner/ Mazel, 1984.

Freud S, Group Psychology and the analysis of the ego. In Journal Strachey (Eds and Trans). The Standard edition of the complete psychological works of Sigmund Freud. (Vol 18), pp 67-143. London: Hoagarth Press, 1955.

Garfield S. Psychotherapy: An Eclectic Approach. New York: Wiley- Interscience, 1980.

Geddes JR, Calabrese JR, and Goodwin GM. Lamotrigine for treatment of bipolar depression: Indepenent meta-analysis and meta-regression of individual patient data from five randomized trials. British Journal of Psychiatry, 94(1), 4-9. 2009.

Geddes JR. Efficacy and Safety of Electroconvulsive Therapy in Depressive Disorders: A systematic review and meta-analysis. The Lancet, 361; 799- 808, 2003.

Giger JN. and Davidhizar RE. Tanscultural Nursing: Assessment and Intervention 4th Edition St. Louis: C.V. Mosby, 2004.

Glasser W. and Wubbolding RE. Reality Therapy. In RJ Corsini and D. Wedding (Eds), Current Psychotherapies 5th Edition. Itasca IL: F.E. Peacock Publishers, 1995.

Goldberg JF and Hoop J. Bipolar depression: Longterm Challenges for the clinician. Medscape Psychiatry, 2004.

Goldstein J. Insight Meditation. Boston: Shambhala, 1993.

Greenblatt DJ, Hamatz JS, Shapiro L. Sensitivity to triazolam in the elderly. New England Journal of Medicine, 324: 1691-1698, 1991.

Greene RA and Feldon L. Dr. Robert Greens's Perfect Balance. New York: Three Rivers Press, 2005.

Haas E.M. Staying Healthy with Nutrition. Twenty-first century edition. Berkely, CA: Celestial Arts, 2006.

Hales RE. and Yudofsky, S. Essentials of Clinical Psychiatry. American Psychiatric Publishing, Inc. 2004.

Hardy JD, Wolff HG, and Goodell H. Pain Sensations and Reactions. Hafner Publishing, New York. Reprint of edition by Williams and Wilkins Co. 1967.

Heide FJ. And Borkovec TD. Relaxation- Induced Anxiety: Paradoxical Anxiety Enhancement Due to Relaxation Training. Journal of Consulting and Clinical Psychology, 51: 171-182, 1983.

Heimburger D and Ard J. Handbook of Clinical Nutrition. Mosby, 2006.

Horowitz MJ. Post-traumatic Stress Disorder, in Treatments of Psychiatric Disorders, Vol. 3. Washington DC. American Psychiatric Association, 1989.

Horowitz MJ. Stress Response Syndromes, 2nd Edition. New York. Jason Aronson, 1986.

Ishihara K and Sasa M. Mechanism Underlying the Therapeutic Effects of Electroconvulsive Therapy (ECT) on Depression. Japanese Journal of Pharmacology, 80 (3); 185-189, 1999.

Jacobson, Edmund. Progressive Relaxation. Midway Reprint. Chicago: The University of Chicago Press, 1974.

Jacobson E. Modern Treatment of Tense Patients. Springfield. Illinois. Charles C. Thomas, 1970.

Jamison DR. Psycho therapeutic Issues and Suicide Prevention in the Treatment of Bipolar Disorders, in American Psychiartic Association Annual Review, Vol. 6. Washingtom, DC. American Psychiatric Press, 1987.

Jenike M. Handbook of Geriatric Psychopharmocology. Littleton, MA PSG Publishing, 1985.

Jones SL and Butman RE. Modern Psychotherapies: A Comprehensive Christian Appraisal, IVP Academic 1991.

Joranson DE and Lietman R. The McNeil National Pain Study. New York: Louis. Harris and Associates, 1994.

Jorissen, BL. Riedel, WJ. Nutrients, Age, and Cognition. Clinical Nutrition; 21, 89-95. 2002.

Kabat-Zinn J. Wherever You Go, There You Are (a good introduction to meditation and mindfulness practice). Tenth Anniversary edition. New York: Hyperion, 2005.

Kaplan H. and Sadock B. Synopsis of Psychiatry, 8th Edition. New York: Lippincott, Williams and Wilkins, 1997.

Karasu TB, Gelenberg A and Merriam A. Practice guideline for the treatment of patients with major depressive disorder. In the American Psychiatric Association Practice Guidelines for the Treatment of Psychiatric Disorders, compendium. Washington, DC: American Psychiatric Association, 2006.

Karasu TB. Psychotherapy for Depression, Jason Aronson, Inc. 1990.

Karasu TB and Bellak L. Specialized Techniques in Individual Psychotherapy. Brunner/ Mael. New York, 1980.

Keck PE., McElroy SL, Strakowski SM, Bourne ML, West SA. Compliance with maintenance treatment in bipolar disorder. Psychopharmacology Bulletin. 33: 87-91. 1997.

Kellner CH. Anti-ECT legislation in Texas. Convulsive Therapy. 11 11: 148. 1995.

Kendell, RE and Zealley AK. Companion to Psychiatric Studies, 3rd Edition. Churchill Livingstone, 1983.

Kendler BS. The Best Kept Secret to Healthy Aging. Purity Research Department, 2006.

Lai TS, Chan DM, Lai SW. "Folie a' deux in the aged: A case report." Clinical Gerontologist 22: 113-117. 2001.

Lasagna L. Clinical measurement of pain. Annals of the New York Academy of Sciences. 86, 28-37. 1960.

Lewis L. A consumer perspective concerning the diagnosis and treatment of bipolar disorder. Biological Psychiatry, 48: 442-444, 2000.

Lieberman HR, Kanarek RB, and Prasad C. Nutritional Neuroscience. Taylor & Francis Group, 2005.

Lichstein K. Clinical Relaxation Strategies. New York: Wiley, 1988.

Lipitt R + White RK. An experimental study of leadership and group life. Readings in social psychology 3rd Edition. New York: Holt, Rinehart + Winston, 1958.

Longmire DR. Tutorial: The Medical Pain History. Pain Digest. 1: 29-33. 1992.

Loo C, Mitchell P, Sachdev P et al. Double-blind controlled Investigation of transcranial magnetic stimulation for the treatment of resistant major depression. American Journal of Psychiatry, 156: 946-8, 1999.

Lutz CA. and Przytulski KR. Nutrition and Diet Therapy 4th Edition. Philadelphia: F.A. Davis, 2006.

Malhi GS, Adams D and Berk M. Medicating mood with maintenance in mind: Bipolar depression pharmacotherapy. Bipolar Disorders, 11 (Supple 2), 55-76, 2009.

Manji HK, Quiroz JA, Payne JL, et al. The underlying neurobiology of bipolar disorder. World Psychiatry, (3); 136-146, 2003.

May P, Simpson GM. Schizophrenia: Overview of Treatment Methods, in Comprehensive Textbook of Psychiatry, 3rd Edition, Vol. 2. Baltimore, MD. Williams and Wilkins, 1980.

Marcus DA. Chronic Pain: A Primary Care Guide to Practical Mangement, Humana Press, 2005.

Marangell LB, Silver JM, Goff DC, and Yudofsky SC. Psychopharmacology and Electroconvulsive Therapy 4th Edition. Washington, DC: American Psychiatric Publishing, 2003.

Mason PHC. Recovering from the War: A Woman's Guide to Helping Your Vietnam Vet, Your Family, and Yourself. Penguin Books, 1990.

McGlashan TH. Schizophrenia: Psychosocial Treatments and the Role of Psychosocial Factors in its Etiology and Pathogenesis, in Amercian Psychiatric Association Annual Review. Vol. 5. Washington, DC. American Psychiatric Press, 1986.

Mc Mahon SB and Koltzenburg M. 5th Edition of Wall and Melzack's Textbook of Pain. Elsevier, Churchill Livingstone, 2006.

Melzack R and Wall PD. The Challenge of Pain. New York: Basic Books, 1983.

Mersky H and Bogduku P, eds: Classification of Chronic Pain, 2nd Edition: Seattle, IASP Press, 1994.

Millan MJ. The induction of pain: an integrative review. In Progress in Neurobiology, Vol. 57 pp 1-164. Elsevier, Amsterdam, 1999.

Nicholi Am. Jr. The Harvard Guide to Psychiatry. The Belknap Press of Harvard University Press, 3rd Edition. Cambridge: Massachussetts, 1999.

Ortberg J. The Life You've Always Wanted. Grand Rapids: Zondervan, 2002.

Patel C. Biofeedback-aided relaxation and meditation in the management of hypertension. Biofeedback and Self-Regulation, 2: 1-41. 1977.

Pies, R.W. Clinical Manual of Psychiatric Diagnosis and Treatment: A Biopsychosocial Approach. American Psychiatric Press, Inc. 2005.

Pies RW. The organic disorders. Hospital Community Psychiatry 42: 199. 1991.

Poplos D. All About ECT. Retrieved Feb 10, 2005 from http: www. Schizophrenia.com/ family/ectl.html.

Powdermaker FB. And Frank JD. Group Psychotherapy: Studies in Methodology of Research and Therapy. Cambridge: Harvard university Press, 1953.

Raj PP. Pain Relief: Fact or Fancy? Regional Anesthesia. 15: 157-169, 1990.

Rammurthy S, Rogers JN, Alanmanou E. Decision Making in Pain Mangement. 2nd Edition. Mosby, Elsevier. 2006.

Reid WH, Keller S, Leatherman M, et al. ECT in Texas: 19 months of Mandatory Reporting. Journal of Clinical Psychiatry 59: 8-13. 1998.

Romero- Gwynn, E; Gwynn DL, Grivetti R, et al. Dietary Acculturation among Latinos of Mexican Descent. Nutrition Today (July/ August): 6-11, 1993.

Rosen R. Inhale, Exhale, Relax. In Yoga Journal Balanced Living. Winter 2004.

Roth N. An Invitation to Christian Yoga. Boston: Cowley, 1989.

Roy R and Tunks E. Chronic Pain: Psychosocial Factors in Rehabilitation. Baltimore, Williams + Wilkins. 1982.

Rummans TA. Medical Indications for Electroconvulsive Therapy. Psychiatric Annals 23: 27-32. 1993.

Rupke SJ, Blecke D, and Renfrow M. Cognitive therapy for depression. American Family Physician, 73(1): 83-86, 2006.

Rush AJ, Beck AT, Kovacs M, et al. Comparative Efficacy of Cognitive Therapy and Imipramine in the Treatment of Depressed Outpatients. Cognitive Therapy and Research. 1: 17-37. 1977.

Sachs G. Barriers to Concordance. Paper presented at the Bipolar Disorder Though Leader Summit, Boston. MA. 2000.

Sackeim HA, Decina P, Prohovnik I, et al. Seizure threshold in electroconvulsive therapy: effects of sex, age, electrode placement, and number of treatments. Archive of General Psychiatry 44: 355-360, 1987.

Sadock BJ and Sadock VA. Synopsis of Psychiatry: Behavioral Sciences/ Clinical Psychiatry 9th Edition. Philadelphia: Lippincott Williams and Wilkins, 2003.

Sampson EE + Marthas M. Group process for the health professions 3rd Edition. Albany: NY. Delmar Publishers, 1990.

Scandrett S. and Uecker S. Relaxation Training. In G. Bulechek an J. Mc Clowskey, Nursing Interventions, Philadelphia: W. B. Saunders, 1985.

Sifneos PE. Short-Term Dynamic Psychotherapy: Evaluation and Technique, Plenum Medical Book Co: New York, 1979.

Silveira IM, and Seeman MV. Shared Psychotic disorder: a critical review of the literature. Canadian Journal of Psychiatry 40: 389-395, 1995.

Slavson SR. A Textbook in Analytic Group Psychotherapy. New York: International Universities Press, 1964.

Smith ML, Glass GV, and Miller TI. The Benefits of Psychotherapy. Baltimore, MD: Johns Hopkins University Press, 1980.

Spar JE, LaRue A. Concise Guide to Geriatric Psychiatry. Washington, DC.: American Psychiatric Press, 1990.

Spotnitz H. Psychotherapy of Preoedipal Conditions: Schizophrenia and Severe Character Disorders. Jason Aronson, Inc. 1995.

Steinberg L. Yoga. In MA Bright (Ed). Holistic Health and Healing. Philadelphia: F.A. Davis, 2002.

Stewart WF, Lipton RB, Ceentano DD, et al. Prevalence of Migraine Headache in the United States. JAMA 267: 64-69. 1992.

Storey P. Psychological Medicine: An introduction to Psychiatry. Churchill Livingstone, 1986.

Taub EA. Managing Your Stress in Today World. Researchers Digest, 2009.

Thase M.E. Pharmacotherapy of bipolar depression: an update. Current Psychiatry Reports: 8(6), 478- 488. 2006.

Thorn B.E. Cognitive Therapy for Chronic Pain: A Step-by-Step Guide. New York: The Guilford Press, 2004.

Tierra M. The Way of Herbs. New York: Pocket Books, 1998.

Townsend RE, House JF and Addario DA. A Comparison of Biofeedback- Mediated Relaxation and group therapy in the treatment of chronic anxiety. American Journal of Psychiatry, 132: 598-601, 1975.

Trivieri L and Anderson J.W. Alternative Medicine: The Definitive Guide. Berkeley, CA: Celestial Arts, 2002.

Turk DC and Melzack R. Handbook of Pain Assessment 2nd Edition. The Guilford Press: New York, 2001.

Umphred D.A. Neurological Rehabilitation 5th Edition, Mosby Elsevier, 2007.

U.S. Department of Agriculture. Food, Nutrition, and Consumer Services, 2004.

Wahlund B and von Rosen D. ECT of Major Depressed Patients in Relation to Biological and Clinical Variables: A Brief Overview. Neuropsychopharmacology; 28:521-526,2003.

Willis WD and Coggeshall RE. Sensory Mechanisms of the spinal cord, 3rd Edition. Kluwer: New York, 2003.

Willis WD, and Westund KN. Neuroanatomy of the pain system and of the pathways that modulate pain. Journal of Clinical Neurophysiology. 14: 2-31, 1997.

Willis WD. The Pain System. The Neural Basis of Nociceptive Transmission in the Mammalian Nervous System. Pain and Headache, Vol. 8. (P.L. Gildenberge, ed). Karger, Basal. 1985.

Wu CH, Lu FH, Chang CS, et al. Relationship among habitual tea consumption, percent body fat, and body fat distribution. Obesity Research 11: 1088-1095. 2003.

Yudofsky SC. Electroconvulsive Therapy in General Hospital Psychiatry: a focus on new indications and technologies. General Hospital Psychiatry 3(4): 292-6. 1981.

Zahourek R. Relaxation and Imagery: Tools for Therapeutic Communication and Intervention. Philadelphia: W.B. Saunders, 1988.

Section 7

Emergency Psychiatry

> *Suicide is a particularly awful way to die: the mental suffering leading up to it is usually prolonged, intense, and unpallated. Madness, or psychosis, represents only one end of the manic depressive continuum. Suicide is the anchor point on a continuum of suicidal thoughts and behaviors. A possible link between madness and genius is one of the oldest and most perisistent of cultural notions. History has reflected in its laws and attitudes at least a measure of the complexity of suicide. During the Renaissance there was a renewed interest in the relationship between genius, melancholia, and madness. An act against the self, suicide is also a violent force in the lives of others.*
>
> *Kay Redfield Jamison*
> *Night Falls Fast:*
> *Understanding Suicide*

Crisis is identified as a sudden event in one's life that disturbs homeostasis, during which usual coping mechanisms cannot resolve the problem. The primary goal of an emergency psychiatric evaluation is the timely assessment of the patient in crisis What constitutes a psychiatric emergency is highly subjective. By definition, suicidal and homicidal patients are dangerous to themselves and to others.

Agitation is a state of increased mental excitement and motor activity. It may occur in a wide range of mental disorders. It can be an emergency because agitation often precedes violence. A group of psychiatric emergencies present with a variety of signs and symptoms, which include confusion, disorientation, hallucinations, and delusions and which are caused by organic mental disorders. The psychiatric conditions most commonly associated with violence include such psychotic disorders as schizophrenia and mania (particularly if the patient is paranoid or is experiencing command hallucinations). These hallucinations are auditory or visual; often they are unpleasant buzzing sounds. The patient may also have delusions and paranoid ideas of reference. Withdrawal form alcohol and sedative- hypnotics, catatonic excitement, agitated depression, personality disorders characterized by rage and poor impulse control (For example, antisocial, borderline, and paranoid personality disorders).

Chapter 30

Suicidal Thoughts and Feelings

Suicide is intentional self-inflicted death. That is why suicidal ideation and attempted suicide are among the most common emergency presentations. Pokorny (1964) investigated the suicide rate among former patients in a psychiatric service of a Texas Veterans' hospital over a 15 year period. Common themes in suicide include a crisis that causes intense suffering and feelings of hopelessness and helplessness, conflicts between survival and unbearable stress, a narrowing of the patient's perceived options, and the wish to escape. Clinicians should be alert to behaviors that suggest suicidal intent: preparing a will, giving away possessions, or purchasing a burial plot.

Suicide Statistics. Suicide is the eight most frequent cause of death for adults and the second leading cause of death for person's between ages 15 and 24. Nearly 30,000 suicides occur each year in the United States about one every 18 minutes. Nearly three times as many men take their lives as women, and whites are more likely than blacks to kill themselves.

Research has shown that more than 90% of suicide completers had a major psychiatric illness and that half were clinically depressed at the time of the act. Nearly one-third of suicides occur in persons with chronic alcoholism; schizophrenia, anxiety disorders, and other psychiatric disorders are less common among suicide completers.

Kinds of Suicide

To understand suicide in general, it helps to know what the several kinds of suicide are. The following definitions should help (Victoroff, 1983):

Intentional suicide: An act or pattern of self-destructive behavior of high lethality, deliberately planned by the subject to result in his death.

Subintentional suicide: An act or pattern of self-destructive behavior or of low or uncertain subject as likely to result in his death.

Unintentional suicide: An act of pattern of self-destructive behavior of variable levels of lethality, not consciously expected by the subject to result in his death.

Parasuicide: An act designed by the subject to stimulate suicide but characterized by low expectation of lethal outcome.

Euthanasia: An act that results in the death of a person by at least one other person; the motive is declared to be more merciful and the means are a painless as possible. Euthananasia may be brought about by the direct request of the patient who consciously directs others to consummate his death.

Chronic suicide: Instances of self-destructive behavior carried over an extended period, resulting in deterioration of health and/or decompensation of mental stability, and eventually ending in death.

Suicide attempters: Person who at any time have made an intentional or sub-intentional suicide attempt.

Suicide Contemplators: Those persons who manifest suicide ideation.

Suicide Ideation: Thoughts, contemplations, reveries, fantasies, and obsessions in which a person invents themes and stories with his suicidal death as an essential element.

Psychosomatic Suicide: Sever ulcerative colitis, bronchial asthma, massive urticarial, hypertension, and anorexia nervosa are some of the diseases that under certain circumstances may be unconscious means of suicide.

Dyadic suicide: The event of murder followed by suicide. Sometimes the mental disturbance contaminates an entire family, which is at risk for one of its members to institute a massacre.

Paradoxical suicidal behavior: Suicidal acts, frequently seen in children, manifest the continual and probably unconscious wish for maternal protection and help and may eventually become the cry for help of a suicidal act.

BOX-30-1: Suicide Risk Factors

An excellent mnemonic for the major factors for suicide risk factors is SAD PERSONS, devised by Patterson et al (1983).

Sex: Women are more likely to attempt suicide; men are more likely to succeed.

Age: Age falls into bimodal distribution, with teenagers and the elderly at highest risk.

Depression: Fifteen percent of depressive patients die by suicide.

Previous attempt: Ten percent of those who have previously attempted suicide die by suicide.

Ethanol abuse: Fifteen percent of alcoholics commit suicide.

Rational thinking loss: Psychosis is risk factor, an 10% of patients with chronic schizophrenia die by suicide.

Social supports are lacking.

Organized plan: A well-formulated suicide plan is a red flag.

No Spouse: Being divorced, separated, or widowed is a risk factor; having responsibility for children is an important statistical protector against suicide

Sickness: Chronic illness is a risk factor.

When a person has been thinking about ending his own life or has made an attempt to do so, the physician must learn details about these thoughts. These details are important to determine if the patient is at serious risk of harming himself or whether it is safe to allow him to be released (BOX 30-2).

BOX 30-2. Risks of Harming Self when Interviewing a Suicidal Patient:

- Presence of a suicide plan?
- Access to means?
- How lethal are means?
- Real desire to die?
- Frequently / Intensity of suicidal thoughts?
- Intrusiveness of thoughts?
- Command hallucinations?
- Anything to live for?
- Patient's likelihood of acting on suicidal impulses.
- Any decrease in preoccupation with suicidal after supportive interview?
- Social support system intact?
- Demographic profile.

Suicide in Mental Illness. The most common and most important suicidal symptoms relate to depression. The patient who us both agitated and depressed is particularly at high risk. Because the patient often has a number of physical manifestations that are part of the depression, the psychiatrist explores problems with sleep, appetite, bowel habits, sexual functioning, and pain syndromes. To assess this, the psychiatrist inquires, "What is it that has kept you from carrying out your plans?" That is why suicide is intentional self-inflicted death.

Alcoholics and all other substance abusers tend to be high suicidal risks. Nearly 40% of suicide completers have alcohol in their blood-stream at the time of death, suggesting that alcohol may have disinhibited them sufficiently to give them the courage to complete the act.

Potential for suicide is a major concern among patients with schizophrenia. Radomsky and associates (1999) report that suicide is the primary cause of premature death among individuals with the disorder. They estimate that approximately 10 percent of patients with schizophrenia die by suicide. Despite seeming to be euphoric, schizoaffective disorder patients are often suicidal.

Suicidal symptoms may also occur with psychotic states. The patient may have delusions, hallucinations, distorted sensory, impressions, loss of contact with reality, disorientation, or highly unusual ideas and experience. As a baseline for assessing psychotic behavior, the therapist should use his own sense of what is real and appropriate. For example, a person in the midst of a manic episode may believe that he or she has superhuman powers or is indestructible.

Patients with personality disorders benefit mostly form empathic confrontation and assistance with resuming a rational, responsible approach to the problem that precipitated the crisis and to which they have usually contributed.

Suicide prevention involves decreasing access to the means committing suicide and increasing access to support systems (doctors, therapists, family members, and friends). If the veteran feels suicidal, the patient should always inform members of the support systems and other significant people in the core circle. Some people feel that their suicidal despair is always in the background even when they distract themselves from it. Suicide prevention can include learning to tolerate feelings of despair when no one can make them go away. What follows are some "improving the moment" strategies for tolerating personal distress (Linehan+Dexter-Mazza, 2007).

Table 30-1: Suicide Prevention Plan

Suicide Prevention Plan

List your typical early warning signs of a depressive episode.

_____

_____

Circle the things you can do if one or more of these early warning symptoms appear, or if you have suicidal thoughts or impulses.

- Get rid of all dangerous weapons.
- Call your psychiatrist and psychotherapist to ask for an emergency appointment.
- Implement your behavioral activation plan by scheduling rewarding or distracting activities.
- Challenge negative thoughts through cognitive restructuring.
- Ask your core circle of friends and family members for support; agree not to hurt yourself if they haven't had a chance to get back to you.
- Practice meditation or relaxation techniques.
- Exercise.
- Rely on input form religious and spiritual sources.
- Review your Reasons for Living Inventory.

Circle the things your doctor and therapist can do.

- See you on an emergency basis.
- Modify your medication regimen.
- Arrange a hospitalization (if necessary).
- Help you understand where your suicidal thoughts are coming from and what effects they are having on you or others.
- Work with you on behavioral strategies for handling your painful thoughts and emo tions.

Circle those things that members of your core circle can do.

- Listen to you, validate your feelings, and offer suggestions.
- Avoid being critical or judgmental.
- Distract you through mutually enjoyable activities.
- Help you take care of responsibilities that have become burdensome or difficult to perform (for example, child care).
- Stay with you until you feel safe.
- Call your doctor to help you arrange an appointment.
- Take you to the hospital (if necessary).
- Agree to store your weapons or pills away from you.

List members of your core circle and put numbers after each indicating which of items 1-8 they are willing to perform (list more than one item, if appropriate).

_____   _____
_____   _____
_____   _____

List your doctors' names and phone numbers.

_____   _____
_____   _____
_____   _____
_____

Familiarize yourself with the warning Signs of Suicide
Call the National Suicide
Prevention toll-free
Hot-line Number 1-800-273-TALK (8255)
Press 1 for Veterans

Now try to put all of this information together into a suicide prevention plan. At the beginning of the exercise, list your self-care prodromal signs of depression. Be sure to list any suicidal thoughts or impulses, including those that seem fleeting or insignificant (for example, "I start thinking about dying, but I would never do anything about it") In working out some plan for prevention, the clinician must first determine the individual's suicidal potential, that is, the degree of probability that the person will try to kill himself in the immediate or near future.

VIGNETTE

A 67 year-old homeless woman with long-standing bipolar illness and alcoholism was brought to the emergency room by ambulance. Concerned neighbor's garbage cans in their neighborhood. Her vital signs were normal, but her level of consciousness was diminished. She agitated manner and refused to cooperate with medical examination. The emergency clinician observed that the patient was drunk and that she had not been taking her usual medication. The patient had no previous history of cardiac problems before this change in mental status.

Her suicidal thoughts often came up in response to food. When depressed, she would ear voraciously and then look in the mirror, thinking she had grown fat and ugly; it was usually then that she felt suicidal. She sought reassurances about her appearance form others at these times, but these reassurances did little to alleviate her suicidal thoughts.

The patient stated that she had wanted to die and that she had herd that the combination of psychiatric medicines and alcohol was lethal. She had not previously made a suicide attempt; however, she was under the ongoing care of a psychiatrist because of panic attacks. Before she had started these medicines, the panic attacks had become disabling.

Discussion. The feelings, thoughts, and behaviors that make up suicidal despair are quite complex. These can be vague at first (for example, "I wonders what it would be like to be dead"), even more serious ("I've thought of various suicide plans and have settled on one, as well as a time and a place"). The assessment of risk is the most crucial component of the formulation because the safety of the patient, the clinician, and others is the foremost concern in any psychiatric evaluation. For those who complete suicide the most common diagnoses are affective disorder and alcoholism.

Strategies protect the patient from carrying out suicidal actions by Miklowitz (2011):

Strategy No.1: Get rid of the means to inflict self-harm. These include guns, sleeping pills, poisons, ropes, and sharp knives or other weapons. To avoid overdosing on psychiatric medications, keep only a couple of days dosages in the house and have a friend or relative dispense them as they are needed.

Strategy No.2: See a psychiatrist and therapist immediately. Call them and let them know you are at risk so that they can help in the development of an integrated plan for managing suicidal impulses, depression, anxiety, stress, and medication. Don't be afraid to disclose information about suicidal impulses for fear that the doctor will (1) immediately hospitalize them, (2) be deeply disappointed in them and feel that the treatment plan has failed, or (3) be uncomfortable with the topic of suicide.

Strategy No. 3: Use your core circle. One theme of this chapter is the value of a core circle of family members, partners, and friends in helping keep safe. Start by reviewing the exercise for identifying your core circle.

Strategy No. 4: Reviewing Reasons for Living. Marsh Linehan and her associates have developed and inventory of reasons for living.

Strategy No. 5: Improving the Moment Tools. Suicide prevention can include learning to tolerate feelings of despair even when they won't go away. When depressed and suicidal feelings are accompanied by significant anxiety, there may be benefit from self-relaxation or mindfulness exercises. This may involve sitting in a comfortable chair; tensing and relaxing each muscle groups, starting with the feet and moving up to the face; and imagining relaxing pleasant scenes (for example, lying on a beach).

Outpatient Detoxification. In a psychiatric emergency situation, the physician's most important role is the ensure that associated medical conditions and medical complications of the abused substance are discovered, diagnosed, and when possibly, treated.

Outpatient commitment, now permitted in many states, is generally reserved for chronically noncompliant patients, most of whom are severely mentally ill. Patients can have an incentive to follow through on treatment plans. Guidelines for treatment of the outpatient suicidal client should include the following: The person should not be left alone. Arrangements must be made for the client to stay with family or friends. If this is not possible, hospitalization should enlist the help of family or friends. If this not possible, hospitalization should be reconsidered. In addition, client should enlist the full names of family or friends to ensure that the home environment is safe from dangerous items, such as firearms or stockpiled drugs.

Be Direct. Talk openly and matter of flatly about suicide. Then listen actively and encourage expression of feelings, including anger. Accept the client's feelings in a nonjudgmental manner. In conclusion, get help for the person. **1-800-SUICIDE** is a national hotline that is available 24 hours a day.

Psychiatric Evaluation. One indication for hospitalization is a serious psychotic or affective disorder that is not responding to outpatient treatment. Of course, any patient who represents a physical threat to self or others should be hospitalized, especially if he is experiencing command hallucinations or is likely to act on delusional ideas. A patient who says that he definitely intends to kill himself and has the means at hand to do so, or one who has strong suicidal feelings and is unable to control these impulses must be hospitalized. Another is a patient so disorganized as to be unable to care for his daily needs.

BOX 30-3 Indication for Hospitalizing a Suicidal Patient

- **Intention to kill self- and means**
- **Strong suicidal feelings he/she cannot control**
- **Medically serious attempt**
- **Repeated serious attempts**
- **Serious attempts associated with substance abuse**
- **Command hallucinations or psychosis**

Is hospitalization the appropriate treatment? Some patients, including those with borderline personality disorder, may become dependent on the hospital and regress when admitted. During crises they may require admission, but hospitalization should be avoided if possible, and a long-term treatment plan should be devised, usually in cooperation with the outpatient therapist. A suicidal patient can also be hospitalized involuntarily if she refuses voluntary hospitalization. The length of time that a patient can be held initially for treatment varies from state to state, but it is often in the range of 72 hours. Also, a severely suicidal patient who resists treatment may require one-to-one observation to prevent escape or self-injury.

Chapter 30: Suicidal Examination Review

1. For every depressed patient, what suicidal thoughts and feelings explore the risk of suicide?

    A. The pace of the interview is rapid, with the patient responding to questions with long answers.
    B. Very often there is a blunted range of facial expressions, and often other times, the patient may cry or fight back tears.
    C. The psychiatrist should never explore anniversary phenomena such that depression occurs on the anniversary of a significant loss.
    D. The patient is not able to control impulses in thoughts or actions.

2. What definition is expressed by an act or pattern of self-destructive behavior of low or uncertain lethality, not clearly perceived by the subject as likely to result in his death?

    A. Intentional Suicide
    B. Sub intentional Suicide
    C. Unintentional Suicide
    D. Psychosomatic Suicide

3. What suicidal acts, frequently seen in children, manifest the continual and probably unconscious wish for maternal protection and help and may eventually become the cry for help of a suicidal act?

    A. Dyadic Suicide
    B. Para suicide
    C. Paradoxical Suicide
    D. Psychosomatic Suicide

4. What methods of attempting suicide are most often completed?

    A. the ingestion of drugs or poisons
    B. Episodes involving firearm

      C. men who tend to hang themselves

      D. all of the above

5.   What biology shows that levels of a neurophysiology is lower in the brains of people who attempt or complete suicide?

      A. Serotonin

      B. Dopamine

      C. Histamine

      D. Gamma-amino butyric acid

6.   How is sex manifested in suicide attempts or competed actions?

      A. Although women are three times more likely than men to attempt suicide, men account for more than 65% of completed suicides

      B. Women tend to choose more violent means of suicide, such as guns or hanging

      C. men more often take overdoses or drown

      D. All of the above

7.   What kind of suicide may be triggered by a sudden change in a person's relations to society?

      A. Egoistic Suicide

      B. Altruistic Suicide

      C. Anomic suicide

      D. Self-annihilation

8.   What personality disorders occur in patients with suicidal behaviors?

      A. Borderline and Antisocial Personality disorders

      B. Schizotypal and schizoid disorders

      C. Narcissi and Histrionic Personality Disorders

      D. Paranoid and passive-aggressive disorders

9. When evaluating a patient who has just made a suicide attempt, how should you assess whether was planned or impulsive?

   A. Was the patient alone, and did the patient notify anyone?
   B. The patient's reactions to being saved; is the patient disappointed or relieved?
   C. Does he link the predominant dysphoric affect and experience of hopelessness to suicidal thoughts?
   D. All of the above

10. According to the suicide prevention plan, what steps can be taken?

    A. Ensure easy access to lethal items
    B. Keep only a couple of days' dosages in the house
    C. Store-up supply of pills, and dispense them as needed
    D. Keep gun in the house loaded for easy access

Chapter 30: Examination Answers

1. B
2. B
3. C
4. D
5. A
6. A
7. C
8. A
9. D
10. B

Chapter 31

Acute Psychosis

Acute psychosis, characterized by thought disorganization, delusions, hallucinations, and inappropriate or agitated behavior, is a medical- psychiatric emergency that requires careful evaluation, safety measures, and prompt treatment.

Acute psychosis is not a diagnosis but a clinical syndromes that may be caused by a wide variety of disorders, such as mania, an exacerbation of schizophrenia, or phencyclidine (PCP) abuse. At a minimum, the emergency evaluation should address the following five questions before any disposition is decided on: (1) Is it safe for the patient to be in the emergency room? (2) Is the problem organic or functional or a combination? (3) Is the patient psychotic? (4) Is the patient suicidal or homicidal? (5) To what degree is the patient capable of self-care?

Differential diagnosis. Acute psychosis is the psychiatric term for psychosis which is triggered by extreme stress. An acute psychotic state can be very short lived, lasting only a few hours, or it may spontaneously resolve itself within two weeks. Much depends upon cause, anility to diagnose, chance of the casual condition going into remission, and availability of effective treatment. The specific etiologies of acute psychosis include major psychiatric disorders (affective disorders, schizophrenia, and schizophreniform disorders), drug-induced psychosis, and medical or neurologic illnesses that can mimic primary psychiatric disorders. Even a person with severe onset of things like hallucinations may have moments of lucidity and be able to participate in treatment decisions.

By definition, signs and symptoms of acute psychosis have developed rapidly, over a period of days or weeks. Diagnosis of acute psychosis may be difficult. The syndrome includes psychotic thinking i.e. delusions, hallucinations, ideas of reference) in which the patient is convinced that ordinary events, such a television programs, people's conversations, or everyday occurrences bear some relation to him or her), or incoherent thought.

If the patient is too agitated to examine, the smallest amount of the safest sedative drug should be used until the diagnosis becomes clear. Depending on the degree of agitation, more may be needed, but over sedation must be avoided or the diagnostic picture will be clouded. Other symptoms may include insomnia, anxiety, psychomotor agitation, hyperactivity, affective derangements (such as elation or emotional ability), and the patient's disregard for the consequences of his or her actions. Agitated, assaultive behavior or failure to comply with treatment recommendations may also result. Command auditory hallucinations may cause a patient to deny symptoms and to throw prescriptions in the garbage immediately after leaving the emergency room.

Box 31-1. Questions that determine the course and nature of the illness:

A. How rapidly have symptoms developed, and what is their total duration?

B. Has the patient exhibited any vegetative signs?

1. How many hours a night is the patient sleeping?
2. Is the patient eating?
3. Has the patient been overactive or had periods of akinesia and mutism?

C. What are the patient's mental symptoms?

1. Are there delusions or auditory hallucinations?

2. Is the patient experiencing visual hallucinations?
3. Does the patient feel frightened, suspicious, or irritable?

VIGNETTE

IF the patient is extremely agitated or violent, restraints may be needed.

Paramedics arrived at her residence and found her screaming and cussing them out. She kept saying that the devil was after her. She also cries out in fear of visual hallucinations, saying "Police are around the corner; they are trying to shoot me!" Her family that was present at her home stated that she had never had anything like this could happen. She was a devout Christian woman with a god job and nice home. The most important immediate medication for this patient would include oral or intravenous glucose. The physician's first task is to ensure the safety of the patient and the staff. A patient who is violent or threatening violence, or is wildly psychotic and agitated, should be put into four-point leather restraints. We ended up havening to restrain her due to her combativeness. Even if violence is not an immediate problem, it is important to remove all potentially dangerous objects from the patient's possession, such as sharp objects, sources of flame, or belts. The need to do this should be explained in a firm way, but with respect for the patient's dignity. She spit, screamed, cussed, and hit all the way to the hospital. The doctors said that she was having an acute psychotic episode. For example, it could be said that "the symptoms of your illness are unpredictable, so it is important that you have nothing that you could hurt yourself with. "Patients benefit from a low stimulation environment. A quiet room is optimal if available if not, the patient should be placed in as bare a room as possible that is free of any potentially dangerous objects (including extra furniture).

Discussion. Vital signs should be obtained immediately. If the patient is febrile or has marked abnormalities of blood pressure, respiratory rate, or heart rate, rapid medical assessment will be needed. It should be recalled that all agitated patients will have some degree of hypertension, tachycardia, tachypnea, and perhaps even a mild elevation in temperature.

Physical Restraints. The physical restraint of paitents may be necessary to prevent violence. Always begin by offering the patient a chance to stop the behavior that is leading to potential restraint. Speak authoritatively, and direct the patient to stop the behavior. Try to provide a quiet space alone (under visual observation), where the patient can try to calm down. Repeatedly explain that the continued behavior will lead to physical restraint. However, do not negotiate with the patient. Simply identify which specific behaviors warrant physical restraint, and if they continue, proceed with restraint. Do not let the patient feel that there is any doubt in your mind regarding what interventions are necessary.

In choosing a restraint, use a type with which the staff members have been trained and are familiar. The improper use of restraints can lead to injury. Avoid restraining only one limb, since thrashing can cause a sprain or a fracture in the patient. Then, once the patient is restrained, offer medication again if the patient has not yet complied. Patients who remain agitated in restraints should be medicated until they are calm. Continue to monitor the patient's vital signs every half hour while the patient is in restraints constantly reevaluate the need for restraints by an objective assessment of the patient's behavior as frequently as possible, preferably every 15 to 30 minutes. Finally, document the reasons for placing the patient in restraints.

Acute psychosis, like delirium, is a medical emergency. The acutely psychotic patient is difficult to treat in the emergency department because he or she is often excited and disruptive and cannot be reasoned with. The patient usually has severe impairments of thought and judgment. Combined with agitation or hyper- activity, these impairments may result in violence, inadvertent self-injury, or suicide. The cardinal points in emergency management are a safe environment, low stimulation, and antipsychotic medication with or without sedation. The patient may threaten job, financial well-being, and relationships with family and friends. Patients may break the law with resultant arrest. Beyond these potentially catastrophic psychosocial difficulties, the psychosis may be the presentation of a medical illness that requires immediate intervention.

Discussion. Mania is probably the most common disorder that presents as acute psychosis. Patients who are manic may display a wide variety of psychotic symptoms, including symptoms that are bot mood congruent. The differential diagnostic manifestations are acute onset (days to weeks) from a normal baseline; a history of prior manic or depressed episodes (with or without psychosis); a history of sleeplessness; hyperactivity; elated, irritable, or a paranoid affect; rapid speech that may also be difficult to interrupt (pressured); and inflated self-esteem.

Drug-induced psychosis may be caused by acute ingestion, chronic ingestion (especially of amphetamines), or withdrawal. It is important to distinguish them from functional psychosis because management will be markedly different. A history of drug use by the patient must raise the physician's suspicion. The patients themselves are often unreliable reporters, making data obtained from objective tests and from friends and family invaluable. If possible, a sample of the ingested substance should be obtained for analysis and toxic screens of serum, urine, and gastric contents should be ordered.

Treatment

A patient suffering from acute psychosis might require restraints or sedation for his/ her own safety the main goal of treatment is to prevent the patient form harming either themselves or others. Treatment can be difficult because a person with acute psychosis may be violent, may be a danger to self or others, and usually is not aware enough to fully consent to treatment. The first goal is usually to use medications that will promote calmer behavior.

In a hospital setting, a person with acute psychosis may need to be treated without their consent. This may mean administering medications that tranquilize the patient and placing the patient in restraints if necessary.

The acute symptoms last about a week, during which the patient is hospitalized for 14 days and returned to normal functioning about six weeks after onset; started to work again. Acute psychosis is looked at as a type of "attack." These attacks are sudden, incomprehensible, uncontrollable, and fortunately, reversible. Many people, according, to Freud, experience these attacks when they have are longing for something they have lost. People are usually able to gradually detach themselves from the lost object and heal.

Patients with acute psychosis may die as a result of stresses related to the acute psychosis, rather than to the treatment.

Antipsychotic medications do have potentially dangerous side effects to include (1) ventricular fibrillation (antipsychotics are not arrhythmogenic); (2) depressed gag reflex, leading to asphyxia form the aspiration of regurgitated food; (3) lowering of the seizure threshold, causing seizure; (4) dystonia of the larynx and pharynx, leading to asphyxiation; (5) orthostatic hypotension, leading to a cerebrovascular event or myocardial infarction; (6) neuroleptic malignant syndrome; (7) anticholinergic effects, reducing gastrointestinal (GI) motility and leading to shock in patients with acquired mega colon; (8) end bronchial mucous plugs in asthmatic patients; and (9) clozapine-induced agranulocytosis, leading to opportunities infection.

Carefully describe the potential side effects of medications to the patients and their families. Instruct them to seek medical care rapidly if side effects occur, especially dystonia, severe rigidity, seizures, and hypotension. Inform patients that antipsychotics in rare cases cause agranulocytosis, so they should be evaluated for any sign of even a minor infection, such as a fever.

Chapter 31: Acute Psychosis Examination Review

1. What is the cardinal point in the emergency management of acute psychosis?

    A. Safe environment
    B. Low stimulation
    C. Antipsychotic medication
    D. All of the above

2. When does psychotic symptoms follow a significant psychosocial stressor and symptoms that last for a period of no longer than several hours to 2 weeks?

    A. Schizophreniform disorder
    B. Brief reactive psychosis
    C. Schizoaffective disorder
    D. Drug-induced psychosis

3. What drug abuse emergencies may include delusions, hallucinations, bizarre behavior agitation, anxiety, panic and aggressiveness?

    A. Hallucinogens
    B. Amphetamines
    C. PCP psychosis
    D. LSD psychosis

4. What medications are used to treat paranoid or hypomanic symptoms as well as marked lability of affect?

    A. Sedative hypnotics
    B. Amphetamines
    C. Hallucinogens
    D. Mescaline and STP

5. What is typical regimen of haloperidol is given intramuscularly every hour until sedation is achieved?

   A. The first maintenance dose is then given orally 6 to 8 hours after the last injection
   B. The low doses of neuroleptics are presented here despite rapid neuroleptization.
   C. If a benzodiazepine is given intravenously, there is no danger of respiratory depression.
   D. High-dose regimen is recommended because drugs such as Parkinsonism are dose-related.

6. Why is the acutely psychotic patient difficult to treat in the emergency department?

   A. Because the patient is often excited, disruptive, and cannot be reasoned with.
   B. Because the etiology of the syndrome can be decided form mental status alone
   C. Because the clinical syndromes may be caused by depression
   D. Because depending on the degree of agitation, over sedation should be applied until the diagnostic picture will be clouded.

7. How does impending violence require immediate intervention?

   A. By negotiating with the patient
   B. Have a minimum number of staff members so that the patient does not feel threatened
   C. Offer a chemical restraint before implementing physical restraint
   D. Once the patient is restrained, do not offer further medication

8. What is the most common disorder that presents as acute psychosis?

   A. The presence of psychotic symptoms on mental status examination derives pathognomonic from schizophrenia

B. Patients who are manic may display a wide variety of psychotic symptoms, including symptoms that are not mood congruent

C. The key differential diagnostic manifestations are acute onset (six to eight months) form a normal baseline.

D. Acute onset, prior history of affective illness, family history of affective illness, and absence of neurovegetative signs (such a sleeplessness).

9. What forms of depression help make clinical diagnosis?

A. Depression frequently presents as acute agitated psychosis

B. Depression rarely present s with paranoia

C. Depression occasionally present with paranoia rather than sadness as the most prominent symptom

D. Depression is characterized each day to deflated self-esteem.

10. Describe the factitious psychosis and malingering that occurs most commonly in patients with underlying personality disorders.

A. Neuroleptics are greatly of proven benefit in all personality disorders

B. The diagnosis requires the identification of some secondary gain or the admission of voluntary control

C. Poor functioning in both social and occupational roles

D. Use of primitive but psychotic defenses, such an acting out or passive aggression.

Chapter 31: Examination Answers

1. D
2. B
3. C
4. B
5. A
6. A
7. C
8. B
9. C
10. B

Chapter 32

Violent Behavior

Violence is one of the most feared yet least likely behaviors of people with mental illness. Violence is physical aggression inflicted by one person on another. When it is directed toward oneself, it is called self-mutilation or suicidal behavior.

Violence can be due to a wide range of psychiatric disorders, but it may also occur in normal people who cannot cope with life stresses in less severe ways. One of the best indicators of whether an individual has the potential to be violent is past history. If a person has never been violent before, it is necessary to examine the circumstances to determine if it might happen again. Was the person taking medication? Did he or she feel threatened? Was the person provoked? Did he or she do harm to another person or property? The answers to these questions will help in determining the likelihood of future violence.

Box 32-1. Model for Assessing Violence Psychiatric Interviewing the Violent Behaviors

- Countertransference or emotional reactions
- Applied role in decreasing violence
- Training in signs and indications
- Biopsychosocial model of 18 risk factors for violence toward others

I.   Psychological domain
II. Social domain
III. Biological domain

Psychological Domain

_____ 1. Male Gender
_____ 2. Age 15-24
_____ 3. Past History of Violence; frequency, severity
_____ 4. Paranoia
_____ 5. Intelligence
_____ 6. Anger/ Fear problems: control
_____ 7. Psychopathy and other attachment problems

Social Domain

_____ 8. Family of origin violence
_____ 9. Adolescent peer group violence
_____ 10. Economic instability or poverty
_____ 11. Weapons history, skill, interest, and approach behavior
_____ 12. Victim pool
_____ 13. Alcohol and / or psychostimulant use
_____ 14. Popular Culture

Biological Domain

_____ 15. History of CNS trauma
_____ 16. CNS signs and symptoms
_____ 17. Objective CNS measures
_____ 18. Major Mental Disorder

When dealing with these types of violence, learn to recognize the cues related to the patient's losing control. This kind of violence is often evoked when a person feels concerned, threatened, or verbally attacked. In addition, the patient stays calm and conveys expectation that the patient will maintain control.

Our model for assessing violence toward others is illustrated in the figure composed of three domains: psychological domain, social domain, and biological domain. The term biopsychosocial model since it draws from current psychiatric and psychological research that suggests that these domains of functioning interact with one another; and should not be assessed in isolation.

Each domain also affects the other, and for those of the family therapy, the concept is similar to systems therapy. This model also contains within the three central questions that should begin every violence risk and threat assessment, although these questions should only be in the mind of the evaluator and not asked directly of the patient or client.

Now put a checkmark beside each of the 18 violence risk factors that are present in the case vignette of symptoms. As the patient familiarizes himself/herself with these variables, they begin to jump out at the patient, which is the point of a practice case in this book. So let's go through each of the domains, and compare the client's scoring with that of the patient.

Some of these correlates are static, and some are dynamic. Those factors which are static are those which are historical or dispositional and do not change, or change very slowly and are not amenable to any intervention. Those factors are dynamic when; they are those which are situational or clinical and do change, often quite rapidly. Probably the most stable factor of many in the prediction of violent behavior is being male. This means that half of the world's population (almost) is substantially at greater risk for violence than the other half. Moreover, the sex ratio averages about 10:1, that is, for every ten males who are violent there is one female who is, but this ratio varies considerably form study to study, ranging from about 2:1 to 50:1.

Biological determinants of violence irregularities in the brain have been associated with aggressive behavior. Violent people commonly have a history of head injury or show abnormal electro-encephalogram (EEG) readings. Lesions of the temporal lobes, frontal lobes, and hypothalamus, as well as abnormal activity in the prepiriform area and amygdala, which are associated with increased aggression. Among the neurotransmitters, dopamine is associated with increased aggression. In acts of aggression, the so-called catharsis hypothesis exists. Although Freud accepted the existence of such catharsis, he was relatively pessimistic about its usefulness in preventing overt aggression.

Most mentally ill persons include patients who are violent under the conditions such as:

Schizophrenic Disorder-This treatment biased ECT forms control of psychotic violence (see chapter 28). Always explain what action is taking place and why. Violent patients are often frightened-find out why and what. The chronically violent patients should receive medication trials. Treat psychosis with antipsychotics, seizures with anticonvulsants, and benzodiazepines which can be useful during times of stress, but paradoxical rages occur in some patients. Teach these patients to recognize early signs of increasing anger and to develop ways to discharge tension. Finally, help the patient to develop a support system and to learn to control environmental stresses. Legal responsibility to maintain a channel of communication with the potentially violent patient-this begins by being available by phone (Beck, 1987). Since most patients with schizophrenic disorders are managed as outpatients, where they are often screening in emergency departments, especially after hours when psychiatric consultants may not be available. Schizophrenic disorders include schizophrenia, schizophreniform disorder, and brief reactive psychosis. These disorders are distinguished by the duration of symptoms. (See chapter 14, 16, and 17).

Brief reactive psychosis, the onset of which typically follows a traumatic event, may occur in someone without a previous psychiatric history and often includes paranoid features acute psychosis also is a characteristic of uncompensated schizophrenia. Patients may exhibit hallucinations, delusions, and loosening of associations. The psychotic patient may be hyperactive, aggressive, agitated, or behaving in an irrational manner. The patient may appear to respond to voices or situations that the examiner cannot hear or see.

Since the patient responds to thoughts or stimuli unknown, unheard, or unseen by the medical staff, the onset of violence can be abrupt and unexpected. Those with paranoid delusions may be attempting to protect themselves from medical staff or other patients who are perceived as threats or enemies. Mute and catatonic patients may be the most potentially dangerous of the schizophrenic patient group and should be approached with caution.

Affective Disorders- Both mania and depression can be associated with hostile or violent behavior. Combative patients may become hostile if they feel that their plans are being thwarted or that they are not taken seriously. Pressure of speech, visible agitation, delusions of grandeur, and long periods of being awake characterize the manic patient. The depressed patient can also be dangerous. Such patients may feel that their lives are not worth much and therefore, neither is anyone else's. Some depressed patients who become suicidal will kill their family before they kill themselves.

Personality Disorder- Personality disorders are conditions in which one's personality traits interfere with normal social and occupational functioning or cause subjective emotional distress. The personality disorders most likely to be associated with hostility or violence include the antisocial, borderline, and paranoid. (Phillips, Yen & Gunderson, 2003).

Antisocial Personality Disorder. Persons with an antisocial personality disorder have a history of trampling upon the rights of others. There is usually an early history of truancy or pyromania and childhood aggression. In contrast, the older patient exhibits failure to maintain a job, drunkenness, and marital chaos. Their history is also remarkable for lying, stealing, cheating, and precocious sexual behavior. Such patients tend to feel little remorse for their actions, so they are among the most dangerous of hostile patients. These patients are notoriously difficult to treat, perhaps because they seem comfortable with their personality.

Borderline Personality Disorder. Patients with a borderline personality disorder have severe problems with interpersonal relationships. These relationships are usually marred by intense and stormy outbursts. The patients are generally unpredictable and have a sudden outbursts of intense anger stimulated by relatively trivial circumstances. They can become intensely angry, often at members of the family or close friends. They frequently have severe problems in their sense of identity. They typically feel chronically empty and bored by appearing odd, strange, or eccentric to others. Under severe stress they may show acute signs of reality distortion, depression, and a clinical picture resembling psychosis. These patients usually have great difficulty maintaining their jobs and rarely have long-term, satisfying relationships. This disorder is far more common among men than women.

Paranoid Personality Disorder. Patients with a paranoid personality disorder feel an all-present an unwarranted suspiciousness of other people. They have a narrow emotional life and are hypersensitive to criticism or perceived rejection. They are constantly looking around them to confirm their expectation that they will be manipulated to used by others. Usually these patients find some kernel of truth to their beliefs, which gives rise to a self-full-filling prophesy: what they believe to be true will become true if only they look hard enough. They often counterattack whenever they perceive a threat but their misperception of the world around them never reaches delusional proportions. This lack of a delusional system differentiates them from persons with paranoid psychosis. The disorder is more often seen in men. They may get into a fight I a bar or at other social gatherings where they feel that they are being laughed at, stared at, or in some way ridiculed. Do not sit close to a paranoid patient, who may feel that you are threatening. They react violently to these perceived threats and provoke a fight. The fight of course, validates their view that others are out to get them.

Substance-Related Emergencies. Patients with some form of substance abuse or its complications require immediate medical treatment:

1) Patients who have overdosed require prompt medical intervention focusing on airway maintenance, monitoring of vital signs, and elimination of any drugs retained in the stomach

2) Patients who have Wernicke's encephalopathy require prompt parenteral administration of thiamine.

3) Patients who are in alcohol or sedative-hypnotic withdrawal should be treated with supportive measures.

Violent Behavior.

A. Rosenberg (1988) described four factors that may precipitate violence. The first is the cultural belief that is=t is acceptable to engage in violent actions. This is reflected in the acceptance of the moral correctness of striking women or children, whether to achieve some goal or to express one's feelings. And then, television reinforces acceptance of violence as a means of expression in life.

B. The second factor is structural stress. This factor refers to the conflict that is introduced in relationships when an individual's goals cannot be obtained because of psychologic, economic, and social concerns. The fact that the highest rates of violent injuries are seen in the poorest communities indicates that in lower socioeconomic groups this factor can be a major contributor.

   a. Cultural belief
   b. Structural stress
   c. Social isolation
   d. Intervene in violent situations

C. The third factor is social isolation, which can add to the potential for violence and is often the result of battering. Part of the pattern of battering includes forced isolation, restricted access to money, transportation, and other resources. Alcohol use makes this isolation worse, because alcoholism tends to isolate women more than men.

D. The fourth factor is the availability of services that can be used to violent situations. Social service agencies, police, church, and medical care providers are the usual source of these services.

In deciding how to proceed in terms of talking to the patient or using physical means of control, the clinician should make an instant differential diagnosis and categorize the patient's condition into one of the four groups (Table 32-1):

Table 32-1. Types of Violent Patients and Emergency Responses

TYPE	RESPONSE
Organic Mental Disorders	Patient generally requires restraint until etiology is known (Not usually amenable to talk)
Psychotic Disorders	Patient generally requires restraint and neuroleptic (Not usually amenable to talk)
Nonpsychotic, nonorganic Disorders	Patient generally responds to talk with de-escalation. Staff for restrain and/or medication should be available nearby.
Personality Disorder or Intermittent Explosive Disorder	Patients are often amenable to verbal intervention without seclusion or restraint

1. Organic mental disorder. For patients with cognitive impairment disorders and substance-related disorders in the middle of a violent episode, it is frequently impossible to intervene effectively and influence them through verbal means. One should treat the underlying medical or other physical disorder rather than only rely on neuroleptics to control violence.

2. Psychotic disorders. The violent patients in this group are usually schizophrenic or manic and are again difficult to influence through verbal means. Neuroleptic medication rapidly administered us usually the treatment of choice for these patients, although they may have to be restrained or secluded until it takes effect.
3. Nonpsychotic, non-organic disorders.
4. This group primarily includes patients with personality disorder or intermittent explosive disorder who are often amenable to verbal intervention without seclusion or restraint. In deciding to use physical means of control, the psychiatrist can assess the patient is degree of impulse control by the patient's compliance with routine requests and procedures in the clinic or emergency.

Let's illustrate this approach with a brief clinical vignette.

VIGNETTE

A 50 year old single male veteran, currently unemployed and homeless, was living in public shelters and on the street. He required considerable assistance with his grooming and dress, and his behavior was frightening because of its unpredictability. A patient at a local mental health clinic, he is seen monthly. He as diagnosed in the Veterans Clinic with advanced Alzheimer's disease, and was admitted for evaluation of violent and unpredictable behavior. As his illness progressed, he became more confused and made more frequent misinterpretations of external stimuli. His symptoms have remained unchanged for about 1 year, but he presented today demanding to go into the hospital. The clinician asks, "Why now?" He replied, "My mother died last year on this day, and since this morning I have been hearing her voice telling me to join her. I almost jumped off the viaduct on the way here, and if you send me home, I don't think I can keep from doing that on the way back."

The patient was cooperative when the medical student interviewed him and appeared rather calm. In the interview his disturbed though processes related to cerebral degeneration evidenced by disorientation, confusion, memory deficits, and inaccurate interpretation of the environment. He was observed to be confused by not knowing the date, his location, or the situation. The interview established risk for other-directed violence related to impairment of impulse control; hallucinations. In addition he was capable of risk for suicide related to depressed mood secondary to awareness in decline of mental and/ or physical capability. His low self-esteem was related to loss of independent functioning evidenced by expression of shame and self- degradation and progressive social isolation. His disturbed sleep pattern related to excessive hyper-activity and agitation, evidenced by difficulty falling asleep and sleeping only short periods. He is able to fall asleep within 30 minutes of retiring. This is because he is able to sleep 6 to 8 hours per night without medication.

Discussion. Preventing Violence. There are three general types of violent behavior, each requiring a different plan of response.

1. A reaction to or expression of psychotic symptoms. It is based purely on delusions and is not responsive to reasoning or discussion. Prompt police intervention or hospitalization is in order.
2. Loss of self-control and subsequent lashing out. When dealing with this type of violence:

    ➤ Learn to recognize the cues related to your relative's losing control –for example, becoming wide-eyed or hyperventilating. This kind of violence is often evoked when a person feels cornered, threatened, or verbally attacked.
    ➤ Stay calm, and convey your expectation that your relative will maintain control.
    ➤ Give as much emotional and physical distance as possible
    ➤ Assure your own physical safety
    ➤ After everyone has calmed down, discuss the incident.

3. Gestures or threats of violence given primarily to control others or to get one's own way. Handle these as follows:

    •   Evaluate the incident, both on your own and in conjunction with a family member.
    •   When everyone is calm, initiate a discussion outlining which behaviors are not acceptable and what their consequences will be.
    •   Be prepared to follow through pm the consequence. These may include a loss of privileges or a call to police, depending on the seriousness of the behavior.

Table 32-2. Diagnosis Associated with Violent Behavior

A. Psychotic Disorders

    1. Schizophrenia (especially paranoid and catatonic)
    2. Mania
    3. Paranoid Disorders
    4. Postpartum Psychosis

B. Organic Mental Disorders

    1. Delirium
    2. Drug intoxication or withdrawal

C. Personality Disorders

    1. Antisocial
    2. Paranoid and others with transient psychosis

D. Situational Problems

    1. Domestic Quarrels (spouse abuse)
    2. Child abuse
    3. Homosexual panic

E. Brain Disorders

    1. Seizure Disorders
    2. Structural Defects
    3. Mental retardation

F. Dissociative States

Treatment

Psychiatric Interview: the answers to these questions will help determine the likelihood of future violence.

- Keep up with daily hygiene?
- Was the person intoxicated?
- Psychotic
- Completely out of control?

    ➤ When dealing with this type of violence, learn to recognize the cues related to the patient's losing control. This kind of violence is often evoked when a person feels cornered, threatened, or verbally attacked. Stay calm and convey expectation that the patient will maintain control.

- Was the person taking medication as prescribed?
- Did he/she do harm to a person or property?
- Consider where the patient is in the cycle and when it is best to intervene.

Obligations: Those who have a neurologic or organic disorder that results in violence and urges as unwanted (ego-dystonic) come for psychiatric help. When an individual is confronted by a patient who has committed or is contemplating a violent act, the psychiatrist has four obligations:

- To ensure the safety of the patient and the staff
- To determine whether violent ideation or behavior stems from a specific psychiatric disorder

- To effect an appropriate treatment plan and disposition, and
- To warn third parties if a serious threat of harm is present

Treatment against violence starts by protecting yourself as you assume that violence is always a possibility, and never allow yourself to be surprised by a sudden violent act. Explore possible psychosocial interventions to reduce the risk of violence. If violence is related to a specific situation or person then the signs of impending violence includes recent violent acts against people and property, clench teeth, verbal threats (menacing), weapons or objects potentially usable as weapons.

If the patient is already taking an antipsychotic, give more of the same drug. If the patient's agitation has not decreased in 20 to 30 minutes, repeat the dose. Avoid antipsychotics in patients at risk for seizures. Benzodiazepines may be ineffective in patients who are tolerant; these drugs may also cause disinhibition, which can potentially worsen the violence. Chronically violent patients with organic disorders sometimes respond to beta-blockers.

Chapter 32: Violent Behaviors Examination Review

1. Staff must be aware of the symptoms associated with anger and aggression to make an accurate assessment.

    A. Prevention is the key issue in the management of aggressive or violent behavior
    B. Anxiety (severe to panic) leading to misinterpretation of the environment
    C. Post-trauma response
    D. Has the individual developed more adaptive coping strategies and have they been effective?

2. Studies show that all neurotransmitters EXCEPT which one plays a role in the facilitation and inhibition of aggressive impulses?

    A. Norepinephrine (associated with the "fight-or-flight" syndrome of symptoms that occur in response to stress).
    B. Dopamine (pathways derived from the amino acidtyrosine and plays a role in physical activation of the body).
    C. Histamine (plays a role in depressive illness).
    D. Serotonin (plays a role in sleep and arousal, libido, appetite, mood, aggression, and pain perception).

3. According to Rosenberg (1988), which factors precipitate violence?

    A. Cultural belief
    B. Structural stress
    C. Social isolation
    D. All of the above

4. What is the accepted by the catharsis hypothesis?

    A. Providing angry persons with an opportunity to engage in injurious behavior
    B. Behaviors that increases their tension

C. Behaviors that reduces arousal and weakens their tendency to engage in dangerous acts of aggression

D. Expressive behavior that hinders some persons discharge aggression

5. What are the indications for seclusion or restraint?
   A. To promote harm to others
   B. As ongoing behavioral treatment
   C. TO increase stimulation
   D. TO promote serious disruption of treatment environment

6. The violent patients in the group of psychotic disorders are usually
   A. Schizophrenic
   B. Major Depressive Disorder
   C. Seasonal Affective Disorder
   D. Generalized Anxiety Disorder

7. This phase is the most violent and the shortest, usually lasting up to 24 hours. It most often begins with the batterer justifying his behavior to himself.
   A. The tension-building phase
   B. The acute battering incident
   C. Calm, loving, Respite phase
   D. The Honeymoon Phase

8. In what way is patients exhibiting violent behavior most frequently seen in a hospital emergency department setting?
   A. One of the first actions is to remove physical restraints
   B. Assess the patient's reality testing and ability to verbalize
   C. Place the patient in a crowded room where he/she can interact with other patients
   D. The interview is conducted without a security officer present

9. When are aggressive behaviors classified as extreme?

    A. During expression of sarcasm
    B. With slamming of doors
    C. With threats of physical violence
    D. With physical acts of violence against others

10. The personality disorders most likely to be associated with hostility or violence include

    A. Antisocial
    B. Borderline
    C. Paranoid
    D. All of the above

Chapter 32: Violence Examination Answers

1. A
2. C
3. D
4. C
5. B
6. A
7. B
8. B
9. D
10. D

Chapter 33

Psychiatry of Drug Abuse

In this Chapter, we apply our biopsychosocial model to three broad groups of substance use disorders: those related to central nervous system (CNS) depressants, to CNS stimulants, and to hallucinogens. However, we will devote most of our discussion to the abuse of alcohol, opioids, barbiturates, and cocaine, because arguably the greatest harm to society (if not the individual) stems from these agents.

Table 33-1.Common Organic Mental Syndromes Associated with Psychoactive Substances

Class of Drugs	Symptoms of Use	Therapeutic Use	Overdose Symptoms
(CNS Depressant) Alcohol	Relaxation, loss of inhibitions, lack of concentration, drowsiness, slurred speech	Antidote for methanol consumption	Nausea, vomiting; shallow respirations; cold, clamy skin; weak, rapid pulse; coma; possible death

(CNS Stimulants) Amphetamines & Related Drugs	Hyperactivity, agitation, euphoria, insomnia, loss of appetite	Management of narcolepsy, hyper-kinesia, and weight control	Cardiac arrhythmias, headache, convulsions, hypertension, rapid heartbeat, coma, possible death
(CNS Stimulant) Cocaine	Euphoria, hyperactivity, restlessness, talkativeness, increased pulse		Hallucinations, convulsions, pulmonary edema, respiratory failure, cardiac arrest, possible death
(CNS Stimulant) Opioids	Euphoria, lethargy, drowsiness, lack of motivation, constricted pupils	As analgesics; methadone in substitution therapy; heroin has no therapeutic use	Shallow breathing, slowed pulse. Clammy skin, pulmonary edema, respiratory arrest, convulsions, coma, possible death

The CNS depressants are a heterogeneous group, consisting of alcohol, opiates, and a variety of so-called sedative-hypnotic agents. The last category includes barbiturates, methaqualone-type agents, and the benzodiazepines. In general, CNS depressants produce varying degrees of drowsiness and impairment of motor coordination, judgment, and memory. Depressants slow down reactions to things. Taken in small amounts they may make the patient feel more relaxed. Taken in large amounts they can cause nausea and vomiting and make the patient pass out as they slow down breathing and heart rate. In large doses, any of the CNS depressants can produce respiratory suppression, stupor, coma, and death.

When the CNS depressants are suddenly withdrawn, a general pattern of rebound hyperexcitability ensues; for example, the user becomes more irritable, restless, and tremulous. In a very gross sense, withdrawal of CNS depressants leads to a state of sympathetic nervous system over arousal.

CNS Stimulants. The most commonly abused CNS stimulants are amphetamines and cocaine. Amphetamines may be taken orally or intravenously; cocaine is most often taken intranasal (snorting) but may also be injected intravenously or smoked (freebasing). Because of their pleasurable effects, CNS stimulants have a high abuse potential. With continued use, the pleasurable effects diminish, and there is a corresponding increase in dysphoric effects. Stimulation of the CNS results in tremor, restlessness, anorexia, insomnia, agitation, and increased motor activity. Many individuals who abuse or are dependent on CNS stimulants began using the substance for the appetite-suppressant effect in an attempt at weight control. These drugs exert a profound effect on the GI tract. Both stomach and intestinal tone are increased, whereas peristaltic activity of the intestines is diminished. These effects lead to a marked decrease in the movement of food through the GI tract.

CNS Stimulant Amphetamines. Amphetamines was first employed clinically in 1935, as a stimulant compound which could counteract the excessive tendency to fall asleep that is found in the medical condition of narcolepsy. The mental effect of amphetamine take the form of increased alertness, and a greater sense of well-being and energy. Confidence is enhanced euphoria develops, together with wakefulness and loss of fatigue. Thought, speech and motor activity become more rapid. There may be increased quantity, though not quality, of output in mental tasks. Appetite is suppressed; patients who began taking amphetamines for its anorectic effect as a treatment for obesity have become dependent on the drug because of its other actions on cerebral processes.

The drug increases systolic and diastolic blood pressure, and elevates the pulse rate, as well as a mild elevation of body temperature.

When the excitatory effects of a dose of amphetamines subside there can follow some hours of depressed mood and fatigue (Hofman, 1975). It is relevant that amphetamine exacerbates the clinical features of schizophrenia; the two conditions of amphetamine psychosis and schizophrenia may have a common neurochemical pathway in the central nervous system (Snyder, 1973).

Stimulant drugs make the patient feel more awake and alert. They increase heart rate, body temperature and blood pressure. But stimulants may make him feel agitated, keep him awake, decrease the patient's appetite and dilate pupils. Large amounts can cause anxiety, paranoia, aggression and stomach cramps. Psychosis form stimulants, can even lead to violence, imprisonment or hospitalization in a psychiatric setting. Thus, moderate doses of amphetamines given orally to normal subjects may produce a spectrum of mood states (e.g. mild euphoria, anxiety, irritability, or even transient drowsiness). In higher doses, the CNS stimulants tend to produce more stereotyped responses. Typically, the user is hyperactive, suspicious, and often frankly paranoid. Some users attempt to antagonize the hyper stimulating effects of these drugs via simultaneous use of opioids-hence, the heroin and cocaine "speedball." Because both amphetamines and cocaine suppress REM sleep, there is also a marked "REM rebound" phenomenon during withdrawal.

Amphetamines Intoxication and Withdrawal. Amphetamine intoxication, a syndrome produced by amphetamine ingestion, is characterized by behavioral effects—including hypervigilance, grandiosity, euphoria, and agitation—combined with physical effects that include hypertensions, tachycardia, and dilated pupils. Why can amphetamines be orally ingested, injected, snorted, or smoked? Many amphetamine abusers are first introduced to the drug as a treatment for obesity or depressions. Other abusers are those most likely to use the drug to prevent fatigue, such as doctors, students, and truck drivers. Episodes of intoxication may last days or weeks, followed by a withdrawal syndrome when the drug supply is exhausted. Withdrawal generally begins within three days after heavy users cease or decrease drug use. Amphetamine withdrawal generally begins within three days after heavy users cease or decrease drug use. Amphetamine withdrawal is characterized by severe fatigue, insomnia or hypersomnia, agitation, anxiety, drug craving, and depression after the discontinuation of heavy amphetamine abuse. Patients may present with suicidality, which can persist with severe depressive symptoms for months. Amphetamines psychosis has often been sued as a "chemical model" for schizophrenia, although phencyclidine (PCP) - induced psychosis may be a closer fit.

Cocaine. Cocaine is vegetable alkaloid derived from leaves of the coca plant. It is often referred to as Coke, C, Snow, happy dust, and white girl. There are over 120 street expressions for cocaine free base, including: crack, rock, white tornado, white cloud, and super white. Cocaine has become the all- American drug. But cocaine can be a very dangerous drug. The euphoric lift, the feeling of being confident and "on top of things"; that comes from a few brief snots, is often followed by a letdown. Regular use can induce depression, edginess, and weight loss. As usage increases, so does the danger of paranoia, hallucinations, and a total physical collapse. Cocaine, like opium, heroin, and morphine, is classified as a narcotic. Opium, heroin, and morphine are "downers," which quiet the body and dull the senses' cocaine is an "upper"- a stimulant, similar to amphetamines. It increases the heartbeat, raises the blood pressure and body temperature, and curbs the appetite. Coming down form a high may cause such deep gloom that the only remedy is more cocaine.

Hallucinogens change the patient's perceptions of reality and cause visual or auditory hallucinations. It's impossible to predict whether hallucinations will be positive or unpleasant. It's not uncommon to experience anxiety, panic or paranoia during a hallucination. It's also difficult to predict the length and frequency of hallucinations. Some people develop a drug- induced psychosis as a result of taking hallucinogenic drugs. Some of the manifestations have been likened to a psychotic break. The hallucinations experienced by an individual with schizophrenia, however, are most often auditory, whereas substance-induced hallucinations are usually visual (Mack, Franklin, & Frances, 2003). Hallucinogenic drugs include LSD, PCP, magic mushrooms, and mescaline. Cannabis may have hallucinogenic effects as well as depressant effects. LSD was first synthesized in 1938 by Dr. Albert Hoffman (Goldstein, 2002). It was used as a clinical research tool to investigate the biochemical etiology of schizophrenia. It's soon reached the illicit market, and its abuse began to over shadow the research effort.

The mental results of LSD are a paradigm for the effects on the mind of the other hallucinogens. Its effects on mental processes develop gradually, reach their height in 2-4 hours, and begin to subside after about 12 hours. Even though it is taken orally, perception is influenced in many ways. On closing the eyes after-images are prolonged, or brightly colored and realistic images may be seen. Self- harm has been inflicted by subjects suicidal depressed from LSD. Users attempting to escape in panic from the effects of the drug have accidently injured themselves. This is why physical dependence to LSD, demonstrated by an abstinence syndrome when the drug is discontinued after regular use.

One of the most commonly abused hallucinogens today is Phencyclidine (PCP, angel dust) which is one of the most dangerous drugs available for abuse. Its unpredictable effects and long clinical course and its association with violence present a challenge to the emergency department staff. Symptoms of PCP intoxication develop within an hour of use (or less when it is smoked, snorted, or used intravenously). Psychological symptoms begin with low doses that produce euphoria, grandiosity, a feeling of "numbness," and emotional liability. Higher doses because symptoms that range from perceptual distortions, anxiety, excitation, confusion, and synesthesia's to a paranoid psychosis, rigidity, and a catatonic-like state to convulsions, coma, and death. A number of deaths have been directly attributed to the use of PCP, and numerous accidental death have occurred as a result of overdose and of the behavioral changes the drug precipitates.

Physical symptoms include tachycardia, hypertension, vertical and horizontal nystagmus, ataxia, dysarthria, myoclonus, decreased pain sensitivity, diaphoresis, and seizures. The patient usually clears from symptoms in 3-6 hours. Long-term organic symptoms may occur (e.g. memory loss, and word-finding difficulty).

PCP is considered one of the most common causes of emergency room admissions for drug-induced psychoses. The psychoses may persist in some individuals anywhere from 24 hours to several months or even years after PCP use. In addition, there has been an increasing interest in using PCP as a model to study schizophrenia. As opposed to amphetamines, PCP- induced psychosis incorporates both positive as well as the negative symptoms of schizophrenia (Javitt and Zukin, 1991).

Cannabis is second only to alcohol as the most widely abused drug in the United States. The major psychoactive ingredient of this class of substances is tetrahydrocannabinol (THC). Marijuana, the most prevalent type of cannabis preparation, is composed of the dried leaves, stems, and flowers of the plant. Cannabis products are usually smoked in the form of loosely rolled cigarettes. Cannabis can also be taken orally when it is prepared in food, but about two to three times the amount of cannabis must be ingested orally to equal the potency of the obtained by the inhalation of its smoke. Hashish is a more potent concentrate of the resin derived from the flowering tops of the plant. Hash oil is a very concentrated form of THC made by boiling hashish in a solvent and filtering out the solid matter (Street Drugs, 2005). Controversy persists as to whether marijuana use leads to the use of stronger drugs, the so-called stepping stone hypothesis. It has been well demonstrated that there is a hierarchy of drug use and that marijuana is generally used before depressants, hallucinogens, cocaine, or heroin.

Research continues in regard to the possible therapeutic uses of cannabis. It has been shown to be an effective agent or relieving the nausea and vomiting associated with cancer chemotherapy, and when other antinausea medications fail. It has been used in the treatment of chronic pain, glaucoma, multiple sclerosis, and acquired immune deficiency syndrome.

Following is a summary of the effects that have been attributed to marijuana in recent years: Cardiovascular Effects. Cannabis ingestion induces tachycardia and orthostatic hypertension (National Institutes of Health, 2003). With the decrease in blood pressure, myocardial oxygen supply is decreased. Tachycardia in turn increases oxygen demand.

Respiratory Effects. Marijuana produces a greater amount of tar than its equivalent weight in tobacco. Because of the method by which marijuana is smoked- that is, the smoke is help in the lungs for as long as possible to achieve the desired effect- larger amounts of tar are deposited in the lungs, promoting deleterious effects to the lungs. Frequent marijuana users often have laryngitis, bronchitis, cough, and hoarseness. Cannabis smoke contains more carcinogens than tobacco smoke; therefore lung damage and cancer are real risks for heavy users (Goldstein, 2002).

Reproductive Effects. Some studies have shown a decrease in levels of serum testosterone and abnormalities in sperm counts, motility, and structure correlated with heavy marijuana use in males. In women, heavy marijuana use has been correlated with failure to ovulate, difficulty with lactation, and an increased risk of spontaneous abortion. Withdrawal symptoms are limited to modest increases in irritability, restlessness, insomnia, and anorexia and mild nausea. All these symptoms appear only when a person abruptly stops taking high doses of cannabis. No treatment is necessary.

Opioids. The development of opioid abuse and dependence may follow one of two typical behavior patterns. The first occurs in the individual who has obtained the drug by prescription from a physician for the relief of a medical problem. The second pattern of behavior associated with abuse and dependency of opioids occurs among individuals who use the drugs for recreational purposes and obtain them from illegal sources. Opiates bind to specific types of receptors in the CNS and elsewhere in the body.

These receptors in turn mediate the well-known opiate effects of analgesia, respiratory depression, constipation, and euphoria. The acute effects of opiates on the CNS include nausea, decreased pain perception, euphoria (probably via limbic system effects), and sedation. In larger doses, markedly decreased respirations; bradycardia; pupillary mitosis; stupor; and coma may result.

Morphine is the most well-known ingredient; the drug was so named in 1803 after Morpheus, the Greek God of dreams and sleep. But the structure of the morphine molecule was not fully appreciated until 1925; its composition was confirmed by synthesis in 1952.

The clinical effects of morphine are numerous. The drug diminishes hunger and appetite. It also produces constipation and urgency or urinary retention. Hypotension can induce dizziness and fainting, although the effects of morphine on the circulatory system are considerably less pronounced than on respiration. Morphine has a depressant effect on many activities of the brain. In small doses the higher cortical functions that promote self-control are impaired first, so that apparent stimulation ad elation sometimes occur, but any effect from disinhibition is transient. Slowing of thought and blunting of affect develop; the subject becomes unable to concentrate adequately or to feel strong or unpleasant emotions. The parts of the brain sub-serving pain and the respiratory center are especially depressed. The vomiting center in the medulla is at first stimulated, so that nausea and vomiting may follow on injection of morphine.

Withdrawal from opiates typically produces diarrhea, rhinorrhea, profuse sweating, muscle twitching, mild fever increased respiration piloerection "goosebumps," and diffuse body pain. With short-acting opiates such as heroin, morphine, and oxycodone, withdrawal signs (lacrimation, yawning, rhinorrhea, sweating) may begin 8 to 12 hours after the last dose, peak at 48 to 72 hours, and subside over 7 to 10 days. With longer-acting opiates such as methadone, withdrawal usually begins 24 to 48 hours after the last dose, peaks at 3 days or so, and lasts up to several weeks (Ciraulo and Ciraulo, 1988).

The basic features of substance dependence are summarized in the following vignette.

VIGNETTE

A 30 year-old physician called his friend, who was a psychotherapist. He was concerned that no one hear their conversation; he wanted to talk to his friend but not at the hospital where other staff members might see him.

The therapist recalled that the patient had a very distinguished background; his father, grandfather, and great-grandfather had been highly respected physicians. When he was in medical school he had married an intelligent and attractive woman, has three lovely children, and had done his residency with a famous cardiologist-surgeon.

The patient began the interview by telling the therapist that he had been indefinitely suspended from the hospital staff. His explanation started with his internship when the hours were long and the physical and emotional demands were constant. He had started using constant. He had started using cocaine then, "not every day or night-just when I was so tired I didn't think I could keep my eyes open from fatigue and complete exhaustion." The therapist asked how he was using it and he replied, "I was just snorting it." She asked about the present, and he said, "Now I'm smoking it-freebasing- and injecting it." He also said that he was not combining heroin with it when he injected it. He had been freebasing for about 2 ½ years and injecting for a little over a year. He had scheduled a triple bypass on a patient for the previous Monday morning. He explained that he never injected himself for three days before surgery, but he did freebase. He made it a pint to be scrubbed early, before anyone else was around, and gowned so no one could see his arms (with tracks form injecting the cocaine). He added that he had been a little shaky that morning (probably because of his heavy use of cocaine). Unfortunately, the chief of staff was in the scrub room when the patient entered. This other doctor apparently saw the tracks on the patient's arm and quietly but firmly asked him to hold out both his arms. The doctor asked the patient what he had been shooting up on, how long, and where he got his supply (by writing prescriptions for nonexistent patients). He was informed that he would have to enter a substance abuse facility and stay there until he was determined "clean" by the discharge clinic staff. During the first night at the clinic, the therapist received a call from the director of the facility. He informed the wife that her husband had died on the train; he had apparently "tanked up" and died in his sleep.

Discussion. Opium, heroin, and morphine are classified as narcotics and are downers, which quiet the body and dull the senses. Cocaine is an upper- a stimulant, similar to amphetamines. All of these drugs affect dopamine, norepinephrine, serotonin, and acetylcholine. It increases the heartbeat, raises the blood pressure and body temperature, and curbs the appetite. It can damage the liver, cause malnutrition, and increase the risk of heart attacks. There is growing clinical evidence that when cocaine is taken in the most potent and dangerous form- injected in solution or chemically converted and smoked in a process call freebasing- it becomes addictive. Peak plasma levels are achieved in this way within about 30 minutes. Most users are ready for another dose about 50 minutes after first inhaling the drug. Intravenous cocaine use is popular among serious abusers. This route causes an intense rush within a minute or two. In contrast, crack is easily and cheaply made by mixing cocaine with baking soda and water. In each case, cocaine is absorbed efficiently through the lungs and goes very rapidly to the brain. Blood levels peak almost immediately, which produces a rapid, intense rush. At a minimum, the emergency evaluation should address the following five questions before any disposition is decided on: (1) is it safe for the patient to be in the emergency room? (2) Is the problem organic or functional or a combination? (3) Is the patient psychotic (4) is the patient suicidal or homicidal? (5) To what degree is the patient capable of self-care?

Extremely high doses can lead to convulsions, but more commonly severe cerebral depression develops, with coma and decreased respiration. Death may ensue. In 1985, there were over 550 cocaine-related deaths, mainly from myocardial infarctions in relatively healthy individuals (Kaplan and Saddock, 1988). That is why treatment of cocaine overdose is a medical emergency, calling for control of ventricular arrhythmias, hypertension, tachycardia, and tonic-clinic seizures (Mendelson and Mello, 1991).

Treatment. How many different types of alcoholism or drug abuse are there? To answer this question, many of the treatment samples that have been studied were drawn from substance abuse treatment programs in VA hospitals. Reducing use of drugs will help to improve mental health.

Box 33-1 includes some things the patient could try:

- Make it difficult to access drugs
- Distract yourself
- Get support
- Talk to someone
- Look after yourself
- Make it difficult to access drugs- don't keep a supply of drugs and avoid spending time with people who use them.
- Distract yourself when you feel like taking the drug- hang out with friends who are not taking the drug, go for a run or walk, listen to music.
- Get support- your family and friends may give you more support if they know that you are doing something about your drug use.
- Talk to someone- talking to a friend, family member or counselor can help you to stay motivated to keep trying.
- Look after yourself- eating well and drinking lots of water that can help you to stay healthy.

Methadone Maintenance. In almost all individuals who are dependent on opioids, properly prescribed methadone substantially reduces and frequently eliminates use of non-prescribed opioids. Methadone has no direct effect on low self-esteem, post-traumatic stress disorder, personality disorders, or the many other forms of psychopathology that frequently accompany opioid dependence, nor does it have any direct effect on unemployment, poor education, or dysfunctional families.

Properly prescribed methadone is not intoxicating or sedating, is effective orally, suppresses narcotic withdrawal for 24-36 hours, and does not have effects that interfere with ordinary activities. Common side effects are sedation, if the dose is too high; constipation, which can be treated by increasing fluid intake and using stool softeners; occasional transient ankle edema in women; excessive sweating; and changes in libido. All these side effects tend to improve with the passage of time, but they may require dose reduction if they are very disturbing to the patient.

A study by the Veterans Administration (VA) carried out a large nationwide study of Methadone Maintenance. Drug use and criminality decreased during treatment, and gains were made in social functioning both during and after treatment. Methadone maintenance is a treatment specifically designed for dependence on narcotic analgesics, particularly the narcotic of greatest concern in the United States, heroin. Outpatient nonmethadone (OPNM) programs range in designed duration from one session of assessment/ referral to virtual outpatient care with daily psychotherapy and counseling for one year or longer. In some OPNM programs, medications are prescribed by staff psychiatrists or other physicians. These include ameliorants for acute withdrawal symptoms, maintenance antagonists to prevent intoxication, medications to control drug cravings after withdrawal, or treatments for psychiatric comorbidities (e.g. depression, mood disorders, schizophrenia). The major conclusion that can be offered about OPNM is familiar: the longer patients remain treatment, the better the outcomes at follow-up.

Chapter 33: Drugs Examination Review

1. What are the most widely used group of drugs that are used for substitution therapy in Alcohol withdrawal?

   A. Benzodiazepines
   B. CNS Stimulants
   C. CNS Depressants
   D. Hallucinogens

2. What CNS stimulants tend to produce a chemical model for schizophrenia?

   A. Sedative-hypnotic agents
   B. Alcohol-Induced Mental Disorders
   C. Amphetamine Psychosis
   D. Amphetamine Psych

3. What do psychosis no longer solitarychosis occur in the presence of stimulant delusion?

   A. Reality testing is rarely impaired
   B. The delusional content is rarely paranoid
   C. Cocaine delusions are usually transient and usually remit after sleep
   D. Cocaine abstinence patterns produces rapid withdrawal

4. What symptoms characterize marijuana intoxication?

   A. Time seems to pass slowly, concentration is altered, and little may be accomplished
   B. Although marijuana smoking is most often done in groups and even individuals are no longer solitary
   C. drug is used to cope with dysphoric feelings of boredom, anxiety, frustration, and inadequacy in relation to the demands or expectations of peers.
   D. All of the above

5. How do stimulants produce euphoria?

    A. high abuse potential activities mesolimbic pathways to produce euphoria
    B. increases in reward are enhanced by dopamine receptor blockades
    C. All of the single neurochemical actions aare responsible for stimulant euphoria
    D. Euphoric stimulation can become dysphoric as the dosage and duration of administration decrease.

6. How is marijuana used to modify the effects of other drugs?

    A. It is used to increase the anxiety of tobacco products.
    B. It is used to reduce the wired feelings induced by cocaine and other stimulants
    C. It is used to decrease the intoxication associated with alcohol use
    D. The anxiolytic and sedative properties of the drug increases painful effects of depression.

7. Describe the persistence as to whether marijuana use leads to the use of stronger drugs.

    A. The so-called stepping stone hypothesis
    B. The use of marijuana is often called a "gateway drug"
    C. This trend contributes to the use of cocaine and heroin rather than marijuana
    D. All of the episodes

8. Describe how stimulants create an activated euphoria

    A. Stimulants decrease well-being form alertness
    B. anxiety is increased
    C. Self- confidence and self- perceptions of mastery increase
    D. Social inhibitions are increased

9. What phenomenon is defined as the need for increasingly larger or more frequent doses of a Substance in order to obtain the desired effects originally produced by a lower dose?

   A. Substance intoxication
   B. Substance dependence
   C. Substance tolerance
   D. Substance withdrawal

10. Identify Research that outlined phases through which the alcoholic's pattern of drinking takes place.

    A. In Phase I the individual has lost control and drinks all day long
    B. Phase II begins with blackouts
    C. In phase II binge drinking is common
    D. In phase IV alcohol is used to relieve the everyday stress and tensions of life

Chapter 33: Drug Review Answers

1. A
2. C
3. C
4. D
5. A
6. B
7. D
8. C
9. C
10. B

Chapter 34

Psychiatry of Alcohol

Alcohol is a natural substance formed by the reaction of fermenting sugar with yeast spores. Although there are many alcohols, the kind in alcoholic beverages is known scientifically a s ethyl alcohol. By strict definition, alcohol is classified as a food because it contains calories; however, it has no nutritional values. Different alcohol beverages are produces by using different sources of sugar for the fermentation process. For example, beer is made from malted barley, wine form grapes or berries, whiskey from malted grains, and rum from molasses. Distilled beverages (e.g. whiskey, scotch, gin, vodka, and other hard liquors) derive their name from further concentration of the alcohol through a process called distillation.

Alcohol effects on Central Nervous System (CNS)

Alcohol everts a depressant effect on the CNS, resulting in behavioral and mood changes. The effects of alcohol on the CNS are proportional to the to the alcoholic concentration in the blood. The body burns alcohol at about 0.5 ounce per hour, so behavioral changes would not be expected in an individual who slowly consumes only one averaged-sized drink per hour. Other factors that influence these effects, however, such as individual size and whether or not the stomach contains food at the time the alcohol is consumed. Most states consider that an individual is legally intoxicated with a blood alcohol level of 0.08 to 0.10 percent.

As alcoholism progresses, minor physical changes begin to occur, including the development of acne rosacea (and enlarged, reddened nose); the development of palmar erythema (reddened palms associated with higher estrogen levels circulating in the blood of alcoholic persons); or the development of painless enlargement of the liver consistent with fatty infiltration, the earliest form of alcoholic liver disease. Advancing signs of liver disease can develop, including jaundice or ascites in alcoholic hepatitis and cirrhosis. The main features of these conditions are summarized in Table 34-1.

Table 34-1. Alcohol-Related NeuroPsychiatric Syndromes.

Syndrome	Pathophysiology	Physical Features	Psychiatric Features
Alcohol amnestic disorder/ alcohol encephalopathy	Thiamine deficiency; impaired absorption of thiamine from gut; lesions in thalamic nuclei and mammillary bodies	Ataxia, opthalmoplegia, nystagmus; may be cerebellar signs, peripheral neuropathy, and hypotension	Quiet global confusion, mild delirium; impaired short term memory; confabulation, emotional lability
Delirium Tremens	Alcohol withdrawal; kindling over time; basis of vivid hallucinations	Elevated pulse and blood pressure; sweating, tremor, fever seizures	Disorientation; perceptual distortions (visual/tactile) paranoia, agitation

Alcohol Hallucinosis	Usually associated with ethanol withdrawal, but may occur while drinking; related to schizophrenia	Tinnitus common; less psychomotor agitation than in DTs	Orientation, sensorium within normal limits; often auditory (sometimes visual) hallucinations of command or derogatory type; paranoid delusions common
Alcohol Idiosyncratic Intoxication	Some patients show temporal lobe spiking on EEG after small amount of ETOH	Markedly increased psychomotor activation; rage, violence, followed by prolonged sleep.	Confusion, disorientation, transient delusions and/ or hallucinations; amnesia for rage episode

Table 34-2. DSM-IV-TR. Diagnostic Criteria for Alcohol Intoxication

A. Recent ingestion of alcohol.
B. Clinically insignificant maladaptive behavior or psychological changes (e. g., inappropriate sexual or aggressive behavior, mood lability, impaired judgement, impaired social or occupational functioning) that developed during, or shortly after, alcohol ingestion.
C. One (or more) of the following signs, developing during, or shortly after, alcohol use:

1. Slurred speech
2. Incoordination
3. Unsteady gait
4. Nystagmus
5. Impairment in attention or memory
6. Stupor or coma

D. The symptoms are not due to a general medical condition and are not better accounted for by another mental disorder.

The excessive use of alcohol that is harmful to physical and mental health has three common forms:

1.   Continuous use of a large quantity of alcohol
2.   Heavy use only on weekends or when job functioning is least likely to be impaired, and
3.   Binges of heavy drinking (lasting days to weeks) interspersed with long periods of sobriety.

Alcohol abuse is manifested by the continual use of alcohol that interferes with a person's overall functioning and that usually evolves into dependence. Generally, this category describes a person whose drinking problem is not yet sufficient to warrant a diagnosis of alcohol dependence.

Why do people drink? Drinking patterns in the United States show that people use alcoholic beverages to enhance the flavor of food with meals; at social gatherings to encourage relaxation and conviviality among the guests; and to promote a feeling of celebration at special occasions such as weddings, birthdays, and anniversaries. Alcohol is the most widely abused drug in the United States today. The National Council on Alcoholism and Drug Dependence (2005) reports:

Alcoholism is the third leading cause of preventable death in the U.S. As the nation's number one health problem, addiction strains the health problem, addiction strains the health care system, the economy, harms family life and threatens public safety.

One –quarter of all emergency room admissions, one-third of all suicides, and more than half of all homicides and incidents of domestic violence are alcohol-related. Almost half of all traffic fatalities are alcohol-related. Heavy drinking contributes to illness in each of the top three causes of death: heart disease, cancer, and stroke. And fetal alcohol syndrome is the leading known cause of mental retardation.

How do we evaluate alcohol consumption? The CAGE and TWEAK can be administered in a self-completion format or can be integrated into a clinical interview. For alcohol dependence, the CAGE questionnaire is often used (Ewing, 1984):

C	Have you felt you should **Cut** back on your drinking?
A	Has anybody **Annoyed** you with comments on your drinking?
G	Have you felt **Guilty** about your drinking?
E	Have you ever had an **Eye-opener** in the morning to get rid of a hangover?

Two or three positive responses should create a high index of suspicion and an affirmative answer to all four is probably pathognomonic for alcohol addiction.

An alternative interview questionnaire, the **TWEAK,** was developed for use with women, particularly inner city African American women (Russell et al, 1994).

The five questions of the **TWEAK** are:

T	How many drinks can you hold? (3+ suggests **tolerance** and is scored 2 points)
W	Have your close friends or relatives **worried** or complained about your drinking in the past year? (2 points)
E	Do you sometimes take a drink in the morning when you first get up? (**Eye-opener,** 1point)
A	Has a friend or family member ever told you about things you said or did while you were drinking that you could not remember? (**Amnesia** or blackout, 1 point)
K	Do you sometimes feel the need to cut down on your drinking? **K** (c)**ut** down, 1 point)

A scale relating various degrees of clinical intoxication to blood alcohol levels demonstrates alcohol overdose. Blood alcohol concentration can be useful in detecting alcohol abuse or dependence. For example, a level of 150 mg/dL in a nonintoxicated person is strong evidence for alcoholism.

Blood alcohol levels can be roughly correlated to level of intoxication:

0-100 mg/dL: A sense of well-being, sedation, tranquility

100-150 mg/dL: Incoordination, irritability

150-250 mg/dL: Slurred speech, ataxia

>250 mg/dL: Passing out, unconsciousness

Greater than 350 mg/dL: comatose and death.

When does alcohol ingestion reach the level of alcohol intoxication? It is defined be recent ingestion of a sufficient amount of alcohol to produce maladaptive behavioral changes.

- Mild-intoxication- may produce a relaxed, talkative, euphoric, disinhibited person, severe intoxication often leads to more maladaptive changes, which can include aggressiveness, impaired judgment, and impaired social or work functioning.

- Tolerance- is both behavioral and metabolic (with an increased rate of metabolism). Withdrawal symptoms are evidence of tolerance. Even the morning hangover in the nonalcoholic may represent an acute tolerance phenomenon.

- Alcohol exhibits cross tolerance with all sedative-hypnotics, (including barbiturates, and benzodiazapines) and general anesthetics.

- Blackouts- periods of intoxication for which there is complete anterograde amnesia and during which the patient appears awake and alert. Occasionally it can last up to days with the intoxicated person performing complete tasks, such as long-distance travel with no subsequent recollection.

VIGNETTE

A 35 year old male veteran present to the emergency room experiencing tremor that a few hours after his last alcoholic drink. He stated that he had not anything to drink in the past 2 days, but that prior to that he had been drinking one quart of vodka per day. He also noticed that his night attire and bed sheets were soaked in perspiration. In addition, he complained of insomnia ("I wake up early and feel weird.") When sleep did occur it was accompanied by frequent and vivid dreams. During the periods while falling asleep and waking, visual and auditory hallucinations were present. His alcoholic abstinence syndrome was remarkable for gastrointestinal shaking, anorexia, nausea, and vomiting. Vitals signs featured blood pressure and pulse rate elevated such that their elevation continued such that their elevation continued after cessation of drinking as a sign of the withdrawal phase.

Thinking, whether irrational or rational, leads your irrational thinking and developing a greater awareness is important in the decision to stop drinking or using, as well as in your ability to follow through with that decision. When the patient learns to recognize irrational thinking, he well find some of these common irrational beliefs again and again. Acknowledging them can help him understand both problems behavior and emotions and how they defeat him.

Since the primary irrational belief is must, when his beliefs include absolutistic and unconditional musts, such as, "I need a drink," or "I can't stand living without booze." He easily defeats himself by feeling miserable and by acting irrationally. He is left with rational thinking that can help him quit; and it teaches him how to manage the problems that he faces in remaining sober.

Discussion. Alcohol withdrawal syndromes may be divided into an early onset, less severe syndrome, and a severe syndrome of late-onset (delirium tremens). Wernicke-Korsakoff **Syndrome** is probably related to thiamine deficiency. It occurs most commonly in nutritionally deficient alcoholics. The acute stage of the syndrome, which is often has a fairly abrupt onset, is referred to as Wernicke' encephalopathy. (Victor et al, 1971) The syndrome is significant for the following mental status abnormalities: most common is a global confusional state; early symptoms include listlessness, inattentiveness, poor concentration, and an inability to sustain a conversation. Drowsiness is common, but stupor or coma is rare. In the alcoholic patient, Korsakoff's psychosis may also be associated with third ventricle tumors and other neurologic disorders. Korsakoff's psychosis is characterized by a striking inability to learn. In addition there is always some degree of disturbance of past memory. Once Korsakoff's psychosis emerges, with prognosis for recovery is poor. With only 20 percent of patients making a substantial improvement.

These syndromes usually are precipitated by the abrupt withdrawal form alcohol, but can be seen in alcoholic persons who simply reduce their usual high intake. Uncomplicated alcohol withdrawal (the shakes) begins 12-18 hours after the cessation of drinking and peaks at 24-48 hours, then subsides within 5-7 says, even without treatment. Minor symptoms include anxiety, tremors, nausea, and vomiting; heart rate and blood pressure may be increased. Alcoholic withdrawal seizures (rumfits) occur 7-38 hours after the cessation of drinking and peak between 24-48 hours. The patient may have a single burst of one to six generalized seizures' status epileptics is rare. Withdrawal seizures occur primarily in chronic, long-term alcoholic patients. Alcoholic hallucinosis-vivid and unpleasant auditory hallucinations begin 48 hours after cessation of drinking and occurs in the presence of ta clear sensorium. The hallucinations typically last about 1 week but have been reported to become chronic. Like withdrawal seizures, they are a sign of severe alcoholism. The most dramatic withdrawal syndrome is alcohol withdrawal delirium (delirium tremens-DTs) Manifestations include delirium (confusion and disorientation, perceptual disturbances, sleep cycle disturbance, agitation), mild fever, and autonomic hyper-arousal. The delirium may begin 2-3 days after the drinking stops or after a significant reduction of in-take. Symptoms peak 4 or 5 days later. (Kahan and Wilson,2000).The syndrome typically lasts about 3 days but can persist for weeks.

Read the following two sets of beliefs and notice how the patient feels after reading each set in

BOX 34-1: Rational Beliefs and Irrational Beliefs

Rational Beliefs

- I failed; that's bad; it means I am fallible and I didn't get what I want.
- I want what I want, and don't like not getting it.
- I want you to treat me better; if you don't, you have blundered.
- I don't like so much work; it's a lot to do.

Irrational Beliefs

- I failed; I didn't get what I want' that's awful; it means I am no good.
- I need what I want, and I can't stand not getting it.
- You must treat me better; if you don't, you're no good.
- I can't stand so much work; it's too much.

Table 34.3 DSM-IV-TR Diagnostic Criteria for Alcohol Withdrawal

A. Cessation of (or reduction in) alcohol use that has been heavy and prolonged.

B. Two (or more) of the following, developing within several hours to a few days after Criterion A:

1. Autonomic hyperactivity (e.g., sweating or pulse rate greater than 100)
2. Increased hand tremor
3. Insomnia
4. Nausea or vomiting
5. Transient visual, tactile, or auditory hallucinations or illusions
6. Psychomotor agitation
7. Anxiety
8. Grand mal seizures

C. The symptoms in Criterion B cause clinically significant distress or impairment in social, occupational, or other important areas of functioning.

D. D. The symptoms are not due to a general medical condition and are not better counted for by another mental disorder.

Alcohol Withdrawal. The management of alcohol withdrawal consist of general support (i.e. adequate food and hydration, careful medical monitoring), nutritional supplementation, and the use of benzodiazepines. Efforts at rehabilitation can begin once alcohol detoxification has been accomplished. Rehabilitation has two goals: (1) that the patient remain sober, and (2) that coexisting disorders be identified and treated. Perhaps two-thirds of alcoholic patients have additional psychiatric diagnoses (including mood or anxiety disorders) that may require treatment. Patients should be encouraged to attend Alcoholics Anonymous (AA), a worldwide self-help group for recovering alcoholic persons founded in 1935. AA uses a program of 12 steps. New members are asked to admit their problems, to give up a sense of personal control over the disease, to make personal amends, and to help others to achieve sobriety. The meetings provide a blend of acceptance, belonging, forgiveness, and understanding.

Chapter 34: Psychiatry of Alcohol Examination Review

1. What substance refers to the need for markedly increased amounts to produce the same physical or psychological effect?

    A. Dependence
    B. Withdrawal
    C. Tolerance
    D. Remissions

2. By strict definition, how is alcohol classified as a food because it contains specific calories?

    A. Beer is made from grapes
    B. Whiskey is made from malted grains
    C. Wine is made form molasses
    D. Rum is made from berries

3. What is the universal and earliest manifestations of alcohol withdrawal?

    A. Tremulousness (shakes)
    B. Status epilepticus
    C. Pancreatitis
    D. Peritoneal dialysis

4. What effects does alcohol have on the body?

    A. Alcohol has to be digested in t he stomach
    B. The blood carries it directly to the brain where the alcohol acts on the brains central control areas.
    C. Alcohol causes increased brain activity
    D. Absorption is increased when the stomach is empty rather than containing food

5. How is peripheral neuropathy characterized in alcoholism?

   A. A reddish tinge in the urine
   B. A gradual wasting and weakness in skeletal muscles
   C. Deficiencies in the B vitamins, particularly thiamine
   D. Paralysis of the ocular muscles

6. What effect does alcohol have on the heart?

   A. Generally related to congestive heart failure
   B. Decreased exercise tolerance
   C. A non-productive cough
   D. All of the above

7. When is the familial association of alcohol dependence strongest?

   A. In the male child of an alcohol-dependent father
   B. In female elderly patients
   C. In groups of Hispanic women
   D. In the presence of gastrointestinal (GI) tract problems

8. What complications characterize alcoholic cirrhosis?

   A. Decreased blood pressure through the portal circulation
   B. B. Continued decreased in serum ammonia that results in progressively impaired mental functioning
   C. Excessive amounts of serous fluid accumulates in the abdominal cavity which Occurs in response to portal hypertension
   D. Veins in the esophagus that shrink because of decreased pressure from blood

9. What effect does alcohol have on the stomach?

   A. Inflammation of the stomach lining characterized by epigastric distress, nausea, and vomiting
   B. Identified by a syndrome of confusion
   C. toxic effects of alcohol on the esophageal mucosa
   D. Enlarged and tender liver

10. Among the personality-disordered patients, when are patients particularly likely to develop long-standing patterns of alcohol dependence?

   A. Paranoid personality Disorder
   B. Antisocial personality Disorder
   C. Schizoid personality Disorder
   D. Borderline Personality Disorder

Chapter 34: Examination Answers

1. C
2. B
3. A
4. B
5. C
6. D
7. A
8. C
9. A
10. B

Reference Section 7

Addington D.E. Reducing suicide risk in patients with Schizophrenia. Medscapree Psychiatry ad Mental Health, 2006.

Adity A, Mohan D, Wig NN. Determinants of Emergency Room Visits for Psychological Problems in a General Hospital. International Journal of Social Psychiatry 34: 25-30, 1988.

Aguilera DC. Crisis Intervention: Theory and Methodology (6th ed) The C.V. Mosby Company, 1990.

Aguilera D.C. Crisis Intervention: Theory and Methodology (8th Ed). St Louis: CV Mosby, 1998.

Albukeirat FA. And Mackler SA. The epidemic of cocaine-related neurologic catastrophies. Resident and Staff Physician 38: 33-40, 1992.

Alterman AI and Cacciola JS. The Antisocial Personality Disorder Diagnosis in Substance Abusers: Problems and Issues. Journal of Nervous Mental Disorders 179: 401-409, 1991.

Andreasen NC, Black DW. Introductory Textbook of Psychiatry. American Psychiatric Publishing, Inc, 2006.

Anderson WH and Kuehnle JC. Diagnosis and Management of Acute Psychosis. North England Journal of Medicine. 305: 1128, 1981.

Anglin MD, Speckart GS, Booth MW, et al. Consequences and costs of shutting off Methadone. Addict Behavior 14: 307-356, 1989.

INSERT 10

AUDIT. The Alcohol Use Disorders Identification Test: Guidelines for Use in Primary Care, World Helath Organization, 1992.

Baird SF. Helping the Family Through a Crisis. Nursing 17(6), 1987.

Bale RN, VanStone WW Kuldau JM, et al. Therapeutic Communities vs Methadone Maintenance. Archive General Psychiatry 37: 179-193, 1980.

Ball JC and Ross A. The Effectiveness of Methadone Maintenance. New York, Springer-=Verlag New York, 1991.

Bassuk EL, Birk AN, editors: Emergency Psychiatriy Concepts, Methods and Practices, Plenum Press, 1984.

Bayuk LL. Nursing families in Crisis: Protecting Yourself. Washington State Journal of Nursing 54(2), 1983.

Bebbington P.E. The Efficacy of Alcoholics Anonymous: the elusiveness of hard data. British Journal of Psychiatry 128, 572-580, 1976.

Beck JC. The potentially violent patient: Legal Duties, clinical practice, and risk management. Psychiatry Annual 17: 695-699, 1987.

Bellak L. A General Hospital as a Focus of Community Psychiatry, JAMA,174, 1960.

Bengelsdorf H and Alden DC. A Mobile Crisis Unit in the Psychiatric Emergency Room. Hospital Community Psychiatry 38(6), 1987.

Beskow J. The prevention of suicide while in psychiatric care. Acta PsychiatricScand (Suppl) 336: 66, 1987.

Besteman KJ. Federal Leadership in Building the National Drug Treatment System, in Treating Drug Abuse, Vol 2. Washington. DC, National Academy Press, 1992.

Bhatia SC, Khan Mlt, and Sharma A. Suicide risk: Evaluation and Management. AM Fam Physician 33 (4): 137.1986.

Bouknight RR. Suicide attempt by drug overdose. American Family Physician 33(4), 1986.

Bowers M.B. Acute Psychosis induced by psychomotomimetic drug abuse. I. Clinical findings. II. Neurochemical findings. Arch Genr. Psychiatry 27, 437-442, 1972.

Brady JV, Fotin RW, Fischman MW, et al. Behavioral interactions and the effects of marijuana. Alcohol, Drugs, and Driving 2: 93-103, 1986.

INSERT 27

Brookoff D, et al. Characteristics of Participants in Domestic Violence. JAMA, 277: 1369-1373, 1997.

Brown SA and Schuckit MA. Changes in Depression Among Abstinent Alcoholics. J Stud Alcohol 49: 412-417, 1988.

Brown SA, Irwin M, Schuckit MA. Changes in Anxiety Among Abstinent Male Alcoholics. J Stud Alcohol 52: 55-61, 1991.

Cadort RJ, O'Gorman TW, Troughton E, et al. Alcoholism and Antisocial Personality: Interrelationships, Genetic and Enviromental Factors. Arch Gen Psychiatry 42:161-167,1985.

Callaham ML. Current Therapy in Emergency Medicine. BC Decker, Inc, 1987.

Caplan G. Principles of Preventive Psychiatry, New York: Basic Books, 1964.

Catherall Dr. Handbook of Stress, Trauma, and the Family. Brunner- Routledge,2004.

Centerwell BS. Teevision and Violence: the scale of the problem and where do we go from here. JAMA 267: 3059- 3063, 1992.

Chance S. Surviving suicide: a journey to resolution, Bull Menninger Clinical 52 (1): 30, 1988.

Cheifetz Dl and Salloway JC. Crisis Intervention: Interpretation and Practice by HMOs. Medical Care 23:(1): 89-93, 1985.

Chiang NC and Hawks RL. Implicaions of Drug Levels in Body Fluids: Basic Concepts, Urine Testing for Drugs of Abuse, NIDA Res Monogr 73, Rockville, MD, National Institute on Drug Ause, 62-83, 1986.

Choron J. An incisive look at self-destruction: Suicide. New York, Charles Scibner's Sons, 1972.

Ciraulo DA and Ciraulo AM. Substance abuse, in Handbook of Clinical Psychopharmacology. Jason Aronson 121-158, 1988.

Clark WD. Alcoholism: Blocks to Diagnosis and Treatment. Am J Med 71: 275-286, 1981.

Clonginger CR. Neurogenetic Adaptive Mechanisms in Alcoholism. Science 236: 410-416, 1987.

Cohen S. The Substance Abuse Problems. New York, Haworth, 1981.

Cole SG, Lehman WE, Cole EA, et al. Inpatient vs Outpatietn Treatment of Alcohol and Drug Abusers. American Journal of Drug and Alcohol Abuse, 8:329-345, 1981.

Cook CCH. The Minnesota Model in the Management of Drug and Alcohol Dependency: Miracle, Method or Myth? Part I: The Philosophy and the Programme, British Journal of Addiciton 82: 625-634, 1988.

Davidson L. Suicide and Season. New York: American Foundation of Suicide Prevention, 2005.

Davis B.L. The PCP epidemic: a critical review. International Journal Addiction, 17, 1137-1155, 1982.

Davis M. McKay M + Eshelman ER. The realxation and stress reduction workbook. Oakland, CA: New Harbinger, 2000.

Davis S. Violence by Psychiatric inpatients: A Review. Hospital Community Psychiatry 42: 585-590, 1991.

Digman JM. Personality Structure: Emergence of the Five-Factor Model. Annual Review of Psychology; 41: 417- 440, 1990.

Dougherty MB. Emergency Room: Fighting a State of Crisis, Nurse Management 15(6), 1984.

Dubin, WR. Violent patients. In G. Bosker (Ed). The emergency Medicine reports textbooks of adult and Pediatric emergency medicine. Atlanta, GA:Thomson American Health Consultants, 2003.

Drye RC, Goulding RL, and Goulding ME. No –suicide decisions: Patient monitoring of Suicidal risk. American Journal of Psychiatry 135: 171-174, 1973.

Eichelman B. Toward a rational pharmacotherapy for aggressive and violent Behavior. Hospital Community Psychiatry. 39: 3-39, 1988.

Ellison JM, Hughes DH, White KA. An Emergency Psychiatry Update. Hospital Community Psychiatry. 40: 250-260, 1989.

Ewing JA. Detecting alcoholism: the CAGE Questionaire. Journal of the American Medical Association, 252; 1905-1907, 1984.

Fadem B. Behavioral Science in Medicine. Lippincott William& Wilkins, 2004.

Fawcett J, Golden B+ Rosenfeld N. New hope for people with bipolar disorder. Roseville, CA: Prima Health, 2000.

Feldman JL, Fitzpatrick RJ. Managed Mental Health Care: Administrative and Clinical Issues. American Psychiatric Press, Inc. 1992.

Finney JW and Moos RH. Matching Patient with Treatments: Coneptual and Methodological Issues. Journal Study of Alcohol 47: 122-134, 1986.

Firestone RW. Suicide and the Inner Voice: Risk Assessment, Treatment, and Case Management. SAGE Publications, 1997.

Galanter M, Talbott D, Gallegos K, et al. Combined Alcoholics Anonymous and Professional Care for Addicted Physicians. American Journal of Psychiatry 147: 64-68, 1990.

Gawin FH and Ellinwood EH. Cocaine and Other Stimulants. New England J Med 318: 1173-1182, 1988.

Gerson S, and Bassuk E. Psychiatric emergencies: An overview. American Journal of Psychiatry 137: 1, 1980.

Glatt KM. Helpline: Suicide prevention at a suicide site, Suicide Life Threat Behavior 17(4): 299, 1987.

Giannini AJ and Miller NS. Biopsychiatric approach to drug abuse. Residen and Staff Physician 37: 47- 52, 1991.

Gilmore KM. Hazelden Primary Residential Treatment Program: Profile and Patient Outcome. Center City, MN, Hazeldon, 1985.

Goeders NE and Smith JE. Cortical dopaminergic involvement in cocaine reinfrocement. Science 253: 195- 203, 1982.

Golan N. When is a Client in Crisis? Social Casework 50: 389, July 1969.

Gold I and Baraff LJ. Psychiatric Screeing in the Emergency department: its effect on physician behavior. American Emergency Medicine, 18: 875-880, 1989.

Goldberg W. and Tomlanovich M. Domestic Violence Victims in the Emergency Department: new findings. JAMA, 251: 24, 3259- 3264, 1984.

Goldstein A. Addiction: From biology to drug policy (2nd edition), New York: Oxford University Press, 2002.

Goodwin DW and Guze SB. Psychiatric Diagnosis, 4th Edition. New York, Oxford University Press, 1989.

Gotlib IH, Hammen CL. Handbook of Depression, The Guilford Press, 2002.

Greene H. Geopgraphical and ethnic differences in heroin use incidence trends. In:Proceedings of the 31st International

Congress on Alcoholism and Drug Dependence. Lausanne, International Council on Alcohol and Addiction, 1975.

Grinspoon L. Effects of Marijuana. Hospital Community Psychiatry 34: 307, 1983.

Gunne L and Gronbladh L. The Swedish Methadone Maintenance Program, in the Social and Medical Aspects of Drug Abuse, Jamaica, NY, Spectrum Publications, 1984.

Hallgrimsson O. Methadone Treatment: the Nordic Attitude. Journal of Drug Issues 10: 463-474, 1980.

Hankoff LD, Einsidler B. Suicide: Theory and Clinical Aspects. Psg Publishing Company, 1979.

Hatrick J.K. Delayed Psychosis due to LSD. Lancet ii, 742- 744, 1970.

Harvard Medical School. Dual Diagnosis: Part II. Harvard Mental Health Letter 20(3); 105, 2003.

Henriksson MM, et al. Mental Disorders and Comorbidity in suicide. American Joural of Psychiatry 150: 935, 1993.

Hillman J Suicide and the Soul. New York, Harper & Row, 1964.

Hirschfeld RM, Russell JM: Assessment and treatment of suicidal patients. New England Journal of Medicine. 337: 910, 1997.

Ho TP: The suicide risk of discharged psychiatric patients. Journal of Psychiatry 64: 702, 2003.

Hofman FG. A Handbook on Drug and Alcohol Abuse: The Biochemical Apects. New York, Oxford University Press, pp 224-240, 1975.

Hoffman JA and Forsmann- Falck R. Emergency Psychiatry Training: The New Old Problem, Gen Hospitalization Psychiatry 6 (2), 1984.

Hughes PH, Concard SE, Baldwin DC, et al. Resident physician substance use in the United States. JAMA 265: 2069-2073, 1991.

Hyman SE and Bierer BE. Manual of Psychiatric Emergencies. Little, Brown nd Company, 1984.

Institute of Medicine: Broadening the Base of Treatment for Alcohol Problems. Washington DC, National Academy Press, 1990.

Isometsa ET, Henriksson MM, Aro H, et al. Suicide in Major Depression. American Journal of Psychiatry, 151:530-536, 1994.

Jacob M, Carlen PL, Marshman J. A., et al. PCP ingestion: drug abuse and psychosis. International Journal of Addiction. 16, 749- 758, 1981.

Jacobs D. Evaluation and Management of the Violent Patient in Emergency Settings. Psychiatric Clinics in North America, 6: 259-269, 1983.

Jacobson G. Crisis Theory, New Dir Men Health Service. 6:1, 1980.

Jaffe JH, Babor TF, Fishbein DH. Alcoholics, Aggression and Anti-social Personality. Journal Study of Alcohol 49: 211-218, 1988.

Jaffe JH. Drug addicition and drug abuse, in the pharmacological. Basis of Therapeutics, 5th Edition. New York, Macmillan: 284-324, 1975.

Javitt DC and Zukin SR. Recent advances in the phencyclidine Model of Schizophrenia. American Journal of Psychiatry. 148: 1301-1308, 1991.

Jellinek EM. The Disease Concept of Alcoholism. New Haven: Hillhouse of Press, 1960.

Jellinek EM. Phases of Alcohol Addiction. Quarterly Journal of Studies on Alcohol, 13; 673-684, 1952.

Jirstad J. some experience in psychotherapy with suicidal patients. Acta Psychiatry Scand (Suppl) 336: 76, 1987.

Johnson J. Psychiatric Nursing in a Crisis Center: Standards and Practice. Nursing Mangaement 17 (8): 81-82, 1986.

Jones RT. Cannabis and Helath. Ann Rev Med 34: 247-258, 1983.

Julien, R.M. A primer of Drug Action: A Comprehensive Guide to Actions, Uses, and Side Effects of Psychoactive Drugs (10th edition) New York: Worth Publishers, 2005.

Kahan M. Wilson L. Alcohol Withdrawal. In E. Brands (Ed) Management of Alcohol, Tobacco, and Other Drug Problems. Toronto: Centre for Addiciton and Mental Health, 2000.

Kaplan HI, Sadock BJ. Pocket Handbook f Emergency Psychiatric Medicine. Williams + Wilkins, 1993.

Kaplan HI and Sadock BJ. Synopsis of Psychiatry, 5th Edition. Baltimore, MD, Williams &Wilkins, 1988.

Kalafat J. Training Community Psychologists for Crisis Intervention. American Journal Community Psychology 12(2): 241-251, 1984.

Khantzian EJ. The Self-Medicaiton Hypothesis of Addictive Disorders: Focus on Heroin and Cocaine Dependence. American Journal of Psychiatry 142: 1259-1264, 1985.

Kleber HD. Cocaine abuse: historical, epidemiological, and psychological perspectives. Journal of Psychiatry 49 (No.2, Suppl), 1988.

Kleesples PM, Dettmer EL. An evidence based approach to evaluating and managing suicidal emergencies. Journal of Clinical Psychology. 56: 1109, 2000.

Leaman K. A Hospital Alternative for Patients in Crisis. Hospital Community Psychiatry 38 (11), 1987.

Lehman AF, Myers CP, Corty E. Assessment and Classification of patients with psyciatric and substance abuse sundrmes. Hospital Community Psychiatry 40: 1019-1025, 1989.

Lewis DO. Neuropsychiatric and Experiential Correlates of Violent Juvenile Delinquency. Neuropsychology Review. 1(2), 125-136, 1990.

Lewis DO. From Abuse to Violence: Psychophysiological Consequences of Meltreatment. Journal of the American Academy of childand Adolescent Psychioatry, 31: 383-391, 1992.

Lindstrom L. Managing Alcoholism, Matching Clients to Treatmetn. New York: Oxford University Press, 1992.

Linehan MM + Dexter- Maaza ET. Dialectica Behavior Therapy for Borderline Personality Disorder. In DH Barlow (Ed), Clinical handbook of psychological disorders (4th ed). New York: Guilford Press, 2007.

Linehan MM, Goodstein JL, Nielsoen SL and Chiles JA. Reasons for staying alive when you are thinking of Kiling yourself: The Reasons for Living Inventory. Journal of Consulting and Clinical Psychology, 51, 276-286, 1983.

Lion JR, Pasternak SA. CounterTransference Reactions to Violent Patients. American Journal of Psychiatry 130: 207-210, 1973.

Lorenz K. On Aggression. New York: Harcourt Brace, 1996.

Mack AH, Franklin JE, & Frances RJ. Substance use disorders. Textbook of Clinical Psychiatry (4th edition) Washington, DC: American Psychiatric Publishing, 2003.

Macnab F Brief Psychotherapy: An Inegrateive approach in Clinical Practice. West Sussex, England: John Wiley & Sons, 1993.

Mann J, Oquendo M, Underwood MD+ Arango V. The neurobiology of suicide risk: A review for the clinician. Journal of Clinical Psychiatry, 60 (Suppl 2), 1999.

Mark VH and Ervin FR. Violence and the Brain. New York, Harper + Row, 1970.

Martin W.R. Jasinki Dr, and Manksy PA. Naltrexone, and antagonist for the treatment of heroin dependence. Arch. Gen. Psychiatry 28, 782-791, 1973.

Mayfield D, Mc Leod G, Hall P. The CAGE Questionaire: Validation of a New Alcoholism Screening Instrument. American Journal of Psychiatry, 13; 1121-1123, 1974.

Mayo DJ. Confidentiality in Crisis Counseling: a Philosophical Perspective. Suicide Life Threat Behavior. 14(2): 96-112, 1984.

Mc Alpine DE: Suicide: Recognition and Management. Mayo Clinic Proc 62: 778, 1987.

McLellan AT, Lubrosky L, woody GE, et al. Predicting Response to Alcohol and Drug Abuse Treatments: Role of Psyciatric Severity. Arch Gen Psyciatry 40: 620-625, 1983.

Mercy JA, and Hammond WR. Preventing homicide: A public helath perspective. Thousand Oaks, CA: Sage, 1998.

Mercy JA, Rosenberg ML, Powell KE, et al. Public Helath policy for preventing violence. Health Affairs, 12: 7-29,1993.

Merker MS. Psychiatric emergency evaluation. Nurse Clinical North America 21: 387-396, 1986

Miller MC. Suicide prevention contracts: Advantages, disadvantages, and an alternative approach. In the Harvard Medical School Guide to Suicide Assessment and Intervention. Edited by D.G. Douglas. San Francisco, CA, Jossey-Bass, 1999.

Monahan J. Mental Disorder and Violent Behavior: Perceptions and Evidence American Psychology 47: 511-521, 1992.

Morey LC and Blashfield RK. Empirical Classifications of Alcoholism. Journal Study of Alcohol. 42: 925-937, 1981.

Morey LC, Skinner HA, Blashfield RK. A Typology of Alcohol Abusers: Correlates and Implications. Journal of Abnormal of Psychology 93: 408-417, 1984.

Moscicki EK. Identification of Suicide Risk Factors Using Epidemiologic Studies. Psychiatric Clinics of North America, 20: 499-517, 1997,

Murdach AD. Decision Making in Psychiatric Emergencies. Health Social Work 12(4), 1987.

National Institute of Drug Absue: Effectiveness of Drug Abuse Treatment Programs. Rockville, MD, National Institute on Drug Abuse, 1981.

National Institutes of Health (NIH). Workshop on the medical utility of marijuana, 2003.

Nelson FL. Suicide: issues of prevention, intervention, and facilitation. Journal of Clinical Psychology 40(6): 1328, 1984.

Nerviano VJ, and Gross HW. Personality Types of Alcoholics on Objective Inventories. J Stud Alcohol 44: 837-851, 1983.

Newman RG. Methadone Treatment In Narcotic Addiction. New York, Academic Press, 1977

Novick DM, Swartz HA+Frank E. Suicide attempts in bipolar I and Bipolar II disorder: A review and metanalysis of the evidence, Bipolar Disorders 12(1), 2010.

O'Conner PG and Schottenfeld RS. Patients with Alcohol Problems. New England Journal of Medicine. 338: 592-601, 1998.

O'Donnell JA, Clayton RR. The Stepping Sotne Hypothesis: a Reappraisal, in Youth Drug Abuse: Problems, Issues, and Treatment. Lexington, MA, Lexington Books, 1979.

Pary R, Lippmann S, and Robias CR. A preventative approach to the suicid patient, Jouranl Family Practitioner 26 (2); 185, 1988.

Patterson WM, Dohn HH, Bird J and Patterson G. Evaluation of Suicidal Patients: The SAD PERSONS SCALE. Psychosomatics, 24: 343-349,1983.

Phillips KA, Yen S & Gunderson JG. Personality Disorders in Textbook of Clinical Psychiatry (4th edition). Washington, DC: American Psychiatric Publishing, 2003.

Phillips LR. Abuse and Neglect of the Fair Elderly at Home: An exploration of Theoretical Relationships. Journal of Advanced Nursing, 8: 379-392, 1983.

Pillemer K. Domestic Violence Against the Elderly: A case-controlled study. Unpublished Doctoral Dissertation, Department of Sociology, Brandeis University, 1985.

Pokorny AD. Suicide rates in various psychiatric disorders. Journal Nervous Mental Disorders. 139: 499- 506, 1964.

Post Rm, and Kopanda RT. Cocaine, Kindling and Psychosis. American Journal of Psychiatry 133: 627-634, 1976.

Puskar KR and Obus NL. Management of the Psychiatric Emergency. Nurse Practicioner 14: 9-23, 1989.

Quinn MJ. And Tomita SK. Elder Abuse and Neglect: Causes, Diagnosis, and Intervention Strategies. New York: Springer Publishing Co, 1986.

Radomsky ED, Haas GL, Mann J.J. And Sweeny JA. Suicideal behavior in Patients with schizophrenia and other Psychotic Disorders. American Journal of Psychiatry, 1999.

Rangell L. The decision to terminate one's life: psychoanalytic thoughts on suicide. Suicide Life threat Behavior 18(1): 28, 1988.

Ratey JJ, and Gordon A. The psychopharmacology of aggression. Psychopharmacol Bulletin 29: 65-73, 1993.

Rawson R.A., Tennant FS and Mccann M. Characteristics of 68 chronic pcp abusers who sought treatment. Drug Alcohol Depend. 8, 223-227, 1981.

Renner JA and Gastfriend DR. Drug Addiction, in Massachusetts General Hospital Handbook of General Hospital Psychiatry, 3rd Edition. St.Louis, MO, Mosby Year Book, 1991.

Roberts WR and Morey LC. Convergent Validation of a Typology of Alcohol Abusers. Bulletin of the society of Psychologists in Addictive Behaviors 4: 226-233, 1985.

Robins LN. The Vietnam Drug User Returns. Special Action Office Monograph Series A, no 2. Washington, D.C.: Government Printing Office, 1974.

Rosen P, Barkin RM, et al. Emergency Medicine: Concepts and Clinical Practice, 3rd Edition, Mosby Year Book, 1992.

Rosenberg ML. Violence is a public Health Problem: The three leading causes of Mortality in America. Philadelphia, 1988.

Ross HE, Glaser FB, Germanson T. The Prevalence of Psychiatric Disorders in patients with Alcohol and Other Drug Problems. Arch Gen Psychiatry 45:1023-1031, 1988.

Rothberg JM, et al. Suicide in United States Army personnel, Military Medicine 153 (2): 61, 1988.

Rounsaville BJ, Anton SF, Carl K, et al. Psychiatric diagnosis of treatment-seeking cocaine abusers. Arch General Psychiatry 48: 43-51, 1991.

Rund DA, Hutzler JC. Emergency Psychiatry, St Louis, the CV Mosby Co, 1983.

Russell M, Martier SS, Sokol RJ, et al. Screening for pregnancy risk-drinking. Alcoholism: Clinical and Experimental Research, 18: 1156-1161, 1994.

Ryan J. The Neglected Crisis. American Journal of Nursing. 84 (10), 1984.

Salloum IM, Moss HB, Daley DC. Substance abuse and schizophrenia: impediments to optimal care. American Journal Drug Alcohol Abuse 17: 321-336, 1991.

Salome A. Crisis Counseling, Nurs, JIndia 75(5), 1984.

Schram PC and Burti L. Crisis Intervention Techniques Designed to Prevent Hospitalization. Bull Menninger Clinic 50 (2), 1986.

Schuckit MA. Drug and Alcohol Abuse: A Cinical Guide to Diagnosis and Treatement, 3rd Edition. New York, Plenum, 1989.

Schuckit MA, Segal DS. Opioid drug use, in Harrison's Principles of Internal Medicine (12 Edition). New York, McGrawHill, 1991.

Segal B. Homelessness and Drinking. Drugs and Society 5: 1-150, 1991.

Selzer ML. The Michigan Alcoholism Screening est (MAST). American Journal of Psychiatry. 127: 1653, 1971.

Scully JH. Psychiatry: National Medical Series for Independent Study, 3rd edition. Williams + Wilkins, 1996.

Slaby AE, Lieb J, Tancredi LR. Handbook of Psychiatric Emergencies: A Guide for Emrgencies in Psychiatry, 2nd edition. Garden City, NY, Medical Examination Publishing, 1981.

Shea SC. Psychiatric Interviewing: The Art of Understanding. Philadelphia: W. B. Saunders, 1988.

Shea SC. The Practical Art fo Suicide Assessment: A Guide for Mental Helath Professional and Substance Abuse Counselors. John Wiley + Sons, 2002.

Simpson DD. Treatment for Drug Abuse: Follow-up Outcomes and Length of Time Spent. Arch General Psychiatry 38: 875-880, 1981.

Smith LL. A Review of Crisis Intervention Theory. Social Casework, 7: 396, 1978.

Smith DE, Landry MJ, Wesson DR. Barbiturate, Sedative, hypnotic agents, in Treatments of Psychiatric Disorders, Vol 2. Washington, DC. American Psychiatric Association, 1989.

Snyder S.H. Amphetamine psychosis: A model schizophrenia mediated by catecholamines. American Journal of Psychiatry 130; 61-67, 1973.

Spittle B. The Effect of Financial Management of Alcohol-Related Hospitalization. American Journal of Psychiatry 148: 221- 223, 1991.

Stapleton S. Treating Domestic Violence. AM Medical News, September 15: 27, 1997.

Steinglass P. Family Systems Approach to the Alcoholics Family, in Alcoholism and the Family. Edited by Ishu T. Tokyo, Psychiatric Research Institute of Tokyo, 103-113, 1989.

Stengel E. Suicide and Attempted Suicide. Baltimore, Penguin Books, 1964.

Stockwell T, Hodgson R, Edwards G, et al. The Development on a Questionaire to Measure Severity of Alcohol Dependence. British Journal of Addiction 74: 79-87, 1979.

Strickler M and Allgeyer J. The Crisis Group: New Application of Crisis Theory. Social Work 12: 28, July 1967.

Strub RL and Black FW. The Mental Status Examination in Neurology. Philadelphia: Davis, 1977.

Sunderland T. Trends in violence and aggression. Online coverage from the 50th annual meeting of the American Psychiatric Association, May 18-21, 1997.

Talbott JA and Teague JW. Marijuana Psychosis. JAMA 210:299-302, 1969.

Talley S and Chiverton P. The Psychiatric Clinical Specialist's Impact on Psychiatric Emergency Services. Geeral Hospital Psychiatry 5(4): 241-245, 1983.

Tardiff K. The Violent Patietn. Psychiatry Clinical North Amercia, Vol II, No 4, 1988.

Tate P. Alcohol: How to Give It Up and Be Glad You Did. (2nd Edition). Sharp Press: Tucson, Arizona, 1997.

Tavani- Petrone C. Psychiatric Emergencies, Prim Care 13 (1), 1986.

Tennant FS. The Clinical Syndrome of Marijuana Dependence. Psychiatric Annals, 16: 225-234, 1986.

Thombs DL. A Review of PCP Abuse Trends and perceptions. Public Health Reports. University Maryland. 104:325-328, 1989.

Thompson S. Internet sites may encourage suicide. Psychiatry Bulletin 23: 449, 1999.

Thompson WL. Management of alcohol withdrawal Syndromes. Arch. Intern. Med. 138: 278-, 1978.

Tueth MJ. Diagnosing Psychiatric Emergencies in the Elderly. American Journal Emergency Medicine, 12: 364-369, 1994.

U.S. House of Representatives. Elder abuse: An examination of a hidden Problem. Select Committee on Aging, 97th Congress Committee Publishers. NO. 97-277. Washington, DC: Government Printing Office, 1981.

U.S. House of Representatives. Elder Abuse. Select Committee on Aging, 99th Congress Committee Pub. NO 99-516. Washington, DC: Government Printing Office, 1985.

U.S. House of Representatives, Select Committee on Aging. Older Americans Act: A staff Summary. Washington, DC: U.S. Government Printing Office, 1985.

Vaillant G. The Natural History of Alcoholism. Cambridge, MA, Harvard University Press, 1983.

Vaillant GE. What Can Long-term Follow-up Teach Us About Relapse and Prevention of Relapse in Addiciton? British Journal of Addiction 83: 1147-1157, 1988.

Van Der Kolk, BA, Perry JC, Herman JL. Childhood Origins of self-destructive Behavior. American Journal of Psychiatry, 148: 1665-1671, 1991.

Veterans with Mental Disorders, 1963- 1967: Mental Health Facilities Report, National Institute of Mental Health, 1969.

Victor M and Adams RD. The effect of alcohol on the nervous system. Res Publ Association Nerv Mental Disorder 32: 526, 1953.

Victor M, Adams RD and Collins GH. The Wernicke- Korsakoff syndrome. Philadelphia: Davis, 1971.

Victoroff VM. The Suicidal Patient: Recognition, Intervention, and Management Medical Economics Company Inc., 1983.

Waldron G. Crisis Intervention: Is it Effective? Br. J. Hospital Medicine 31(4) 1984.

Walker J.I. Psychiatric Emergencies. Philadelphia: Lippincott, 1983.

Walker LE. The Battered Woman. New York: Harper& Row, 1979.

Weiss RD, Mirin sm, Michael JL, et al. Psychopathology in chronic cocaine abusers. American Journal Drug Alcohol Abuse 12: 17-29, 1986.

Weissberg MP. Emergency Room Medical Clearance: an Educational Problem. American Journal of Psychiatry 136: 787. 1979.

Wekstein L. Handbook of Suicidology: Principles, Problems, and Practice. Brunner Mazel, Inc. 1979.

Woolis R. When Someone You Love Has a Mental Illness: A Handbook for Family, Friends, and Caregivers. Penguin Group (USA), 2003.

Appendix

Professional Medical Writer
Deborah Y. Liggan, M.D.
6550 Meyer Forest Dr. #1012
Houston, TX 77096

Dear Clinician,

The importance of the VA hospital system as a provider of inpatient psychiatric services is evidenced by the fact that in November 1967, 52,000 male veterans with psychiatric disorders were resident in this system.

I would like to introduce you to my most recent text, titled, "The Veteran's Guide to Psychiatry." Please review the Preface to familiarize yourself with the seven sections and their thirty-four chapters. Based on this information, you can choose which text you would like to edit.

We hope that, using this book as a tool, students of all ages and types will learn to enjoy working with psychiatric patients and with the art and science of contemporary psychiatry as much as we do.

In conclusion, please review the list of contributors and update your personal information for credit.

Deborah Y. Liggan, M. D.
Dr. Liggan @ yahoo.com

Index

T

V

W

Y